# Facial
# Reflexology

- Acupressure Traing Flashcards
- Intermediate
- Acupressure Course Book
- Acupressure institute
  510 -845 -1059

# Facial Reflexology

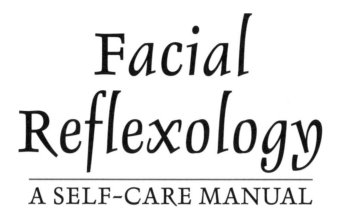

## A SELF-CARE MANUAL

MARIE-FRANCE MULLER, M.D., N.D., PH.D.

Translated from the French by Ralph Doe

Illustrated by René Maurice Nault

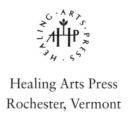

Healing Arts Press
Rochester, Vermont

Healing Arts Press
One Park Street
Rochester, Vermont 05767
www.InnerTraditions.com

Healing Arts Press is a division of Inner Traditions International

Originally published in French in 2004 under the title *Le grande livre de la réflexologie faciale* by Éditions Jouvence
First English edition published in 2006 by Healing Arts Press

*Note to the reader: This book is intended as an informational guide. The remedies, approaches, and techniques described herein are meant to supplement, and not to be a substitute for, professional medical care or treatment. They should not be used to treat a serious ailment without prior consultation with a qualified health care professional.*

**Library of Congress Cataloging-in-Publication Data**

Muller, Marie-France.
   [Grande livre de la réflexologie faciale. English]
   Facial reflexology : a self-care manual / Marie-France Muller ; translated from the French by Ralph Doe ; illustrated by René Maurice Nault
     p. cm.

   Includes bibliographical references and index.
   ISBN 1-59477-013-1
   ISBN 978-159477013-5
   1. Reflexology (Therapy) 2. Acupressure. 3. Face.    I. Title.
   RM723.R43M85 2006
   615.8'224—dc22

                                       2005023601

Printed and bound in Canada

10  9  8  7  6  5  4  3  2

Text design and layout by Priscilla Baker
This book was typeset in Sabon, with Delphin and Agenda used as display typefaces

To send correspondence to the author of this book send a first class letter to the author c/o Inner Traditions • Bear & Company, One Park Street, Rochester, VT 05767, and we will forward the communication to the author.

*I hereby dedicate this book to my American family:*
*To Teresa and Eugene Mougin, Viviane Tyrell, Lenny Gauthier,*
*and Ed Miller; to Dona Rice, Marcy Brennan, and Lynn*
*Jambora, with a special mention for Meaghan Brennan, at last*
*home from Iraq; to Jimmy and Robert Gauthier; and to all their*
*children and grandchildren. I am sorry not to be able to name*
*you all! Thank you for the space you have so generously made*
*for me in your hearts!*

—·—

*For René Nault, my husband, best friend, collaborator, and*
*favorite illustrator. This book is the last book we completed*
*together and marks the end of a rich and fascinating quarter of*
*a century. We shared everything and created so much! Thank*
*you for your love and support—which I now miss so much—and*
*of course all those interesting discussions we never did without*
*for more than a few hours. And my gratitude, finally, for all the*
*work accomplished with loving care for this book to be a success.*

—·—

*My thanks too go to Nhuan Le Quang, who initiated me to the*
*marvelous technique of Dien' Cham' with so much enthusiasm.*

# Contents

# Introduction

# Managing Your Own Health with Facial Reflexology

We are living in the strangest of times! In modern societies we try to teach our children to assume responsibility for themselves and to manage their lives in the best possible way and we also try to stay masters of our lives and our choices. There is one area, however, where we do not retain control much of the time, and where officialdom intrudes increasingly . . . our health!

In modern times, the importance of going to see the doctor at the first symptom has often been asserted. The natural consequence of this advice is that we end up taking all kinds of medicines or drugs with well-known toxic effects. It is certainly true that large-scale adverse effects are starting to become evident, such as the steadily growing ineffectiveness of antibiotics, to which a great part of the population has become resistant during repeated courses of treatment over the years, and related contamination of the food chain. Although warnings about these possibilities were given decades ago, few people took notice and the "antibiotic reflex" became systematic: as soon as the first symptoms appeared or temperature rose, the pills came out.

It has been the same thing with other medicines and drugs, and abuse of them is one of the causes of the current degeneration of our bodies, made evident these days by the widespread appearance of new pathologies. Our immune systems often find themselves powerless when confronted by new viruses and other pathogens, often caused by misuse, including in the domain of healthcare: too many vaccinations, too many medicines and foods that are incapable of giving our bodies what they need to keep functioning smoothly. The impoverishment of soils[1] as well as repeated errors in our diet or nutrition over the years have resulted in higher toxic loads, which our bodies are unable to deal with, especially when we consider increased vulnerability caused by the daily race against time and ensuing stress.

This weakening of our natural defenses—which prevents us from living out our life choices—is characteristic of our times. We have come to the point where most of us can no longer continue without medicine but still are not in perfect health. It has become difficult to ignore the great numbers of people around us suffering from and succumbing to heart disease and other disorders, not to mention the sword of Damocles hanging over the heads of everyone—the fear of cancer. Regarding our body as the enemy always ready for treachery has placed us in a state of permanent war against it. We should not be surprised if it throws the towel into the ring, giving up the unequal and unjust battle!

In spite of all these difficulties, the old dream that we all have is within our reach, as it always has been: the one where we escape illness and gain back our good health that we lost for a while, and learn to preserve it like a precious gift. Our ancestors knew how to do this and transmitted their knowledge, but it often became dilapidated during the times when human beings thought they knew everything and looked upon this precious, ancient, and ancestral knowledge with scorn. Happily nature is rich with resources that allow us to recapture lost health and to conserve it. This is the basis of alternative medicine.

A few of the old methods with known virtues that Mother Nature has placed at our disposal for free are: different breathing techniques, various methods of nutrition, use of plants with therapeutic value (phytotherapy), use of essential oils (aromatherapy), use of various clays, sun radiation, and mineral waters.

However, the search into our environment often misleads us, and we forget that within ourselves, in the substance of our very nature, there are untapped sources of health, balance, and well-being. In the same way as our planet still has many unexplored areas, we remain remarkably unaware of our hidden inner natural resources. Our body has a wide range of methods of self-healing. It is almost as if nature has supplied us with the means to do something to help ourselves or someone else, whatever the situation, whatever happens.

It has to be recognized that if we are capable of creating computers, and equipping them with self-protection and self-repair, it would be strange if our bodies were not thus endowed. But it is important for us to re-educate ourselves because it seems that the instruction manual has been lost for quite some time! This lack of information is being remedied and we will again have access to all of the ancient techniques that allowed our ancestors to survive in much more difficult and demanding circumstances than we have to endure in the modern world.

It is possible for us to rekindle our confidence in our own body, enabling it to pass from being the potential enemy, always ready to let us down, to that of being our friend, which wants to do us good. This recognition is paramount: to know that our body is always doing what it can to maintain us in good health, full of energy! Second after second it silently struggles against any poison or pathogen likely to cause problems, most often without our realizing it or being conscious of the phenomenon. Our body destroys viruses and bacteria, cancerous and abnormal cells, day after day; at the same time it restores vital balances and ensures internal harmony.

Personally, as a practicing therapist, I have always considered that the main part of my work was to teach my patients a certain number of essential points:

- that their body as well as their mind was their faithful and loyal friend
- that they could and must have confidence in it
- that any basic therapeutic action consisted in underpinning their body's efforts—and not fighting against it

To accomplish this there are several methods, which are all effective and which can be used at the same time. None is exclusive; everything depends on the situation at the time and the individual in question.

This book focuses on Dien' Cham'—an amazing method of treatment from Vietnam—which makes it possible for us to discover and develop a part of the enormous potential for self-healing and self-regulation concealed within ourselves. Dien' Cham' is a precious aid you will learn to use on any occasion, as soon as a problem arises, without waiting for the symptoms to develop into a sickness. Dien' means "face" and cham' means "acupuncture;" quite simply, Dien' Cham' is "facial acupuncture," with the implied meaning of "facial reflexology."

Facial reflexology is one form of "reflexology," a series of therapeutic techniques in which simple massage is used to stimulate certain zones of the body, called reflex zones. The major types of reflexology are:

Foot reflexology, which is performed on the reflex zones on the soles of the feet
Hand reflexology, which uses mainly the reflex zones of the palms of the hands
Iridology, which is above all a method of diagnosis based on the interpretation of the reflex zones in the irises of the eyes
Auriculotherapy, which uses the reflex zones of the ears
Thorax and abdominal reflexology
Endonasal reflexology
Facial reflexology

There are many other forms of reflexology, which will be the subject of further publications.[2]

It could be said that nature has placed multiple resources at our disposal, allowing us to maintain good health and restore it if need be, without having recourse to instruments other than our hands or common household objects. Reflex zones can be found on virtually the entire surface of the body. This multiplies the possibilities of self-healing incredibly, even in the case of lesions or injuries to several parts of the body at the same time. From this can be understood the

enormous interest that knowledge of these zones can have for us and the possibilities open to us.

When I first heard about Dien' Cham'—at a Health and Nature fair in Toulouse, France—I was already practicing several types of reflexology, and had heard about other facial reflexology systems. Still, I was rather skeptical when the man who introduced me to this method for the first time, Nhuan Le Quang, claimed to be able to relieve any pain, sometimes permanently, using two or three strokes of the rounded end of a ballpoint pen. Although I knew the kind of "little miracles" reflexology techniques could work, I found it difficult to believe it could be done in such a spectacular way.

However, I was interested, so I agreed to let Nhuan Le Quang experiment on my face, which was not a big risk to take! He started by asking me if I was suffering from anything or if I felt any pain. I was not. However, after thinking about what I could complain about, I remembered the nasty paresthesia of my right fingers caused by an accidental manipulation of the cervical bones in the neck twenty-seven years before. The right arm had remained paralyzed for several months and only reflexology had succeeded in restoring its use, with the exception that I had not regained the sensitivity of the ends of the fingers.

"That's no problem," he exclaimed, to my surprise. My growing skepticism must have shown.

"At any rate let's have a try!" Using the rounded end of an ordinary ballpoint pen—the part of the pen that clicks in and out, opposite the writing end—he rubbed my face and brushed me here and there for a few minutes.

"How do you feel now?" he asked, holding the pen ready to go at it some more. To my amazement I had to admit that energy was again beginning to circulate in my "dead" fingers. Only an area of my index finger was still insensitive. When I told him this, he again gave several areas of my forehead a vigorous rub for ten seconds or so and asked me again. Everything had come back to normal and I could again feel my fingers, for the first time in twenty-seven years!

The story does not stop there! Quite naturally I registered for the next course that Nhuan Le Quang was giving in my area, which was a few weekends later. As there were no books or manuals on it, we simply learned what Dien' Cham' is all about, including the basic techniques and philosophy. Using a single diagram of the projection of the body on the face (**Diagram 1** in chapter 2) we had only studied, in fact skimmed, a few pressure points. I certainly did not have the impression of knowing a great deal on the subject!

The next morning was a Monday. I had an appointment with my dentist, with whom I also had a professional relationship. When I went into the waiting room I found a man sitting on the floor next to an armchair and he looked like he was suffering a lot. I hurried to his side to help him up but he put his arm up to stop me and said: "I'm having a bout of sciatica and it's hurting too much for me to get up!"

Then my dentist came in and asked: "I have called the emergency service. Do you know something that could give him temporary relief while we are waiting?"

"Why not? If you're OK with it, I will try something."

The man readily agreed, so I decided to try some foot reflexology. I attempted in vain to remove his shoe. My "patient" could not even stand me touching his shoe! I was a little disconcerted and wondered what I could do. A hand massage perhaps? Suddenly I remembered the previous day's diagram, which represented the shape of a person projected onto a face. One advantage is that once you have seen it, it is impossible to forget! I could not remember a single pressure point but the diagram had lodged in my mind somehow, just because it had seemed so unlikely that it could be of use!

From the desk I pulled out a pen with a rounded end and found myself rubbing the face of

my "patient" with it, softly, because the zones all looked very painful. I quickly massaged the zones corresponding to the pelvis and the affected leg. As he was in great pain I had to stop after a few seconds. I resumed brushing the zones four or five times and then again left time for the "patient" to catch his breath.

To my great surprise he decided to try to sit on the armchair from which he had slipped. He succeeded after some effort; that was already a promising outcome! Several minutes later the emergency services had still not arrived and I decided to try the short session again, at the end of which my "patient" was able to stand up! In all I gave four short sessions of about twenty seconds in less than half an hour and at the end the "patient" was walking, albeit with pain. What a result! Although it was obvious to the dentist and I that a short session like that would not be enough, the man decided, against our advice, to leave the dental surgery and drive back home! This he managed to do.

I was flabbergasted! Just four brief sessions lasting twenty to thirty seconds, given by someone without experience, were enough to relieve someone having an acute bout of sciatica. Furthermore, conscious of my shortcomings, I knew that I had only used the strict minimum of the zones which could have been useful. That was how I became enthused about this extraordinary technique, which is so simple that anyone can learn it in a few hours and is harmless in case of error. On the spot I decided that it was necessary to spread the news about this amazing method and to write a book.

That book, *Le Dien' Cham', une étonnante méthode de réflexologie faciale vietnamienne* (Dien' Cham', An Astonishing Vietnamese Method of Facial Reflexology)—the first ever devoted to Dien' Cham'—was published by Editions Jouvence, France in 2000. After its publication, it featured in many reviews and articles in the press, radio shows, and television programs, and was also translated into several languages. The keen interest with which this book was greeted throughout Europe can be attributed to the fact that the technique of Dien' Cham' can, in certain cases, really be described as "magic." Once you have learned this method of healing, it helps you to feel in top form anywhere and everywhere without medication and without gadgets! To relieve your aches and pains and those of your friends and family, all you need are your fingers, or a simple instrument, such as a round-ended ballpoint pen, which you use to stimulate the pertinent facial reflex points.

Nothing could be easier! Particularly since the result is never long in coming. A headache disappears in a few seconds, and with a backache an improvement is just as quick. It is preferable not to take my word for it, because you only have to give it a try to convince yourself.

In fact there are very few methods that have so many positive aspects and permit you to:

• heal common complaints without automatically having to go to see your physician
• relieve aches and pains in such a simple, rapid, and effective manner
• recover your health by inducing the effect of a medicine, without it being necessary to take one
• gain self-sufficiency in the field of sickness prevention, in a simple way with a minimum of time and effort, and without expense

Facial reflexology offers all this, as you will soon be able to check out for yourself.

But even the best techniques in the world—and you will quickly see that these are some of them, because they are so simple to practice with rapid effect—are of little help unless the basic rules of a healthy and balanced life are applied at the same time. Of course you will be able to obtain momentary relief remarkably quickly, but until you correct your lifestyle it is impossible to restore health

long-term. In addition, try to remember that even when the advice given in this book produces results without enormous effort, it would have a further-reaching effect if it were allied to a healthy diet and a balanced lifestyle.

It is a strange age that we live in. It has become almost a commonplace idea to want to replace a damaged part of our body with one removed from another human body, or perhaps an animal. Mad scientists foresee a world where it is possible to switch any organ as has already been done in experiments. Any part of the body can be removed or perhaps all of it, except the head or more simply the brain, which could then be grafted on another body. (How would this "removal" take place, from whom, and in what circumstances?)

Animal cloning has already been accomplished and we will soon see the first human clone. Some see this as the solution to the fertility problems we have in our stressed out Western civilization, which is in fact polluted by hormones used in food production and various kinds of medical treatment. It could also be seen as the solution to the lack of donors of organs, with all of the terrible but easily imaginable consequences.

All of the above is possible because the simple laws of staying in good health and healing sickness are not taken into account. Human beings are falling victim to a bad case of megalomania at the beginning of this millennium, believing themselves above natural laws, which they want to govern, or even purely and simply ignore. Of course there are great economic interests at stake in this affair. A few years ago one study showed that in the eyes of some governments, an unhealthy or sick population was more profitable than a healthy one! Consequently certain lines of research are repeatedly plugged, generally those producing a result in ten or so years' time, and those implying the use of drugs with devastating effects. Many other areas of research are neglected. Force is used to gag the "discoverers" who have the audacious attitude of healing without official approval, using cost-effective means and innocently believing this to be an opportunity for their fellow beings.

Indeed, physicians and healers are faced with a lot of pressure, including depressing discoveries resulting from the torture of defenseless animals and probably also experimentation on human beings, possibly not always with their consent, as has happened in recent history. Just thinking about these experiments chills the blood. Can it be that survival is at this price? Consequently it is a real lungful of fresh air to see that there are easy ways to remain in good health and heal problems when they arise, before they degenerate and become chronic.

Dien' Cham' is one of these new techniques, or rather old techniques that have recently been rediscovered. It is likely that it qualifies for the "Oscar" for simplicity and efficiency.

It is a long-held axiom that if you do not want to become sick it is better not to start. And this is the main object. Facial reflexology makes it possible for each and every one of us to be capable of preventing problems from arising and relieving existing troubles. Of course this technique is not a substitute for medical advice but complements it harmoniously. The study of the simple basics of this exciting method will permit you—in just a few hours—to apprehend about sixty reflex points and several reflex zones, all located on the face. You will also be able to apply this knowledge to many common cases.

On the other hand, if a sickness is already declared, Dien' Cham' can also largely contribute to relieving it, or even healing it. With the exception of an accident, it is impossible to fall seriously ill unless you have neglected preliminary signs of the problem. Sickness is not determined by fate, which just happens to you for no reason. If it is possible to restore internal harmony at the first sign of imbalance, quite simply the sickness cannot affect you! It is just a case of knowing what to do.

Facial reflexology has many advantages over other techniques, including effectiveness, speed of execution, and simplicity, because the face is always available and easily accessible. Just remember that you will usually be able to obtain results in just two or three minutes of massage! In addition, it is a technique that can be learned easily and by everyone. Even children can learn to practice it on themselves in case of need. I hope that you are motivated to launch yourself into this new adventure, which will take you toward more independence in the management of your own health and that of your family and friends.

Therapists and healthcare workers will be interested in this technique, which will allow them to bring relief to their patients in just a few minutes before moving on to other methods. I know many nurses who do not hesitate to practice on their patients as well as to teach them a few reflex zones or points to enable them to attenuate their own unpleasant symptoms and pain of various kinds.

After the publication of my first book on Dien' Cham'—in the course of replying to questions from readers and audiences as well as from students of my training courses—I established that a certain number of important elements were missing from it. This I have attempted to correct by writing this work, the scope of which amounts to a full-scale encyclopedia on Dien' Cham', Facial Reflexology.

Chapter 1 of this book presents the history and theory of Dien' Cham', giving important background for its successful practice.

Chapter 2 uses thirteen fundamental Diagrams to present the major facial reflex zones and points, which will prepare you to optimize your sessions.

As you would expect in a do-it-yourself training manual to use at home, this book presents, in Chapter 3, all facets of a Dien' Cham' session, including instruments, stimulation techniques, the selection of reflex points, sequence, length, frequency, and precautions. It also gives specific instructions for both the Basic Session for general relaxation and toning up and a more elaborated Standard Session that can be tailored to particular conditions.

Your practice of facial reflexology will be guided by Chapter 4, a Practical Dictionary of Therapeutic Sessions, organized by specific health problems and the corresponding points to be used for treatment.

Chapter 5 lists the fifty-seven Dien' Cham' points covered by this book, with detailed guidance regarding location, effects, correspondences, indications, and advice on massage technique for each point.

After you have acquired a certain level of practice and obtained your first results, Chapter 6 offers a description of the advanced technique of personalized reflex zone and point determination, which can be practiced on yourself and any other person. Three Reference Lists of points, organized by parts of the body, functions of points, and specific symptoms, appear at the end of the chapter to assist you in your advanced point selections.

Chapter 7 will guide you in extending the benefits of Dien' Cham' to animals too!

Appendix 1 on Chinese facial reflexology offers you the possibility of enriching your knowledge with an introduction to therapeutic techniques of accupressure, such as Do-in and Ji-jo.

Appendix 2 offers a simple Japanese massage of the crown of the head. The scalp mirrors the entire body just as the face does, with corresponding zones for organs and energy pathways.

The book concludes with a Therapeutic Index of Dien' Cham' Point Correspondences: an outline of the information pairing specific health problems and pertinent points given in Chapter 4.

As the main intent of this book is to allow you to directly practice the Dien' Cham' method, I have above all designed it to be practical and clear. From the start I wanted you to be implicated, even if you do not believe me. Just follow the instructions step-by-step and you will see the results! It is as easy as that. Now to your pens!

# I

## The History, Theory, and Practice of Dien' Cham'
### A Surprisingly Effective Vietnamese Method of Facial Reflexology

*This therapy is a form of community medicine. It can be used on a large scale for a wide public in the field of healing by medical first aid.*

BUI QUOC CHAU

## A SHORT HISTORY OF DIEN' CHAM'

Facial reflexology has long been known in all Far Eastern countries such as China and Japan. But it was in Vietnam that the art was to express itself wholly and where the main developments were made in the 1980s. The amazing method of Dien' Cham' has its roots in a technique developed by Professor Bui Quoc Chau and a team of doctors, research scientists, and acupuncturists in Ho Chi Minh City (the modern name for Saigon), which he named "Facytherapy."

### Facytherapy: From the I Ching to Modern Medicine

Professor Bui Quoc Chau, a doctor who specialized in acupuncture, became interested in the principles of reflexology while he was practicing in a hospital environment. Already familiar with the tenets of reflexology—according to which each part of the body can reflect and treat the whole of the body—he had the idea of studying possible correspondences between the face and the body. To him, there seemed to be no logical reason why the same would not apply for the face as for the soles of the feet, the ears, the hands or any other area of the body. This was his basic hypothesis.

To that, he added his knowledge of the I Ching, also called the Book of Changes. Although it is above all known as a method of divination, its use is more extensive than this brief definition would have us believe. There is even a very serious branch of medicine based on the study of it, some aspects of which are founded on the correspondence principle. According to Professor Bui Quoc Chau, everything in nature obeys this law. In music, for instance, we know that the sounds within a melody correspond, and that if a certain note is played on an instrument, another instrument close by will enter into resonance and emit harmonics of this note. This is also one of the principles of the Kybalion, the bible of hermetic philosophy attributed to great Hermes himself. He expressed himself in these terms: "Everything in nature corresponds."

Guided by this principle oriental medicine resolves physiological problems by prescribing the consumption of plants, minerals, or animals that present a correspondence with the part of the body or organ in question. Even if this goes against our Western, Cartesian instincts, one is obliged to acknowledge that it works rather well!

Following both the I Ching hypothesis and the analogy principle—according to which everything with the same form has some correspondences—Professor Bui Quoc Chau started considering the face from this new angle. "Since the line of the nose recalls the curvature of the spinal column, it must correspond to it and allow me to treat it," he said to himself. One day he examined a patient with back pain and decided to explore the bridge of his patient's nose with an instrument. He found a very painful point where he inserted an acupuncture needle. The back pain disappeared instantly! He repeated this experiment several times and each time the results were excellent.

This promising beginning persuaded him to continue. He said to himself that if the curve of the nose corresponds to the spine, the nostrils must correspond to the buttocks because they resemble them. In this case the legs would be represented on both sides of the nostrils, along the creases toward the corners of the mouth; the eyebrows would correspond to the shoulders and arms. This is how he discovered the first projection of the body on the face (see **Diagram 2,** chapter 2). More work enabled him to draw twenty-two diagrams showing projections of the body on the face, and discover more than five hundred reflex points.

With the help of his team, he elaborated a new reflexology that was more complex and effective than acupuncture. It could be seen as a synthesis of reflexology, massage, and acupuncture. He gave the name "facytherapy" to it. This term is derived from two others used by his disciples, which are: facio-diagnosis and cybernetic therapy.

Facio-diagnosis, meaning facial diagnosis, combines the determination of points giving pain and so-called "silent" or insensitive points, which allow a diagnosis to be arrived at. Cybernetics—the highly complex modern science that deals with both electronics and mechanics—relates to facytherapy in that Professor Bui Quoc Chau understands the face as a control panel or computer keyboard. By pressing on a facial "pushbutton" we can obtain a remote response from an organ, the regulation of an organ's function, or relief from pain! It is almost magic!

Facytherapy draws from oriental medicine, in particular acupuncture, as well as from Western medicine, especially in the domain of anatomy, physiopathology, and neurology. It also includes domains as varied as chemistry, physics, geometry, cybernetics, the notion of the energy body, and even oriental culture and philosophy as it is inspired by the basic principles of Buddhism, Zen, Taoism, Confucianism, and the I Ching. There are also elements of Vietnamese indigenous traditions: popular medicine of course, but also language, maxims, folklore, and other manifestations of this ancient culture. The sum total of this knowledge serves as the starting point for the description of rules such as the principles of correspondence, similitude, symmetry, that of the "silent point" and that of opposite effects.

It is important to note that while facytherapy is based on traditional oriental medicine, it is not the same as Chinese medicine's facial acupuncture. It is a completely original method. Although early in the development of facytherapy Bui Quoc Chau made use of traditional acupuncture instruments such as needles, moxas, various rollers, flexible hammers, and so on, it rapidly moved away from acupuncture as it developed its own very different techniques. As far as pressure points are concerned, facytherapy uses over five hundred as opposed to only thirty in acupuncture! Each facial reflex point is also the image of one or several acupuncture points on the meridian in question, and according to precisely determined rules. For example, points **50** and **233** correspond to the liver meridian.

While facytherapy has certain similarities with the other healing and diagnosis methods based on reflexology—such as iridology and foot, endonasal, or vertebral reflexology—it is only distantly related to them. As Professor Bui Quoc Chau himself stipulated, whereas classical reflexology is unidirectional, one organ corresponding to one reflex zone, facytherapy is multidirectional and acts on many systems. This is why it is unique. He has since broadened the principles of facytherapy to the whole body.

Facytherapy cannot be presented as a pure product of medicine but rather as a synthesis of several disciplines: "It is the spiritual child of the Vietnamese civilization, expressing its synthetic and eclectic characteristics, and the correct middle path," as Professor Bui Quoc Chau remarked.

Although facytherapy has proven to be very effective, it is such a highly complex method that only specialists with several years of study can hope to use it. It is particularly difficult for a West-

erner to understand the structure of facytherapy, unless he or she tries to penetrate to the heart of the great traditions. Luckily, Nhuan Le Quang—who was originally Vietnamese and now lives in France—has developed the simplified, accessible method of Dien' Cham', based on this basic theory and work.

## Nhuan Le Quang: A Remarkable Life

It all started for him in a very strange way. While he was still in Vietnam twenty years ago, a medium predicted that one day he would heal people, that he would travel around the world, become famous, and launch a method that was different from any known so far. This strange prediction surprised Nhuan Le Quang enormously and he was very skeptical. At the time he was an architect and lived in a communist country in the south of Vietnam, which offered little hope of this kind of destiny. Much of his family had emigrated to France in 1975 following the "communist events." However, family circumstances prevented him from doing the same, and he had regretfully resigned himself to staying in Vietnam. It should be added that he also suffered from chronic asthma, which made the prediction seem totally absurd.

However, what on the surface appeared to be unfavorable circumstances were the same factors that gave him the opportunity to be introduced to facytherapy, which, as he later said, "was well worth the eleven years I spent in a communist country."

In 1985, having heard of facytherapy, he thought of trying it to rid himself of his asthma, which was a serious handicap. He went to the center directed by Professor Bui Quoc Chau where this method was practiced. At that time acupuncture needles were used to treat facial reflex zones, which was far from pleasant! But he decided to undergo the experience anyway, saying to himself that if it could give him relief, it would be worth it.

One day, aware that he was developing a common cold, which usually quickly produced an asthma attack, he allowed needles to be inserted into his face. They immediately had a surprising effect. To his astonishment his nose stopped running and the cold disappeared instantly, without a trace!

Of course the method appeared extraordinary to him. The same day, he went to look for some acupuncture needles, as well as a book detailing the technique. He wanted to be able to heal himself when necessary, without having to wait for an appointment.

However, the complexity of the method was such that at the beginning he understood very little. The principles of yin and yang, the "five elements," and the multiplicity of the tenets of facytherapy seemed to him to be an inextricable labyrinth, where he was desperately and irretrievably lost. With a lot of time and patience, however, he managed to identify the points that seemed to have the clearest correspondence to his conditions. When a cold appeared a few weeks later, he decided that he would not lose anything by trying the technique. He placed himself in front of a mirror and inserted needles into his face. The cold ceased immediately!

With this result he decided to use all means at his disposal to understand this astonishing method, in the hope that he would be able to heal himself as well as his family. He describes that time in this way: "Since it was my destiny to dedicate my life to this, I learned it all alone. My experience brought me to discover two very simple techniques, so simple that you have to see to believe. I continued on my path, and whether you believe me or not, the techniques actually work. That's the main thing!"

**Warning**

Although Nhuan Le Quang first experimented with acupuncture needles, the subject of this book is reflexology and absolutely not acupuncture, which is reserved for experienced practitioners. In fact there are points on the face that can be fatal if punctured! Please do not imitate the sorcerer's apprentice, and instead use the techniques for simple stimulation of the reflex zones and points that are given in these pages, which are fully effective and bring no risks.

### A Simplified Method

In 1986 Nhuan Le Quang decided to reunite with the other members of his family in France. This is where he had another piece of luck. Having spent several months fruitlessly searching for work, he remembered that he knew an extraordinary method for healing easily and without danger. Consequently he decided to widen his field of experimentation and to perfect the studies he had begun, just armed with his book. It did take him quite some time, of course, given the extensive philosophical and medical foundations of facytherapy. Over a period of several years he moved from the complexity of the theoretical background toward the development of the easy to use, simple techniques of the future Dien' Cham'. As a result of his work, a person who wishes to experience and share the benefits of Dien' Cham' does not have to penetrate the difficult notions of yin and yang or the philosophy of the I Ching, or even have to know the meridians! This represents a singular advantage for Western minds.

Although in Vietnam a steel point instead of needles is used for the stimulation of points, Nhuan Le Quang knew that even this could not be the case in France or in other Western countries, where patients generally refuse this kind of painful treatment. With this in mind he developed more comfortable techniques. Happily, the results were in no way inferior to that of needles or steel points.

In fact, he discovered that with any round-ended instrument, such as a simple ballpoint pen (see Figure 1.1), it is possible to obtain excellent results with minimum effort. As French law banned the use of therapeutic needles to non-physicians, this new technique allowed relief without danger for the patient or for the doctor.

He eventually started to receive invitations to give conferences and show his way of proceeding, especially at alternative medicine fairs. The first time he was invited, the announcement of the results he had obtained spread like wildfire around the event and he ended up practicing Dien' Cham' for free on several hundred people! (It should be noted that a session hardly lasts one or two minutes.) He received more and more invitations and, the more he practiced, the more he realized that results could be obtained using very simple means, just by committing to memory a few pressure points. In this way he succeeded in considerably simplifying the method of facytherapy and reducing it to a manageable set of basic pressure points that could be stimulated using an original and very effective technique.

Then Nhuan Le Quang decided to teach this new kind of simplified facial reflexology. As the name "facytherapy" meant nothing special for him, and hardly seemed to correspond to his structural definition, he decided to call it by the more evocative name of Dien' Cham'. This is how Dien' Cham', "Facial Reflexology," came about. It is a technique limited to fifty-seven reflex points on the face, identified and numbered according to

a fictive grid, and restricted to a few projection systems of the body on the face, showing the various reflex zones.

## Dien' Cham' Training and Practice for All

As I mentioned earlier, I was so impressed by Nhuan Le Quang's restoration of feeling to my fingers in just a few moments that I had decided to learn the method and write a book about it that would allow my readers to use the Dien' Cham' techniques immediately without having to undertake specific additional training. The responses I received to my first book showed me that I had attained my purpose. I have received many personal success stories in relation to treatment given by people who are not therapists. I am happy when I receive such encouragement. The satisfaction expressed by therapists who have used the techniques brings warmth to my heart. However, I realized that many useful indications and elements were missing from the first book. These became evident during my therapeutic practice, conferences, and training courses over many years. I have used this information to enhance the presentation of Dien' Cham' in this book, making it a complete home-training manual.

While the method described here is mainly drawn from the works of Professor Bui Quoc Chau and Nhuan Le Quang's subsequent simplifications, I have also taken into account my own knowledge, observations, and questions. My main goal has been to enable all therapists and patients—in fact, any person desiring to maintain good health—to use this technique. As I was aiming for a practical book, I have avoided including certain notions that are difficult for the Western mind to appreciate. I have also limited myself to techniques that are both simple and effective and, in my experience, have given the best results. Certain diagrams have been redrawn to foster this and I have created others to make things clearer and to simplify the work of memorization.

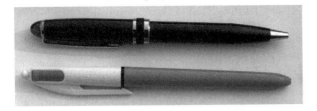

Figure 1.1. Sample of ballpoint pens used for Dien' Cham'. The larger end is most commonly used to rub the reflex zones of the face. The writing end (only when out of ink) is sometimes used to stimulate a specific reflex point.

Naturally, reading a book can never replace a direct experience, which is my only regret. That is why I usually give a quick demonstration of how to stimulate the face at book-signing sessions. In this way I know that the person is immediately going to be able to practice effectively and be able to teach others. Many people hesitate to start out alone in this adventure and ask me to organize practical training sessions. As the method is described in detail in this book, such courses are not essential. However, I do offer weekend courses, particularly to reinforce correct practice of the various types of stimulation. I limit the number of participants to a small group, which enables everyone to receive and give several treatments. I also regularly train all kinds of therapists—physicians, physiotherapists, osteopaths, reflexologists, and nurses—who all want to relieve their patients effectively in one or two minutes without changing other elements in their treatment. I am very happy to do this!

Even so, this manual will provide you with complete instruction for the successful practice of facial reflexology.

# THE BASIC THEORY OF DIEN' CHAM'

*This method consists in stimulating the facial reflex points with, as a main instrument, . . . the rounded end of a ballpoint pen! In less time than it takes to write it down, your aches and pains disappear as if by magic. It is simple, effective, and spectacular.*

To understand this method, which has some strange aspects, it will be useful and interesting to take a brief look at the basic principles which preceded its development.

It seems amazing to certain people that it is still possible to have an interest in the "backward" ideas contained within traditional medicine systems. However it seems obvious that if our ancestors survived without modern medical science, allowing us—I writing this book and you reading it—to be present on the earth in this century, here and now, it is because they possessed and used some effective knowledge. This allowed them not only to survive, but to evolve and transmit thousands of years of experience.

Looking upon them with scorn and laughing at them is just one of the major aberrations of our modern world, which is proud of its own science, based on an inflated sense of the importance of the mental process and denial of all other faculties. Nonetheless commonsense commands that we listen to what the ancients had to transmit to us, as had been done for thousands of years. That is just what Professor Bui Quoc Chau did and look what he succeeded in doing!

## The Basic Principles

There are several main ideas that serve as a foundation for the structure of this method. A minimum of understanding with respect to the main principles will enable us to see how they are applied and allow us to memorize them more easily. As Professor Bui Quoc Chau said, "These principles were like a magic wand or a miraculous key, which helped me to find the secret door opening into the mysteries of the human body."

### The Form Correspondence Principle

Most of the facial diagrams are based on this principle. Professor Bui Quoc Chau mentioned that it reflects the wisdom of a proverb found in the I Ching: "That which resembles assembles." This principle also means: "Whatever has the same shape is similar and corresponds." We have already seen the analogy between the bridge of the nose and the spinal column, the shape of the nostrils and that of the buttocks. Later in this book, the form correspondence principle will be broadened to a more generally applicable principle in numerous domains, harking back to the philosophy of the alchemists!

> "When the flamingo sings, somewhere in the shadows, another flamingo sings in harmony."
>
> I CHING

### The Nature Function Correspondence Principle

The nature function correspondence principle indicates that objects of a similar kind have a tendency to associate easily. Let us take an example that illustrates the principle in a concrete way: the neck links the body to the head; likewise, the wrist links the hand to the forearm and the ankle links the foot to the leg. In Vietnamese the parts of the body that link two others are all designated as *co*. In this way the neck is *cai co*, the wrist *co tay*, and the ankle *co chan*. According to this correspondence principle, the root of the nose, located between the eyebrows and the eyes, is considered as being of the same nature, as it links the nose to the forehead. Of course it is by stimulating this zone that we are able to release the tension in the cervical area and treat sore throats, but the same result can be obtained by massaging the wrists and ankles!

For example, points such as **8** and **106**, which are of the same nature, can be associated with good results. However these notions of a complex character will not be very useful in your day-to-day practice. We will therefore leave them to the specialists.

### The Principle of Homogeneity

This principle establishes a link between the sick parts of the body, their functions, and their manifestations on the level of the face as points known as "soft" points, meaning that a lack of firmness can easily be determined by touching and even visually. The number of these "soft" reflex points, their extent and degree of "softness," is also an indicator of the seriousness of the sickness or imbalance.

### The Principle of Symmetry

According to this principle the parts of the body located on the right hand side are found on the right side of the face, and the same with the left hand side. There are exceptions to this rule, which concern the points located on the forehead, some of which are inverted. This is the case with **Diagram 10** (in chapter 2), which details the forehead and internal organs.

### The Principle of Interconnection

Everything in the universe is interdependent. It is the same with the human body. Are you suffering from a migraine or headache? Have a look at the state of your liver or gall bladder. Do you often have sore throats? Check on the state of your intestines, and so on.

The principle of interconnection governs all reflexology: pressure points, organs, functions, reflex zones, and parts of the body are all connected to one another. This interconnection is particularly pronounced in the field of facial reflexology because of the proximity of the face to the brain. The face is therefore particularly well irrigated and innervated. This is why the face can express all of the emotions, which no other part of the body is capable of doing. The neck establishes the connection between the body and the head. Everything is concentrated in this "bridge," which is the passage for blood circulation and nervous impulses. It is the same for meridians, which converge or start from this region, in particular the yang meridians.

Therefore it should not be surprising to find on the face such a high density of reflex zones and points, which are extremely sensitive to signals sent by the organs and various parts of the body. Their response to stimulation is quickly transmitted to the part of the body concerned and this is why the method is so effective.

## The Principle of the Opposite Effect

According to the kind of sickness, each reflexology point requires a well-defined frequency of stimulation, length, and intensity. If we do not bear this in mind and the stimulation is insufficient, the results we counted on will not be obtained. On the other hand, if the stimulation is too strong or too long—meaning beyond what was necessary—there will be no result. We risk seeing the opposite effect and the situation getting worse.

To avoid this happening the rule is simple: stimulate points that are not painful very briefly and stop stimulating a zone or point that has stopped being sensitive. As I generally advise short sessions, there is little likelihood that you will be faced with this type of problem.

## The Principle of the Painless Point

This theory has allowed precise determination of the points on the face. This too was inspired by a famous I Ching saying, "In yang there is yin, and in yin there is yang." The logical sense of this in terms of facial reflexology leads to the observation that "within the painful zone, there is a point that is painless." Clinical experience, renewed on many occasions by a great number of therapists and conclusive results, have proved the truth of this phrase.

This is how point **1**—the first of a long series of more than five hundred in facytherapy—was located on the bridge of the nose. (Please note that the numbering of the points only corresponds to the order in which they were discovered and their order has no other implication.) This principle was also applied to the determination of other body-to-face correspondence points and zones.

There are many other principles such as that of the triangle or the poetically named one: "water flows to the river." But these complex notions are not necessary for the practice of Dien' Cham'.

## The Face: Mirror of the Body

If the human can be said to be the microcosm of the universe, the same must be true for each of its parts. This is the concept of holography. Our face, as part of ourselves, symbolizes us and therefore represents us wholly. Everything that we are is projected onto our face, in particular our physiological, psychological, and even pathological state. This is where the notion of "mirror" comes from, which is at the base of all reflexology: the organ or other body part is in a subtle relationship with its corresponding zone, here a point on the face. Dien' Cham' consists in the stimulation of the reflex zones that are found easily. Using this technique energy is roused and circulated, allowing organs to naturally recover their vitality and correct functioning. With both curative and preventive qualities, this method maintains good health and energizes the body's essential functions. It reinforces the body's natural immune system defenses, allowing the body to heal itself.

### A Natural Facelift!

A very important secondary benefit: if you do it regularly, stimulation of the face improves circulation. The effect of this is to combat wrinkles and make the face youthful again by giving you a natural facelift.

## Source of All Sickness: the Nervous System

It is quite possible to affirm without being contradicted that all sicknesses have, at their origin, a form of fatigue or exhaustion of the nervous system. That is why first obtaining some relaxation is a notion essential to Chinese medicine and also in Dien' Cham'.

Lack of sleep, overwork, almost constant stress, repeated stress, inadequate physical exercise, sadness, depression, psychological shocks, moral or emotional solitude are states we are all familiar with, which lie at the root of sickness. They all weaken our immune defenses. When our defenses are low, energy decreases, and the body is no longer able to fight off attacks by viruses and bacteria, which are present everywhere in the body itself and in the environment. A sickness will generally take hold in the weakest spot.

When the body is weakened, the outcome is almost always the same. First the person catches a common cold or becomes stiff, which is blamed on the cold or damp, but this only proves that the body's vital energy is blocked. At this point the remedy is simple and should be applied before the situation worsens. Thus the first recourse is stimulation of the pressure points for relaxation and for toning up. This first step, called the Basic Session, will be described in detail in chapter 3. Once the nervous system is relaxed, energy can start to circulate more freely, the organs are reinforced, and the body becomes more capable of self-healing. This automatically dissipates pain and feelings of weakness.

It should also be noted that sicknesses can arise due to energy stagnation. In every case, the importance of maintaining a good energy level in the body must be understood, because this is the best method of prevention. This notion is perfectly clear in Chinese medicine, where pain and suffering are always considered to be caused by blocked energy, which only needs freeing for all pain to disappear. This is why there is no need to treat the target organ directly. A sickness is always caused by a problem with the affected organ's energy. It is therefore the totality that has to be treated. In Chinese medicine this is accomplished by recuperation of the energy balance using acupuncture, a change in diet, the use of plants, and focused breathing. With facial reflexology the same result is obtained much more easily, and, for the nonprofessional, without going through the laborious business of learning Chinese medicine.

### An Example: Backache

A backache—a very frequent complaint these days—is a sign of blocked energy. Move the energy around again and the pain will disappear: it is as simple as that. A backache can be relieved by a few strokes with a pen. If the pain is recent, the relief can be conclusive on the first session. On the other hand, if the pain has been present for years, several sessions spaced regularly will be required. The result will be long lasting, as long as the person takes responsibility for him- or herself and learns the technique well enough to treat the pain when it reappears. Moreover, the more the body is stimulated, the more it is regenerated.

## THE PRACTICE OF DIEN' CHAM'

Years of personal practice have led me to affirm that this reflexology technique is genuinely, surprisingly effective. At health fairs or in demonstrations following my conferences and training courses, I have so many times had the opportunity to bring relief to people with different complaints, just using a few movements with a pen. This has been true for people suffering from all kinds of ailments, sometimes for years, to the astonishment of everyone! In many common cases, especially those concerning pain, even those with a long history, the results are not only satisfactory but spectacular, even magical, above all in the eyes of the one suffering. Sometimes he or she had already tried all kinds of methods without success over many years.

For example, during my conferences, I regularly ask if someone is suffering from scapulohumeral periarthritis (inflammation of the shoulder joint), or epicondylitis of the elbow (such as "tennis elbow"). These two afflictions are at best only improved by cortisones, and generally persist for years, spoiling the lives of those who have to put up with them. Most often, it only requires two minutes of massage of the appropriate facial reflex points to obtain the relief sought for so long! I will leave you to imagine the enthusiasm of an audience confronted with people relieved so quickly and easily! A sure success!

> It is easy to relieve a person effectively. All you have to do is relax the nervous system, free up the energy, and stimulate the natural defenses. Nature will do the rest!

Is the result long-lasting? Yes, in certain benign cases. Some chronic cases also react well to the stimulation of several well-chosen reflex points, which procures long-lasting sedation of the symptoms. A few examples are: a lumbar pain caused by tiredness or a bad position; cervical pain in the neck caused by a chill, tiredness, or small accidents; a headache linked to fatigue or worry or bad digestion; a common cold following a chill or an allergy. In most of the above cases a single session is often enough, even after years of suffering. In certain chronic cases several sessions are necessary and they tend to last longer, but this is rare. I have often advised people to practice the session on themselves four or five times a day until complete and long-lasting sedation of the pain is obtained. Most of the time an outcome is acquired in two or three days!

It seems incredible but it really works. With a few strokes of a pen, a migraine vanishes magically, and it is the same thing with a backache, a bout of asthma, or the beginning of a common cold, which can be stopped at the outset. If you are not suffering from anything in particular, this technique will at least allow you to recover an optimum energy level and relax more easily. Do you suffer from insomnia? Just a few strokes with a pen on a specific zone will give you back the sleep of a baby!

Let me underline the inexpensive nature of this therapy, which can be extremely useful to you or your friends and relatives, and can also allow you to help someone in the street or at your workplace in the case of an accident, for example, while they are waiting for professional help. The method is also without danger. You just stimulate using a pen or the fingers, never needles.

If you are already a therapist, facial reflexology can be of great use in allowing you to procure immediate and effective relief for your patients. Just think: your patient who came to see you doubled up in pain with lumbago could very well leave your office or clinic walking tall, thanks to a few strokes with the rounded tip of a ballpoint pen or a special toothed roller!

Using just thirty or so basic pressure points, everyone can learn to heal in the simplest fashion. The face is always readily accessible and so all points can be stimulated in all circumstances. You just have to acquire the habit of using the technique whenever you feel a pain or a symptom of some sort, then you will readily be able to observe the results of the stimulation. Once I had the simple experience of twisting my ankle while walking a little too quickly on a wet surface. I remembered to stimulate the corresponding zone on the face with the joint of my finger and not only did the pain disappear immediately, but I was able to start running! You can use facial reflexology to quickly relieve any pain, at any time, and in any place, with your fingers or the rounded tip of a ballpoint pen as simple instrument, and you can apply it to yourself, or anyone in your circle.

The advantage of this method resides in the fact that it is possible to learn how to heal yourself. However, it is also necessary to correctly appreciate that there are other factors interfering with your good health. It is normal for pain to return and problems to resist whatever treatment is chosen if the following factors persist:

- If you do not pay enough attention to your breath, diet, and surroundings, avoiding all kinds of pollution
- if you allow yourself to be consumed by worry or unbalanced by your emotions
- if you take no notice of physical or psychological tiredness

*No* miracle method exists to put you out of the reach of sickness, especially if you take no notice of these environmental factors.

## What Kinds of Problems Can Facial Reflexology Help?

The great attraction of facial reflexology is that it is capable of preventing and giving relief from many of the little ailments and pains that diminish your quality of life and that modern medicine often cannot cure, except with stronger and stronger medicines, usually more toxic. Although it will not be practical to give a complete list of all the possibilities here, chapter 4 provides a comprehensive list of treatable conditions. Just to give you a preliminary idea of conditions you can expect to gain relief from:

*Problems with the back, joints, and muscles:* pain in the lower back, back of the neck, shoulders, knees, spine, arms, legs, hands, fingers, feet, ankles, osteoarthritis, rheumatism, polyarthritis, sprains, sciatica, lumbago, and related conditions

*Sexual and genital problems, hormonal upsets:* painful, overabundant, or insufficient menstruation, amenorrhea, white discharge, vaginitis, prostate trouble, sterility, contraception, impotence, frigidity, pain during sexual intercourse, premature ejaculation, pre-menopause, menopause, hot flashes, vaginal dryness, ptosis of the womb, fibroid tumor, ovarian cyst, mammary cyst, breast-feeding difficulties, over or under active thyroid, and related conditions

*Skin problems:* various kinds of inflammation, acne, pruritis, eczema, psoriasis, burns, herpes zona, hives, urticaria, allergies, and related conditions

*Problems of digestion, assimilation, and elimination:* colitis, gastritis, diabetes, constipation, diarrhea, hepatitis, gall stones, kidney stones, water retention, obesity, cellulitis, migraines, and related conditions

*Troubles of the nervous system:* nervous depression, insomnia, anxiety, irritability, nervous or hyperactive child, apathy, chronic tiredness, headaches, travel sickness, and related conditions

*Circulatory troubles:* bad circulation, varicose veins, high or low blood pressure, dizziness, troubles of concentration, and related conditions

*Respiratory troubles:* bronchitis, asthma, sinusitis, common colds, and related conditions

*A few specific or chronic disorders:* Parkinson's disease, certain tumors, hemiplegia, paralysis, paresthesia

*Other:* poor vision, poor hearing, sore throats, and related conditions

Results are generally excellent in all the above cases, both in redressing the condition and in relieving pain and various types of inflammation, especially when the problem is recent, the patient's energy is intact, and he or she is motivated. In the case of chronic sickness it is possible for symptoms to reappear when treatment is discontinued. Therefore this method is designed above all for patients to practice on themselves.

If you practice Dien' Cham' as soon as the first symptoms appear, you will prevent the problem from establishing itself or worsening, and usually avoid having to have recourse to doctors or medicines. Therefore it is better to get to the root of the trouble and get rid of it as soon as possible.

Where more serious or complex conditions arise, or in the case of psychosomatic sickness, results are more limited, and require long-term treatment combined with other therapeutic methods. Dien' Cham' cannot replace classical medical treatment in the case of serious injury, or when pain persists after stimulation. However, Dien' Cham' can be combined with other treatments to activate their effects and contribute notably to putting you on your feet quickly. Nothing stops you from using it while also following a standard allopathic treatment or looking after yourself using plants or other methods like acupuncture, Qi Gong, Reiki, or faith healing, if you think that it is necessary.

Dien' Cham' is a special complementary therapy, which can be used in conjunction with any other kind of treatment. Your immune system and your emunctories will be boosted, and any toxic effects from medicines and drugs taken will be attenuated. People with serious conditions have nothing to lose and everything to gain by combining therapies.

### A Special Case: Cancer

Encouraging results have been recorded with certain cancers treated early on. The method can also greatly assist a patient in coping with the secondary effects of chemotherapy and other painful treatments, by stimulating the immune system, eliminating tiredness, attenuating pain and other unpleasant symptoms, as well as calming anxiety through relaxation and good energy circulation.

Secondary effects and tiredness caused by chemotherapy can be such that patients often do not have the will to stir themselves. With the shock of the news of their sickness and thinking themselves condemned, they literally let themselves die of desperation. Dien' Cham' can help such persons feel better by eliminating secondary effects caused by the treatment. That will allow a certain confidence to be restored, and push them to respond and be more positive. When allopathic treatment is complemented with more natural means, it can thus help a patient decide to pull through. Hope is reborn in this way!

### More Serious Problems Too!

Please do not believe that this method's simplicity and harmlessness mean it can only be used for the most common and benign of complaints. This is not the case. It is also recommended for the treatment of serious sicknesses, as a complement to classical means of course. However, it is impor-

tant for each person to take responsibility for his or her own Dien' Cham' treatment, or, if this is impossible, to be treated by a member of the family circle or a friend, so that the person does not become dependent on a therapist. Even though it is initially advisable, when possible, for a patient to receive treatment from a competent therapist, it is far better that he or she learns to treat him or herself. It is only this autonomy that allows the treatment to be applied as often as needed, in many cases, several times a day. The stimulation of pressure points relaxes the nervous system, restores energy, and revitalizes all of the body functions, allowing it to heal itself. Only regular sessions enable these results to be obtained.

## ENERGY-GIVING MASSAGE

Dien' Cham' is also an extremely effective method of therapeutic massage. I would like to share with you a simple technique that will be of great service. This simple massage ensures that you are fully awake and full of energy for the day. It can remove the tiredness of a sleepless night as well as the beginnings of wrinkles by relaxing the face and improving facial blood and energy circulation. It is a good idea to get into the habit of giving yourself a short session of energy-giving massage every day as soon as you get up in the morning to give yourself a boost. It is also useful during the day, even though it has the slight drawback of messing up your hair! It is so agreeable that soon you will not be able to do without it.

This massage only requires a few minutes and your hands as sole instruments.

In the morning you may have the bad habit of jumping out of bed as soon as the alarm clock rings. This is bad for your health because your energy is resting during the night. To reactivate it properly, start by stretching yourself like animals do, but softly, because contracting the muscles too strongly can have the effect of a blockage, and you risk having cramps and pain.

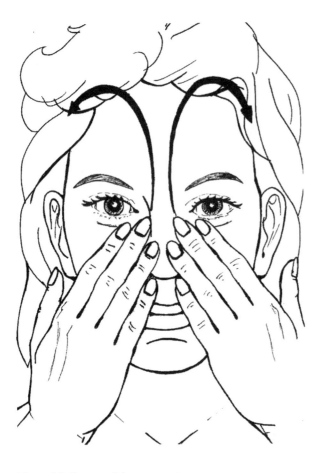

Figure 1.2. Energy-giving massage

- Push your hands upward, sliding your middle fingers to the root of the nose, then to the middle of the forehead and from there into the scalp and the top of the head. The palms and the other fingers should smooth all of the forehead.
- Then the two hands descend on either side of the head massaging the ears to warm them up, and the palms link up at the tip of the chin.
- Replace your hands in the initial position and repeat the circuit twelve times or so in a continuous movement. The pressure of the hands and the fingers on the face must be firm and constant.

When your short session is finished take a minute to sense the heat and circulation of energy on the face. You will have but one desire, which will be to jump out of bed, full of enthusiasm to start the new day!

Are you up at last? You can finish the massage in the bathroom by washing your face with hot water and then splashing it with cold. Your face and whole body will feel invigorated.

This massage is especially good to use to restore your energy when you are on a tiring trip in an automobile. By giving yourself time to rest and rejuvenate you will quickly recover any time "lost" through greater efficiency and focus. You could also perhaps avoid an accident.

This exercise also helps you to better withstand the chill of winter and you will be less susceptible to head colds!

- While you are still in bed, rub your hands one against the other to warm them up. Then place them on your face at either side of your nose with the middle fingers on the upper part of the nose and the other fingers firmly in contact with the face.

# 2

# Reflex Zones and Points: Main Diagrams

## THE FACE: A COMPLEX SYSTEM

While other types of reflexology—such as foot, hand, or ear—only work with one schematic diagram of the projection of the body and the organs onto the zone concerned, facial reflexology is quite different. The face could be compared to a kind of layer cake, one with several strata of flaky pastry. As a result, several compatible projection systems are found on the face. As has already been pointed out, the particularity of facial reflexology is that it is multi-system and multi-directional. Professor Bui Quoc Chau has thus far elaborated twenty-two diagrams showing the projection of the body onto the face! Please do not be worried: the system of Dien' Cham' I am presenting in this book only uses thirteen diagrams. I have also added a few diagrams in order to simplify your study by presenting certain information from the original diagrams separately.

Please do not say "It's too complicated, I'm going to get lost!" Take it easy! You are going to see that there is a kind of internal logic to the system. Everything makes sense. You only have to follow me step by step and all will be well. You will get through the few complex areas quite easily.

Of course the upshot of this is that each point and zone corresponds to many targets, unlike in foot reflexology, where, for example, the liver would be stimulated by a single exact point on the sole of the right foot. In Dien' Cham' the liver has several corresponding zones and points.

This will bring you to ask yourself the following questions at one time or another:

### How can you tell which point or zone to stimulate?

This one is easy: the sensitive ones! If all of them are sensitive, you can stimulate all of them. But most often you will only find one or two that really react. They are the ones, that particular day, which will be the most effective. However in later sessions it is quite possible that other points will take their place. Do not stick to one point or zone thinking, "That's the one for me!" It can be true for that instant and nothing more.

There is a certain advantage to multiple correspondences. If you have a spot or other skin lesion right in the zone that you are interested in, no problem, there is a choice of several others! So there is no excuse to miss out on your session!

*One pressure point seems to correspond to my symptoms but some other indications do not correspond to me. What do I do in this case?*

This can happen quite frequently. Among the various indications for each point, it is quite likely that many of them do not fit with your case.

For example, you have a liver upset and point **233** corresponds. When you look in the indications you will also see "piles" or "hemorrhoids," which you do not have, and "excess perspiration," but you know that you do not perspire or sweat easily. What do you do then? If this point is slightly painful, simply stimulate it. A liver problem can be the origin of the determined symptoms but it is the body that controls the energy freed in this way and which self-heals!

You can understand with this example the simplicity of the method beyond its apparent complexity. Your work is just to free up the energy blocked in certain zones and points and the body does the rest! As long as you respect the very simple basic rules, you do not run the risk of an unwise action or unwanted complications. In Dien' Cham' there are very few possible bad effects and these will be clearly explained at the pertinent moment. So there is no cause for hesitation! Get started!

There are two main ways to use these diagrams in the practice of facial reflexology: one is to focus on corresponding pressure points; and the other is to massage an entire zone. Generally both are used together in a complementary way. The complete practice of Dien' Cham' implies the consideration of the different diagrams of the body's projection on the face, and then use of one for determining the pertinent reflex points.

In order to be able to practice Dien' Cham' in all circumstances, it is necessary to know by heart the main reflex zones and points likely to be able to help. At the beginning some of my readers, especially those of you who are more "visual," will find it easier to memorize one of the main body-on-face projection diagrams, or part of it. It is better to start by learning and practicing one diagram at a time, otherwise there is a danger of mixing them up! Be reassured however, nothing serious can result from this, just a lack of results!

### *Exception:*

**Diagram 1** (figures 2.2a and 2.2b) summarizing the various reflex points is the only exception to this rule regarding the importance of memorizing the various diagrams. Do not attempt to learn this one by heart. It will not serve any purpose. The points on it are drawn in no specific order. You will learn these, little by little, while you practice.

## Use Analogy

To assist you, here is a tip: analogy! If you use this frequently it will enable you to have an excellent practice of facial reflexology without having to take this book with you everywhere. Thanks to it you will never need to overburden your memory or doubt yourself all the time. All you need to do is to refer to your own body for it to refresh your memory of the main correspondences you are going to need.

---

**Basic Rule 1**

There is no inversion—or only exceptionally, and this will be detailed at the correct time.

- right side of the face = right side of the body
- left side of the face = left side of the body

What could be easier?

---

# THE FICTIVE GRID

This grid enables the reflex points to be located with accuracy. The vast majority are found at the intersection between a horizontal and a vertical line. This is why it is important for you to know it well. You need not worry about having to work on faces with different morphologies—long, thickset, thin, broad, and so on. This grid is based upon constants in the face and therefore is adapted to everyone.

## Vertical Lines

From the centerline which cuts the face into two equal parts, right and left, the vertical lines are determined as a function of the eyes, and only the eyes! Therefore ask the person you are working with to look straight ahead.

- The first line separates the face into two equal parts through the bridge of the nose.

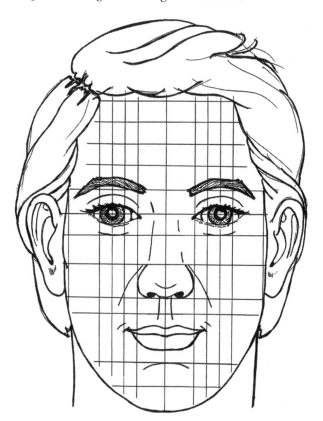

Figure 2.1. Blank Diagram

- The second line, on both sides, crosses the inner corner of the eye.
- The third line touches the inner edge of the iris, the colored part of the eye.
- The fourth line crosses the center of the pupil.
- The fifth line touches the outer edge of the iris.

## Horizontal Lines

Let us start with the forehead: from the hairline to the eyebrows, it is separated into four equal parts.

- The first line follows the hairline.
- The third line separates the forehead into two equal parts.
- The second line passes halfway between the first and the third.
- The fifth line goes through the eyebrow roots.
- The fourth line passes between the third and the fifth.

Let us continue downward from the eyebrows to the chin

- The sixth line crosses the center of the pupil.
- The seventh line touches the lower edge of the orbit.
- The eighth line goes through the upper creases of the nostrils.
- The ninth line touches the base of the nose.
- The tenth line crosses halfway up the upper lip.
- The eleventh line goes through the crease in the chin.

Certain points do not correspond to lines on the grid, especially on the temples and around the nose. These points are easy to locate using the side view of **Diagram 1** (see Figure 2.2b below) and it did not seem necessary to overload the grid for the sake of a few points.

# DIAGRAM 1: PROJECTION OF REFLEX POINTS ON THE FACE

As I mentioned earlier, Professor Bui Quoc Chau has identified over 500 points on the face, but in this book we will work with only fifty-seven for the purposes of simplification. These points are depicted on **Diagram 1 (front view and side view)** (Figures 2.2a and 2.2b). Just imagine a face with 600 points, compared to this one, which must already appear difficult!

To avoid later confusion between the two systems, I have retained the original numbers assigned to these points by Professor Bui Quoc Chau. As a result, the numbers range from "0" to "560," even though there are only fifty-seven points. Do not look for the missing points; you will not find them! Also, do not expect any closeness between adjacent numbers. The points are numbered in the sequence that Professor Bui Quoc Chau determined their properties and correspondences.

**Diagram 1 (side view)** shows the location of the points outside the grid on the temples, around the ears and even those around the nostrils. Do not forget to consult this when you make your first attempts! It will help you avoid mistakes.

Please note that point **14** is to be found just at the base of the earlobe, and **15** is located in the hollow behind the ear.

For further details please refer to chapter 5 where each point is studied separately: correspondences, properties, and precise location.

## Point Stimulation Direction

In **Diagram 1** small arrows give an indication of the best direction for stimulation of each point, according to the specifications of Professor Bui Quoc Chau. This is given as a guide and generally reserved for persons with good knowledge of the technique.

In practice it is not really necessary to be so precise. However these indications are logical. For example, to stimulate point 34 situated at the inside end of the eyebrow, it will be more comfortable to do it by going with the direction of the hairs, rather than the other way, although it will hardly change the result. In the same way, point **26**, located between the eyebrows, can be stimulated by rubbing or by sweeping movements from the top down and from the bottom up.

It all depends on the instrument that you are using (which will be discussed in the next chapter). If you are massaging with a steel instrument the points should be stimulated by rubbing and turning on the spot gently. If you are using a pen, a roller, or a rod it will be easier to stroke the zone where the point is.

## Facial Massage Direction

There is another simple rule to remember concerning the choice of direction for a facial massage, depending on the desired result:

For relaxation, proceed from the head to the feet: from the forehead to the chin.
For toning up, proceed from the feet to the head: from the chin to the forehead.

Beginners would do well not to take into consideration such details as this for their first attempts, as results can be excellent with the simplest of procedures. However, once you have a little practice, this rule can be of real help to you and really boost your results.

### My Advice

Do not try to memorize these points. You will learn them little by little while you practice. Happily you are soon going to be able to use reflex zones and that will allow you perform a session if required, even if you have only retained a few points. The best progress is step-by-step!

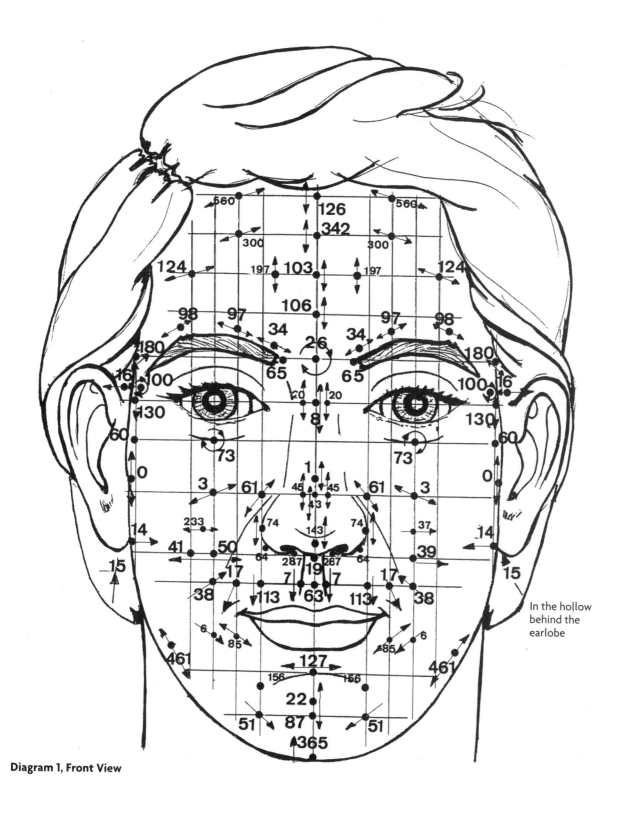

**Diagram 1, Front View**

Figure 2.2a. Reflex points on the face (may be photocopied for personal use)

In the hollow
behind the
earlobe

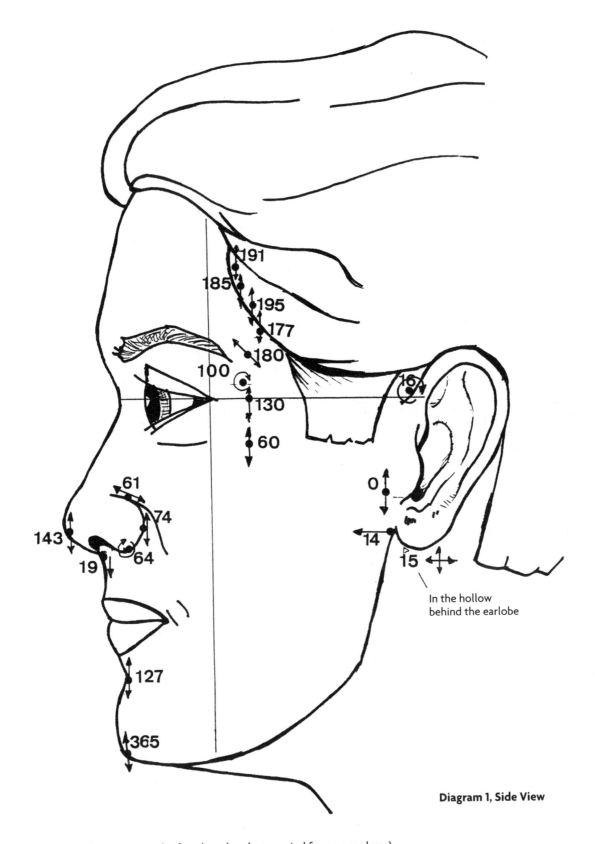

191

185

195

177

180

100

130

60

61

74

143

64

19

127

365

0

14

15

In the hollow
behind the earlobe

**Diagram 1, Side View**

Fig. 2.2b. Reflex points on the face (may be photocopied for personal use)

# DIAGRAM 2: GENERAL PROJECTION OF THE BODY ON THE FACE

Let us now look at the way it is possible to visualize the correspondences of different parts of the body and your face. We will start with the diagram that is the easiest to memorize and the one that will be the most useful in the case of a wound, sprain, accident, or problem with a joint, on any part of the body. **Diagram 2** (Figure 2.3) represents the outer body schematic diagram; said in another way, it shows each body part's correspondence with parts of the face.

The figure shows a human form projected onto the face. The basic idea is to represent in an analogical way the whole body on the face.

- In this way it is easy to see the pelvis or hips in the nostrils, as well as the buttocks!
- The nose reminds us of the torso and the bridge

of the spinal column. The coccyx is at the end of the nose, and as we move upward along the bridge we can recognize first the lumbar, then the dorsal vertebrae, and finally the neck vertebrae, located in the hollow at the root of the nose.

- Following on naturally from this, after the cervical vertebrae, the head is projected in the center of the lower part of the forehead. This head contains everything; brain, eyes, ears on each side of the projection zone, the mouth, teeth, etc. Do you see the logic that you need to follow?

At present we have a torso and a head. What do you think could represent the upper limbs consisting of shoulders, arms, forearms, wrists and hands? Referring to the diagram you can see where the neck vertebrae are—at the nose root. The limbs start from here on each side following the eyebrows. In this way we obtain:

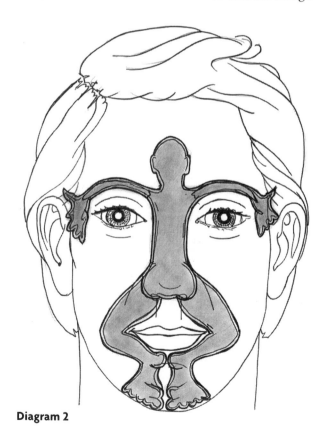

**Diagram 2**

Figure 2.3. General projection of the body on the face

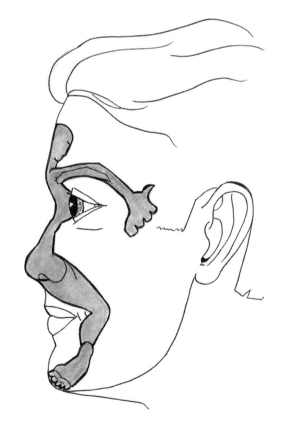

- The shoulders at the root of the eyebrows, right shoulder on the right side, left shoulder on the left. Nothing could be easier! The zone is not represented by a simple line following the curve of the eyebrows. The whole arch of the eyebrows is concerned, and you will sometimes find the painful point on the eyebrows, but also slightly below or slightly above. Some shoulder pains originate in the upper part of the back. In this case do not be surprised to find a painful reflex zone toward the nose at the level of the first dorsal vertebrae on the slope (but not on the bridge).
- Leading on from the shoulder zone, in the same way as for the arm on the body, you will find the zone corresponding to the arm.
- The elbow can be found at the top of the eyebrow, near the center, just before it descends. In case of pain in the elbow, search for the exact point—the most sensitive point—not only on the eyebrow itself, but also a little above and below.
- Following on from the elbow, the forearm is projected on the part of the eyebrow that curves downward.
- At the natural end of the eyebrows—bearing in mind that some women pluck their eyebrows—you will find the zone corresponding to the wrist at the end of the arch.
- From here, over the temples, you will find a projection of the whole of the hand, with the five fingers spread out.

At present we have the projection of the torso, head, and upper limbs. Where do you think we will logically find the projection of the lower limbs? At the base of the torso obviously. Look at your face.

**Basic Rule 2**

In any given reflex zone try to find the most painful point! To do this it is often necessary to feel around a little! Do not hesitate to do this.

You will see two creases, more or less marked, according to your age and type. These "nasogenian creases" start from the side of each nostril, and link up with the corners of your mouth where the lips meet.

Do you not agree that they could well represent the legs slightly apart? So we now have:

- The thighs beginning along the side of each nostril, and running along the nasogenian creases.
- At the corners of the mouth, we find the knees.
- Then the legs along a fictitious line from the corners of the mouth to the chin, on each side of the mouth.
- You will find the ankles projected toward the hollow in the chin on either side.
- Then there are the feet. The soles are found along the middle line of the chin.
- As for the toes, they are projected along the edge of the jaws, with the big toe toward the center of the chin and the others along the jaw. In case of need you will easily find the point corresponding to the one causing problems.

**Basic Rule 3**

The joints always represent a break in the alignment of the limbs or other parts of the body. It is therefore logical to find them projected on zones with the same kind of break, such as top of eyebrow, corner of mouth, hollow in chin, end of eyebrow, edge of scalp, and so on.

Wherever a line of the face is interrupted or changes direction, there is every chance that the spot corresponds to one or more joints, and these will correspond to each other!

If you are able to remember this, it will help you greatly!

To sum up, you will find the body projection in the following descending order:

- The head, represented on the middle part of the forehead.

- The root of the nose corresponds to the neck vertebrae.
- The shoulders and rest of the upper limbs follow the lines of the eyebrows, with the hands represented on the temples.
- The spine represented from the lower forehead, along the bridge of the nose.
- The buttocks and hips represented by the nostrils.
- The thighs following the nasogenian crease.
- The knees at the corners of the mouth.
- The lower legs following a line to the chin.
- The feet together on the chin level.
- The big toes toward the center of the chin.
- The other toes in order along the edge of the jaw.

These indications will allow you to find the zone to be massaged. However, please take notice of the fact that you will have to search for the most sensitive points in the zone of correspondence. After stimulating the whole reflex zone, you will need to spend some time stimulating these points, until the painful sensation disappears. The same rule applies for all projection zones.

# DIAGRAM 3: PROJECTION OF INTERNAL ORGANS ON THE FACE

This newer system of projection can be deduced from the preceding one, and can help memorization enormously. For this you are going to compare your face to a body.

Start by considering your torso. It is composed of two main parts; the thorax and the abdomen. What is the difference between the two? In the thorax is found the rib cage, protecting the organs inside. The abdomen is the soft part, carried by the pelvis.

Now you can consider how your face is also constituted of two main parts: an upper bony part, cheekbones and forehead, and the lower, softer part, carried by the skull.

This basic analogy checks out when we go into detail:

- The thorax and everything within it is projected onto the bony parts of the face; cheekbones and forehead.
- The abdomen and everything inside is projected on the lower part of the face, below the cheekbones.

Let us continue with the analogy referring to our own body. Remember the right side of the face corresponds to the right side of the body and the same goes for the left side!

What do you find in the rib cage?
The lungs, bronchial tubes, the heart.
What are we going to find on the cheekbones and forehead?
The lungs, bronchial tubes, the heart, also!
What is under the ribs on the right side?
The liver and the bile duct.
Where are we going to find the projection of the liver and bile duct on the face?
On the right below the cheekbone!
What do you find under the ribs on the left?
The spleen and the pancreas.
What are we going to find under the left cheekbone?
The spleen and the pancreas.

This analogy is consistent and allows you to deduce what you are going to find below the cheekbones and in what order. Consider your abdomen for example. Under the diaphragm you will find the intestines—the small intestine and the colon—on each side, the kidneys with the adrenal glands above. Lower you will find the bladder, and the genitals at the base of the torso. You will find these organs in the same order as projected on the face!

Let us again take the example of the colon. In your body the colon rises on the right side, turns and passes under your diaphragm, turns again and descends on the left before reaching the rectum and the anus, in the center at the base of the torso. In the same way, on the face you will find the intestine rising on the right of the mouth, following the nasogenian crease, and crossing the upper lip toward the left. The colon then descends via the left nasogenian crease, continues to the center of the chin and terminates in the zone corresponding to the rectum and the anus at the base of the face.

The kidneys are projected on both sides at the corners of the mouth, and above are found the adrenal glands.

Now glance at **Diagram 3** (Figure 2.4), which shows the projection of the internal organs on the face. Keeping this analogy in mind will make remembering so much easier! It should be noted here that all of the internal organ reflex zones are located between the eyebrows and the base of the chin.

### Note:

Please do not be astonished to find the genital organs projected on the upper lip, in addition to the projection on the chin. Remember that the body has several projection systems, overlaid somewhat like a layer cake, as well as the reflex point system!

**Let us recap**, following the order given in Figure 2.4.

1. From the root to the center of the nose, on the left side: **heart and pulmonary artery.**
2. From the eyebrows to the cheekbones: **lungs and bronchial tubes.**
3. Just below the cheekbone on the right: **liver.**
4. Included in the lower part of same area: **gall bladder and bile ducts.**
5. Just below the cheekbone on the left: **stomach and pancreas.**
6. To the left of the nostril, next to the stomach: **spleen.**
7. Just below the nose: **stomach, pancreas, transverse colon, ovaries, prostate.**

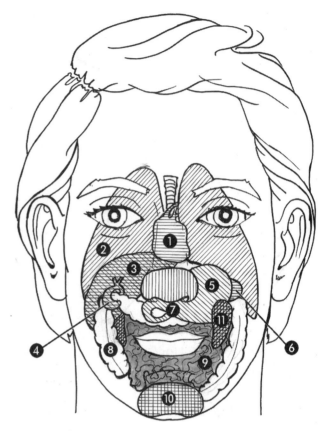

**Diagram 3**

Figure 2.4. Projection of internal organs on the face

8. The area corresponding to the **colon** starts from the edge of the chin on the right, rises to the upper lip (**ascending colon**), crosses the area between the nose and the lip (**transverse colon**), and descends to the point of the chin (**descending colon**).
9. Around the lips: **the small intestine.**
10. The area around the upper part of the chin: **womb, ovaries, prostate gland, testicles, bladder, rectum.**
11. On each side of the mouth: **kidneys and adrenal glands.**

Please note that the zones corresponding to the stomach and the pancreas are on the left of the nose and on the upper lip, because of their more or less center-left location under the rib cage. The presence of the nose prevents us from using all of the reflex zone. However the projection can be found in endonasal reflexology.

## DIAGRAMS 4, 5, AND 6: PROJECTION OF THE LIMBS ON THE FOREHEAD

**Diagram 4** (Figure 2.5) shows a man leaning forward with his hands over his head. These locations of the limbs on the forehead are in accordance with the various parts of the homunculus drawn in the 1920s by the Canadian neurosurgeon Wilder Graves Penfield on his maps depicting the different functions of the human cerebral cortex.

Start by visualizing an imaginary vertical line linking the point between your eyebrows and the center of the hairline. The forehead is now bisected.

On either side of this vertical line, we will be able to find the projection of the corresponding half of the body; right to right, left to left. Along the length of this vertical line we have a projection of the legs; right leg to the right of the line, left leg to the left.

- The buttocks and the pelvis are represented with left and right parts side by side, at the center of the hairline, at the top of the forehead.
- The projection of the knees is at the center of the forehead above the eyebrow roots.
- Then we can find the thighs in between the two above.
- Then we can find the reflex zones of the legs, down from the knees toward the eyebrows.
- A little further down, you will find the ankle reflex zones.
- And then the feet and toe reflex zones, which are projected starting from the point between the eyebrows. The big toes are represented at the root of the eyebrow, whereas the fifth toe is located at point 26 (shown on **Diagram 1**).

From the center of the hairline toward the outer angle, a projection of the torso can be found:

- The back and the spinal column along this line starting with the coccyx in the center, then the lumbar vertebrae, the dorsal vertebrae, and finally, the neck vertebrae between the external angle of the temple, descending along the hairline.
- The abdomen is found in the same order between the projection of the pelvis and halfway along the hairline.
- Then you will find the chest.
- And finally, the shoulder articulation at the external angle of the forehead.

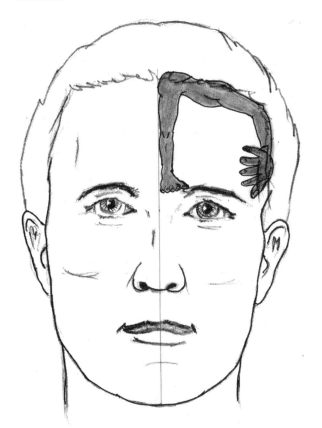

**Diagram 4**

Figure 2.5. Projection of the limbs on the forehead

Then, the projection of the arm descends toward the temple starting at the projection of the shoulder.

- The shoulder, located at the external angle of the hairline.
- The arm descending toward the temple.
- The elbow in the middle of the forehead.
- The forearm.
- And finally the hand and fingers following the hair roots. The thumb is represented on the temple, the little finger on the forehead center-line and the other fingers in between.

**Diagram 5** (Figure 2.6) shows the projection of the left leg on the forehead. The right leg is pro-

jected in similar fashion on the right side of the forehead. The numbers indicate the various parts of the leg:

1. Foot, with the toes projected between central point and the eyebrow root
2. Ankle
3. Calf
4. Knee
5. Thigh
6. Hip and pelvis

**Diagram 6** (Figure 2.7) shows the arm projections on the forehead.

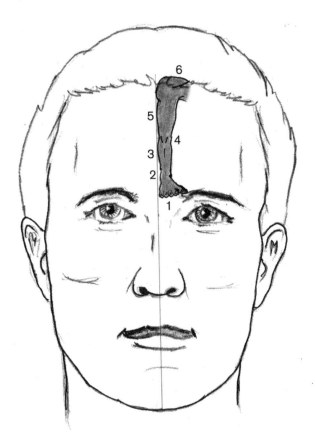

**Diagram 5**

Figure 2.6. Projection of the legs on the forehead

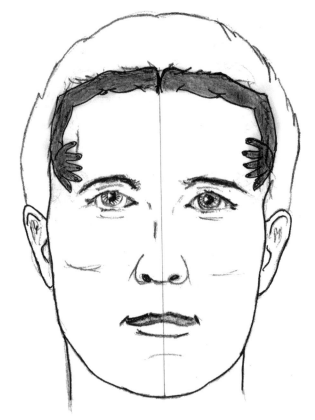

**Diagram 6**

Figure 2.7. Projection of the arms on the forehead

# DIAGRAM 7: PROJECTION OF THE FACE ON THE EAR

Keeping in mind the image shown in **Diagram 4** (Figure 2.5)—of a man bending down, two arms over his head, his head dangling—the head and face reflex zone would be located in the prolongation of the shoulder reflex zone, in front of the temple. That places the neck and nape of the neck above the ear in the hair.

The head and face reflex zone also has another aspect and projection on the ear lobe and just forward of the ear, where we find:

- The eye, at the junction of the upper part of the ear and face, at the level of the end of the eyebrow and in the upper part of the auricle, or outer ear.
- The nose, projected onto the tragus, the small flap of cartilage in front of the ear, and the lower part of the anthelix at the level of the nose median line.
- The mouth and the tongue are projected at the point where the lobe is attached to the face, with projection of half of the mouth, the teeth and the relevant half-tongue on the ear lobe itself.

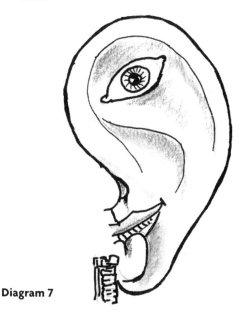

**Diagram 7**

Figure 2.8. Projection of the face on the ear

- The trachea or windpipe, esophagus, larynx, throat, as well as the thyroid glands and para-thyroid glands are projected on the zone below the ear lobe, at the junction of the lobe and the jaw.

# DIAGRAM 8: PROJECTIONS OF THE SPINAL COLUMN ON THE FACE

In **Diagram 8** (Figure 2.9) you will find several reflex zones corresponding to the spinal column. There are four projections of the spinal column on the face, represented in this diagram.

1. On the bridge of the nose (**Diagram 2**), the coccyx is at the tip of the nose and the neck vertebrae are in the hollow between the eyebrows

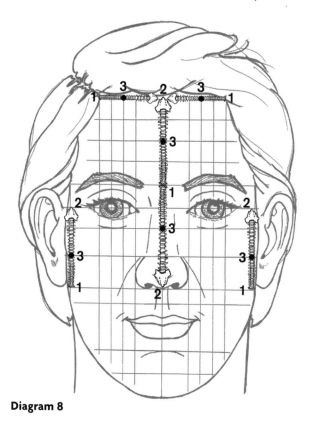

**Diagram 8**

Figure 2.9. Projections of the spinal column on the face
1. Neck vertebrae
2. Coccyx
3. Solar plexus

and the root of the nose. The solar plexus is halfway up, and constitutes the point of separation between the thorax and abdomen.

2. Along a vertical line from the root of the nose to the roots of the hair, in the center, we again have the neck vertebrae between the eyebrows, logically prolonged by a spinal column with the coccyx located at the root of the hair. The solar plexus can be found in the middle of this line, at point **103** (as shown on **Diagram 1**). This point also marks the separation point between the thorax, on the level of the dorsal vertebrae, and the abdomen, located between point **103** and the hairline. Obviously these organ correspondences can be extended to the whole of the forehead, as per **Diagram 9** (Figure 2.10).

3. As the root of the hair is a coccyx zone, a spinal column can again be found starting from this point in the center of the hairline. This time the projection zone is cut into two and so we find the following: the right part of the spine which goes from the coccyx at point **126** (see **Diagram 1**), to the neck vertebrae at the angle on the right of the scalp; the left part of the spine which also starts at point **126**, and ends at the neck vertebrae at the angle on the left of the scalp.

4. The line starting at the lower ear lobe attachment point and continuing to the upper ear-to-face attachment point also represents another spinal column correspondence zone. Please try to remember that at the base of the lobe you will find points **14** and **15** (see **Diagram 1**), which are analogical to the throat, thyroid, and so on. Wherever a throat correspondence can be found, there will also be a correspondence with the neck vertebrae. Therefore the following are found: from point **14** to point **0**, the neck and dorsal vertebrae; from point **0** to point **16**, the lumbar vertebrae and coccyx. The right side/left side rule applies as usual.

With a little practice you will easily be able to locate each vertebra. The alarm signal of your body showing you the exact point is of course the most painful spot!

These spinal column zones are important because very often one of the corresponding zones is more painful than another, and this can vary from one session to the next. For this reason good knowledge of them can prove extremely useful. In practice it is best to test all of them systematically and only use the ones that appear to reacting well.

You would also do well to recall our analogical method:

- Wherever you are able to find a zone or point corresponding to the neck or throat, you will also find the neck vertebrae and therefore the rest of the spinal column.
- In the same way, if you find the projection of the pelvis or the buttocks, you will necessarily find a coccyx and the beginning of a spinal column!

Furthermore, wherever you find a spinal column, that is to say dorsal and lumbar vertebrae, you will also find a thorax and an abdomen. Whatever is behind is similar to what is in front and vice versa. This will enable you to deduce easily the correspondence zones of organs without having to make an effort to remember:

- The lumbar vertebrae and coccyx are in correspondence with an abdomen with all the organs contained in it.
- The dorsal vertebrae correspond to the thorax with its organs.

Always remember that your own body is the best reference and reminder you have. If in any doubt refer back to it immediately and ask questions in the following vein.

Where is my liver?

Under the ribs, on the right, just below the thorax.

Where am I going to find the liver with respect to a projection of the spinal column?

On the right, just below the thorax.

And so on.

You will quickly find this way of remembering highly effective! Thanks to it you will be able to practice Dien' Cham' in any circumstances, with an improvised instrument, and without always having to refer to this book!

## DIAGRAMS 9 AND 10: FOREHEAD REFLEX ZONES

As a starting point let us take the spinal column reflex zone located along the forehead center line, between the root of the nose and the center of the hairline. Remember that between the eyebrows at the root of the nose is a neck vertebrae reflex zone, which is very useful in cases of stiff neck, or crick in the neck! And in the center of the hairline you will find a projection of the pelvis, on the left and on the right, respectively.

From this we can deduce the presence of a new projected person analogous to the one in **Diagram 2**, but this time with his head down! The shoulders and the arms remain in place but the body is upturned. This is what we find projected in **Diagram 9** (Figure 2.10).

This projection results in locating:

- The head on the upper part of the nose, with points corresponding to the eyes, ears, mouth teeth, and so on.
- The shoulders, arms, elbows, forearms, knuckles, hands, and fingers along the eyebrows and on the temples.
- The dorsal vertebrae above the neck vertebrae (points **26** to **103** as shown on **Diagram 1**).
- The solar plexus in the middle of the forehead (point **103**).

- Then, the lumbar vertebrae (points **103** to **342**).
- To finish, the coccyx (points **342** to **126**).

We find the hips and the buttocks at the hairline, and a new projection of the lower limbs on each side, exactly where we found the upper limbs in **Diagram 4** (Figure 2.5). It is as if this man is balanced on his head with arms and legs spread, with a curious pliability of the knees! Here we have:

- The pelvis in the center of the hairline, with right side to right side.
- The thighs along the line of the scalp, from the center to the outer angle.
- The knees at the outer angle.
- The legs from the outer angle, down toward the temples.
- The ankles, feet, and toes still following the hairline to the temples.

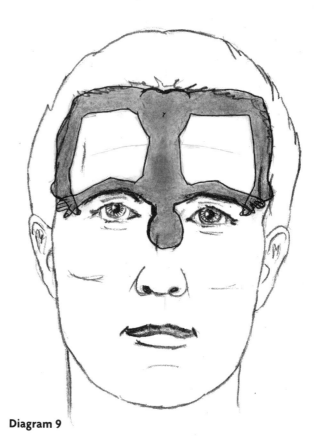

**Diagram 9**

Figure 2.10. Forehead reflex zones

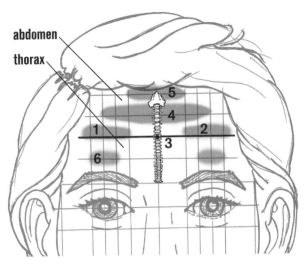

**Diagram 10**

Figure 2.11. Projection of internal organs on the forehead

1. Liver and gall bladder
2. Spleen and pancreas
3. Solar plexus and stomach
4. Lumbar vertebrae, intestines, and kidneys
5. Coccyx, genitals, bladder, and rectum
6. Breasts, heart on the left side, bronchial tubes, and lungs

**Diagram 10** (Figure 2.11), shows the thorax and abdomen projections that are, as usual, on the level of the dorsal and lumbar vertebrae, respectively. All that it is necessary to do to locate them is to draw a horizontal line from the solar plexus (point **103** on **Diagram 1**), which separates the forehead into two parts:

- The eyebrows (at the line between points **124-103-124** on **Diagram 1**) correspond to the thorax, with all that it contains: trachea, esophagus, bronchial tubes, lungs, heart, coronary arteries.

- Above that line (points **124-103-124**) to the hairline is the abdomen with all that is found within: liver, stomach, pancreas, spleen, small intestine, colon with ascending, transverse, and descending sections, kidneys, adrenal glands, ureters, bladder, and genital organs.

It will be easy for you to locate these internal organs using the analogy with your own body, and this also avoids having to give too much detail on this diagram. Furthermore, in case of a problem, the relevant zones will show you their exact location by a very specific pain. The impression is sometimes that of a cut into the skin.

# DIAGRAM 11: PROJECTIONS OF THE JOINTS ON THE FACE

**Diagram 11** (Figure 2.12) contains all of the various projections of the joints on the face. You will notice that they are most often located in a zone where there is a break in a line, for example the various "angles" formed by the hairline, or in a zone which is subject to constant creasing or folding, such as the corners of the mouth. This is analogical to the function of the joint, the role of which is to allow the limb, or other part of the body, to change direction. Please do not be surprised to see the shoulders and the pelvis, the elbows and the knees, the ankles and the wrists, the hands and the feet in the same areas!

Better still, remember that all of the joints correspond. This being the case, you can stimulate all of the joint reflex zones at the same time, giving more attention to the more sensitive ones. It is not by chance that people with arthritis rarely suffer from one joint. Most of the time it is all of the zones that are affected, but some more than others.

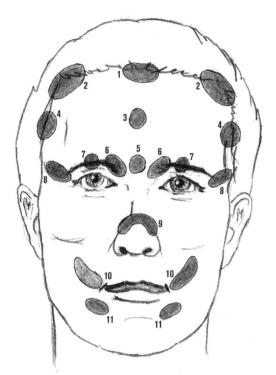

**Diagram 11**

Figure 2.12. Projections of the joints on the face
1. Coccyx, hips, and pelvis
2. Neck vertebrae, knees, and shoulders
3. Knees
4. Knees and elbows
5. Neck vertebrae, ankles
6. Shoulders and toes
7. Elbows
8. Wrists and ankles
9. Pelvis and hips
10. Knees
11. Ankles

# DIAGRAM 12: REFLEX ZONES IN FRONT OF THE EAR

**Diagram 12** (Figure 2.13) depicts the spinal column on a line just in front of the ear, starting from the ear-to-face attachment point, at the level of the eyes, and descending to its base, at the level of the ear lobe. Point 0 (see **Diagram 1**) is located in a little hollow, in the center of this line.

As I mentioned earlier concerning the spinal

column projections, as soon as a coccyx or neck zone has been identified, the rest is easy to deduce. We thus start with points **14** and **15** (see **Diagram 1**) at the base of the ear lobe and in the hollow behind, which correspond to the throat. Considering that the parts of the body are linked in a whole organism, if points **14** and **15** correspond to the throat, the zone in which they are located can only correspond to the neck and the neck vertebrae!

From this we can deduce that from the base of the ear lobe to point **0** (representing the solar plexus) are to be found the neck vertebrae and the dorsal vertebrae, and from point **0** to point **16**, the lumbar vertebrae; finally the coccyx is projected.

Do you remember what was said before about the projection of the spinal column? Once it is established, the thorax and abdomen projections can also be deduced. The same is true of the reflex

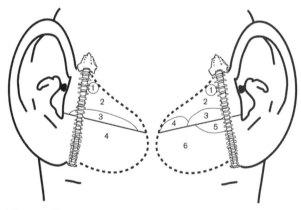

**Diagram 12**

Figure 2.13. Reflex zones in front of the ear
Right ear
1. Bladder and genital organs
2. Intestines
3. Liver and gall bladder
4. Lungs and bronchial tubes
Left ear
1. Bladder and genital organs
2. Intestines
3. Pancreas and spleen
4. Stomach
5. Heart
6. Lungs and bronchial tubes

zones located just in front of the ear at point 0. This allows us to determine the projections of the thorax, from point **14** to point **0**, and the abdomen, from point **0** to point **16**. The analogy remains true with the liver on the right, just after point **0**, the spleen and pancreas at the same level on the left ear, and the intestines above. Obviously you will find the reflex zones of the bladder, rectum, and genital organs toward the top. All of these zones stretch out a few centimeters toward the cheekbones.

As there are two ears you will find:

- In front of the right ear, the projections of the right part of the torso.
- In front of the left ear, the projections of the left part of the torso.

These zones are small but easy to stimulate. Do not search for absolute precision. Just go over the more sensitive corresponding reflex zones as a complement to the forehead and other facial stimulation.

## DIAGRAM 13: PROJECTION OF THE SOLES OF THE FEET ON THE FACE

This figure is given mainly for interest's sake. This diagram is above all for reflexologists who will be surprised at the strange analogy between the reflex zones of the hands, the soles of the feet, and the ears, and their projection on the face!

For those who are familiar with foot or hand reflexology, please note that everything is in place. Briefly here are some of the correspondences:

- The toes, which correspond to various zones of the head, sinus, and so on, and certain psychological and emotional functions, are found at the level of the eyebrows, just at the level of the sinuses. The big toes, which represent the head

as a whole, are together at the root of the nose and above, exactly on the head projection in Dien' Cham'.

- The mounts under the toes correspond to the lungs and bronchial tubes. They are also found in the same correspondence zones in Dien' Cham'.
- It is the same thing for the internal organs, liver, spleen, pancreas, and stomach, which are also found in their correspondence zones.
- Lower down on the soles of the feet, we find the intestine reflex zones which are at the level of the mouth and therefore in place. The ascending colon on the right sole, the transverse colon, which goes from one foot to the other, and then the descending colon on the left sole of the foot, all in the correct order.

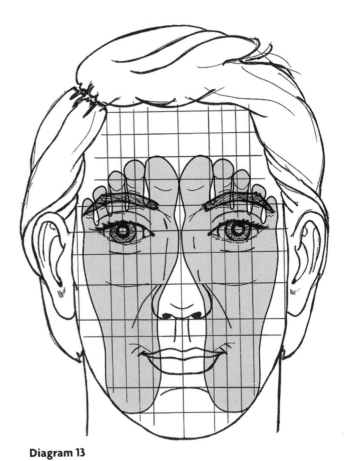

**Diagram 13**

Figure 2.14. Projection of the soles of the feet on the face

- On the heel we find the rectum, anus, and genital organ reflex zones, at the same level as the chin.

The same analogies are found in similar projections of the palms of the hand or the ears on the face. In the latter case, the right ear is projected on the right half of the face and the left ear on the left. Each ear lobe is projected on the level of the chin, and the upper edge of the outer ear follows the line of the eyebrows. The tragus is found at the level of its correspondence, which is the nose.

# 3

# Beginning the Practice of Dien' Cham'

This chapter will show you how to use some of the basic points, with descriptions of the instruments and techniques used to stimulate them. After mastering these basics you will be able to supplement them with further points or reflex zones as you progress.

## THE "INSTRUMENTS"

Unlike acupuncture, for which needles are used, facial reflexology only uses the simplest instruments: your own fingers or the rounded end of any suitable object, such as a ballpoint pen. There are also specific instruments that will give you excellent results. It is obvious that if you are a therapist your clients would be surprised to see you using a simple ballpoint pen! In this case a special roller or a flexible hammer will look more professional! However, bear the following in mind and you will not go wrong:

> **Basic Rule 4**
>
> The type of instrument matters little. What makes the difference is the correct choice of reflex zones and points, as well as the stimulation technique!

Your fingers will be your favorite tools as they are always with you, flexible and easy to direct! With them you can perform massage in two main ways:

- With the joint of the bent thumb or index finger. The end of the finger is too soft for a Dien' Cham' session; a certain pressure has to be exerted if you want results. You can rub reflex zones with the articulation of the fingers but it is difficult to locate pressure points with precision.
- With the index, the middle, or the ring finger, or all three at the same time, you can friction, rub, or tap on all the hard bony areas like the forehead. We will see more about this in detail later.

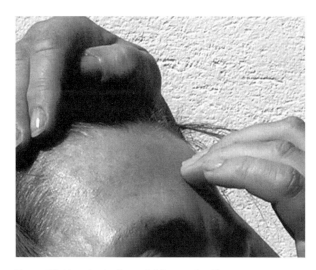

Figure 3.1. Use the index, middle, or ring finger to massage hard, bony areas such as the forehead.

Any other object with a rounded end can serve to perform this stimulation, such as:

- A simple ballpoint pen with a well-rounded end (the end opposite to the inked point). I especially recommend the two- or four-color type of ballpoint that has a little ball of plastic at the end. This ball constitutes a really good instrument for Dien' Cham' (see Figure 3.4). In addition, once the ink is used up, the rounded steel

ball of the writing point can be used to work on reflex points with more precision. You will no longer throw away your ballpoints, above all those with a nice rounded or spherical end!

- A simple wooden chopstick, usually used to eat Chinese meals, which can be bought for a few cents in your local store! You just have to file down the two ends to the shape you want, possibly with an emery board or nail file. The finest end should be filed to form a rounded off point the size of the tip on a ballpoint pen. The other should be rounded off and not too flat.

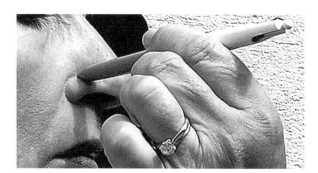

Figure 3.3. The writing end of an empty ballpoint pen can be used to work on the individual points with more precision.

- A glass probe, which is sometimes used in beauty parlors. It is very practical and smooth to touch, with one blunt end, which is practical for the stimulation of reflex zones, and another, slightly sharper but still rounded end, which allows work to be performed on many points.
- Some stones of your own choosing. You will find many at very low cost. Select ones with a long shape, if possible, with rounded ends; about an inch and a half long and half an inch in diameter. The advantage of stones is that they take up no room in your bag and you can choose the color according to your own taste. Some of my readers and students have chosen stones according to their astrological signs or own specific health problem. Personally I have several that I use according to my

Figure 3.2. The rounded end of a ballpoint pen is good for stroking Dien' Cham' reflex zones.

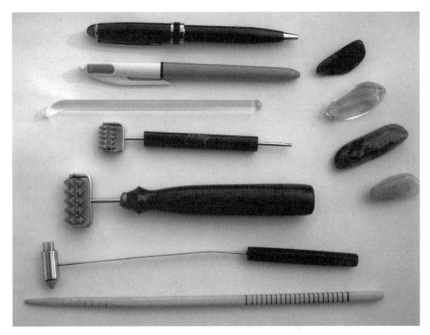

Figure 3.4. Instruments
From top to bottom
• Pens with rounded ends
• Glass probe
• Small roller
• Big roller
• Flexible hammer
• Chopsticks with filed ends
• Various stones

mood and impulse. I love working with stones that are smooth and soft to touch. It is a noble and living substance! You have the choice of all sorts of fine stones, just simply polished. On the beach you will find pebbles polished by the sea and it can become a pleasant game on holiday to look for the one that is precisely suited to your needs!

Professor Bui Quoc Chau's catalog proposes many kinds of instruments of all shapes and sizes, designed for use on all parts of the face and body. Some are specially designed for use on animals and one even allows facial reflexology to be performed on horses! (The basic technique that you can use for treating your pets is presented in chapter 7.) From this variety of rollers of all kinds, my preference goes to three instruments:

• The small facial roller called "ridoki" in Japan. The handle is a steel bar with a rounded end, allowing precise stimulation of certain points. At the other end there is a small-toothed roller. The teeth have filed edges, which makes them comfortable. To stimulate reflex zones you only have to pass the roller over the face. It is simple

and effective. This is the multi-purpose instrument I usually recommend and is also useable on cats and small dogs.

• The big roller, which allows treatment of bigger animals like horses and big dogs. It can also be used for a quick back massage, which is very relaxing. Just roll it over both sides of the spinal column for a few moments. It is a real treat!

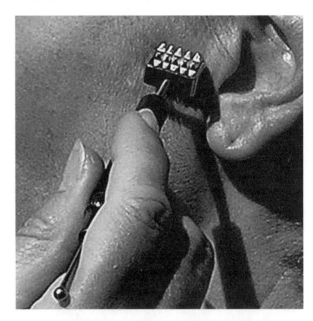

Figure 3.5. The ridoki rolls over the face to stimulate whole reflex zones. The round ball on the other end stimulates individual points precisely.

- The flexible metal hammer. This name prepares you for its use, which is rather painful on the face! I reserve it for special cases that make its use necessary, such as various kinds of paralysis and paresthesia. I recommend its use primarily for professionals. Therapists may already be familiar with the use of the sharp points of flexible hammers to stimulate the skin. Please rest easy, this one is specially designed for the face and the ends are blunt, which attenuates the sensation and avoids all risk of bleeding. The handle of the instrument is made of flexible steel. The head has two sides: one is equipped with seven small points with rounded off ends used for lightly tapping facial reflex zones; the other has a soft rubber end which is useful for massaging children and older, more fragile people or patients. It really does not hurt!

It is certainly not necessary to procure these special instruments because the others are just as effective and cost you nothing! It is very important to learn how to use common objects to stimulate the face so that you will never be found wanting. You will never have to refuse your help to someone in pain with the following sort of excuse: "Oh I am sorry! I would have been able to help with your lumbago, but I left my roller on the bedside table!"

You can also invent your own instruments following the indications that I have given above. Some of my readers and students have shown me all sorts of objects that they have made or found: wood, glass, metal, cut and ground or polished stone, and so on. Some were even creatively decorated, which adds to the pleasure. You should not hesitate further! Go and get started!

# STIMULATION TECHNIQUES

It is much easier to show these techniques than explain them. But do not worry: you will manage just fine and your intuition will allow you to complete my explanation.

## With the Fingers

Here are a few possibilities:

- Rub or make sweeping movements with a joint of your folded finger. This simple technique is very useful as it can be used anywhere with discretion. If you suddenly have backache at your desk, just a few seconds of sweeping movements over the corresponding zones will enable you to rid yourself of it. If you feel a pain in your ankle while running or suffer from muscular tension, there will be no need to stop your exercise because you can obtain relief in just a few seconds. Can you think of anything as practical or easy?
- Stimulate certain points with your fingernail. This method can't be used quite so commonly but certain points—such as point **19** located just under the nose—can be stimulated by pushing the nail in and then making a slight vibratory movement on the spot. In the case of point **19** this will give you a boost that can be useful during the day. Please take care not to use this on pregnant women or people with high blood pressure!
- Lightly tap certain facial reflex zones. You can use your wrist like the rod of a flexible hammer. First test the movement. Raise your right arm with the forearm bent and move your arm back and forth. Make sure that the gesture is supple and unrestrained. Repeat the movement, but this time lightly folding your fingers so that they practically form a right angle with the palm, like a claw in fact. Now open the palm of your raised left hand opposite the right one and tap it as was indicated previously, just once per second, not more. Once this supple movement has been well integrated, try performing the same on your face, and then on

someone in your close circle. The sensation should be agreeable!

Note: This appears to be easier for women to practice than for men, because the simple notion of a "supple wrist" seems difficult for men to integrate. Please be reminded that it is not a question of hitting with a voluntary gesture; you simply use the rebound effect natural to your wrist. With a little practice everyone can manage this!

# FOREHEAD MASSAGE: A QUICK REVITALIZATION SESSION

Straight away we shall put into practice what has just been explained. In thirty seconds you can rid yourself of some stress if necessary and feel in top form again.

## On Yourself

Stand in front of a mirror. Later, when you have a little practice, this will no longer be necessary. With one hand pull back your hair. Holding the fingers of your other hand in the shape of a hammer, regularly and softly tap the whole forehead, from the center to the sides passing through the temples, leaving no area untouched. Persevere on the eyebrows, the center line, and the hair roots.

## On Another Person

Ask the person to sit with his or her back pressed against a chair back, hands gently placed on the knees. You stand opposite. With one hand, lift the hair from his or her forehead if necessary and stimulate as follows with the other. Lightly tap with a regular movement the whole forehead of the person. You can begin in the center, then go to the sides and the temples. The important thing is to go everywhere without hitting with a firm movement. Remain supple and fluid.

This massage is well appreciated. It is pleasant and leaves the person feeling relaxed, invigorated, and with the mind alert. It is the equivalent to a siesta in just thirty seconds or so!

## Using an Instrument: Roller, Pen, Chopstick, or Stone

There are several ways of stimulating. First you should make sure that you are comfortable and, if you are going to remain standing, check that you are in good balance. Your hand should have a good point of purchase on the face, generally the wrist or one or two fingers, the little and ring fingers. This condition should always be respected so that you will not slip into the wrong direction, especially when you are working around the eyes. It is easy to slip if you work without support.

> ### Friendly Advice . . .
> It is best to work on yourself first, in front of a mirror. Then you will see what it feels like during a session.
>
> Most of the time we use our family or friends as guinea pigs, and this is not always as appreciated as we like to think.
>
> After your first attempts have allowed you to get the knack, both you and they will feel more relaxed, your results will be better, and their gratitude will be forthcoming.

Is your position correct? Are you holding your instrument firmly? Now you can proceed as follows:

- Sweep or rub a large zone around a reflex point, collection of points, or a zone, with the same instrument, following the arrows in **Diagram 1**, horizontally, vertically, diagonally, or in a direction that you determine to be logical. Remember that it is disagreeable to have the eyebrows stimulated in the direction opposing the growth of the hairs! Press down firmly but not too hard. The skin should redden a little. Even if the treatment hurts a little, especially to begin with, it should at least remain easily bearable, even comfortable. With a little practice you will be able to better judge the right amount of pressure for yourself. If the stimulation is too light, it will be ineffective. If it is too hard your guinea pigs will disappear forever. You need to find the middle ground.

- Perform a rubbing movement over a point or group of points with either the writing tip of an empty ballpoint pen, the finest tip of a stone or chopstick, or even the special steel end of a roller (make sure that it is rounded off well!) To do this correctly, you must press the instrument on the area to be massaged and turn it on the spot, making sure that the skin moves as well, as if you want to squash the tip. This technique applies to the stimulation of specific points.

- Stimulate a point or zone with a special roller. Pass the toothed roller over the selected zones using light pressure. Ten or twenty strokes are usually enough.

- The rubber hammer can be used to stimulate either a reflex point or a zone with regular light tapping, using the natural rebound of the flexible rod. This rubber end of the flexible hammer is comfortable for children and sensitive people.

- The face can be lightly tapped with the flexible metal hammer using a calm rhythm. As most people find massage with the metal end of the hammer a little painful I personally use it only for cases where it is really necessary, like paralysis or paresthesia. Nevertheless, this instrument is a lot less painful than an equivalent instrument used in other therapies. The ends are not sharp but it allows good stimulation of sleepy, energy-starved zones. As before, use light and regular tapping.

## Correct Stimulation: Repetitions and Pressure

A dozen movements over a given zone or point will usually be enough most of the time. When a

> **Please Note**
>
> Normally even vigorous stimulation of reflex points and zones only leads to a passing redness, which tends to lead to some amusement during my Dien' Cham' courses. Everyone comes out of them with a healthy-looking face!
>
> Sometimes, however, there are cases where the stimulation can provoke a slight detachment of the skin, which gives the appearance of having been scraped. This situation, which is common to people with a severe immune deficiency, should not worry you unduly. It is of course necessary to let the skin heal but at the same time you can continue the Dien' Cham' sessions on other areas that do not react so markedly. You will adapt your stimulation to the reaction you perceive and make it softer. You will find that the state of the skin of your patient will improve at the same time as his or her health.

zone or point is highly sensitive, it is most effective to perform three or four movements while pressing hard, then pause, and start over a few minutes later. I have obtained results on very fragile subjects with just two or three sweeping movements over the relevant zones.

You can rely on the results obtained or lack thereof! Relief should be immediate or almost. If not it can mean just one of two things:

- Bad choice of points or zones
- Insufficient pressure

Occasionally it is necessary to wait from five to ten minutes for the full result to come. That is why I usually have a chat with the person for a few minutes after the session; this gives the person time to see what has happened. If nothing has changed after five or ten minutes, recommence the session choosing other reflex zones and press a little harder perhaps. Adapt your strategy according to results obtained!

## The face can be compared to a neglected indoor plant

One morning you realize that you have forgotten to water a house plant. There is a great tendency to give the plant much more than it can cope with to compensate for the drought! You say to yourself that the plant is also under the weather and that you must give it some fertilizer at the same time. Any experienced gardener will tell you that this is exactly what you must not do! Fertilizer on a plant suffering from drought risks burning it and it is better to water it progressively without flooding, which can damage it further!

It is the same with the face for the first sessions. Train yourself in gentleness and go carefully!

### *How much pressure should I use?*

It is difficult to reply to this one in writing and much easier to show! Let us try all the same:

Test the sweeping and the rubbing motions on the palm of your hand as described before. Press without hurting but enough to really feel the pressure. So far so good!

Now do the same thing on a zone of your face in front of the mirror, trying to exert the same amount of pressure. If you have a doubt come back to your hand and start again.

How do you feel about it? Probably it will be a disagreeable surprise to note that what seems harmless on the hand, is much less pleasant on the face! Oh yes, the face is much more sensitive, above all during the first sessions.

Please console yourself with the thought that the first session is generally the worst, because energy has never been stimulated in this region. Your successive attempts will become less and less unpleasant as your condition improves. Adjust the pressure you exert and the length of the sessions according to your observations. You will find that the stimulation quickly becomes more bearable, and this opens the door to more in-depth work.

This short experiment should enable you to understand easily that it is better to adjust the

pressure to the condition and disposition of your "patient" who sometimes will lack that very necessary quality of "patience." Working on someone who is thin and fragile requires a light and skillful hand to begin with. Use your commonsense too: it is obvious that you must not stimulate a baby, an older, thinner person, and a muscular sportsman or woman in exactly the same way!

## THE BASIC SESSION

You are now at the threshold of your first Dien' Cham' session. It will only take you about thirty seconds, at the end of which you can already expect to feel some of the benefits. The Basic Session includes the stimulation of points promoting relaxation and those toning up. Therefore it is convenient for all situations. Every Dien' Cham' session should start with this Basic Session, which you will later be able to complete by adding points related to the specific health problem that you wish to address.

### Basic Rule 5

Count between twelve and fifteen sweeping movements over each point!

You will need to refer to both views of **Diagram 1** so I suggest that you make a photocopy of the diagram (Figures 2.2a and 2.2b) for ease of reference. Eventually you may want to photocopy each of the diagrams given in chapter 2 for your personal use. Some of my students have even made themselves a small plastic notebook with one diagram per page, allowing them to have it on them always.

It is often easier to start by practicing on someone else, which will allow you to follow the advice in this chapter and consult the corresponding diagram at the same time.

When you start to practice on yourself, it is essential to do this in front of a mirror, to ensure that you have chosen the correct points and zones. Later on you will be able to sense them well enough to locate them without the help of a mirror.

## Relaxing

**Points 124, 34, 26, 0** (please note that all of these points are located on the forehead with the exception of point 0, located in front of the ear).

Disorders of the nervous system are at the origin of all sicknesses, whatever their seriousness, so we always start by relaxing this system. A disturbed nervous system creates constant tiredness, tension that is difficult to bear, and energy loss, which decreases the body's natural immunity. In this kind of a situation, the first virus that comes along finds a suitable host and does not hesitate to set up shop.

- Start with point **124**, located above the eyebrows, in the middle of the forehead. If you are working on someone else, the left hand holds the hair clear, while the right with spread fingers rests on the little and ring fingers. Use the three other digits of the right hand to hold your pen (or other instrument of choice such as a glass rod or stone). Rub this point from left to right following the forehead's curve over a few inches or so, using ample movements and taking care to use sufficient pressure.
- Make fifteen or so of these rubbing movements.
- Continue with point **34**, which is at the root of the eyebrows. Perform wide sweeping movements over this point fifteen times or so, advancing along the eyebrows a little (in the direction of the growth of the hairs). Press down well! This point is excellent for all those who suffer from insomnia.
- Then stimulate point **26** located centrally between the eyebrows. This is done by rubbing the point of your ballpoint pen right on the spot, making small circular movements or by sweeping the whole zone vertically.

- Terminate this first sequence using point **0** (located in front of the ears). Every sequence should end with this point. Its regulatory action will compensate for any errors you have inadvertently made. If, for example, you stimulate a point tending to increase blood pressure and you suffer from high blood pressure, stimulating point **0** will temper that effect. The simplest way is to make a series of twenty energetic sweeping movements up and down over the whole zone located in front of the ears.

This terminates the first part.

**To assist your memory . . .**

Please note that the points for relaxation are approximately disposed in the shape of a cup:

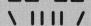

## Toning Up

**Points 127, 19, 26, 103, 126, 0** (vertical axis, in the middle of the face).

These points allow the release of blocked up energy; they also boost inadequate energy, which is necessary for the renewal of the body's immune system. A body that is exhausted and suffering from tiredness cannot defend itself. Consequently it is important to liberate blocked energy and stimulate the life force, which is the only source capable of revitalizing the functions of deficient organs.

- Start with point **127**, located in the center of the chin. Perform fifteen or so small sweeping movements with your instrument, preferably up and down, to improve the tonic effect.
- To boost vital energy, continue with point **19**, located centrally, under the nose. Tap it vertically. Do not hesitate to repeat the stimulation in case of tiredness.

- Return to point **26** between the eyebrows, and stimulate it as described above for a few seconds.
- Then it is time to go to point **103** in the middle of the forehead. Stimulate it using small sweeping movements, top to bottom, and back and forth.
- Now comes the turn of point **126**, in the center of the hairline. This point must also be treated with fifteen or so small sweeping movements, top to bottom.
- Finish as usual using point **0**. You are starting to get into the habit now! Energetically sweep the zones in front of the ears up and down twenty times or so.

**To assist your memory . . .**

Note that all these points are located on a vertical axis from bottom to top

These two procedures constitute the Basic Session, which I advise you to practice every day, when you get up and when you go to bed. This will keep you fit and remove tiredness. This short session can be repeated as often as necessary during the day, as soon as you feel that tiredness or stress is overcoming your resistance.

It is quite common for this simple session to be enough to eliminate minor problems. You can

**All sicknesses are based on poor circulation of energy.**

If you only seek to heal the affected organ, the subject can never be truly healed.

The only true recovery is said to be holistic, which is to say the person taken as a whole.

Let us learn to look after our body as a totality, considering not just the parts that need treatment or are fragile. Good results will quickly be forthcoming!

practice it lying in your bed, sitting, or standing. Your position is of no importance. Teach it to your children, family, and friends and it will be of great help to them.

At the beginning I advise you to regularly use this Basic Session to practice on yourself and your family and friends. Only when this Basic Session is familiar, and you can perform it easily, should you think about making personal additions. Try to make steady progress and correctly assimilate new notions before going on to other steps. This is the key to success!

## PRECAUTIONS AND INADVISABILITY

There are only a few contraindications for Dien' Cham' but it is important to bear them in mind.

### *Pregnancy*

Just like any manipulation of energy and any reflexology practice, Dien' Cham' must be used on pregnant women with caution and good judgment. In fact this period of profound physiological change must be respected as much as possible. On the other hand, in the case of troubles it is better to stimulate certain points rather than take medicine, but only after using chapter 5—which gives clear contraindications for each reflex point—to confirm that the use of a particular point is not inadvisable.

Several reflex zones and points are very useful at the time of delivery, as they assist labor and speed up expulsion. It is obvious that stimulation of the same points during a pregnancy would risk provoking a miscarriage or premature birth! Be very careful, then, when you are performing massage on a pregnant woman. Even the Basic Session is ill-advised during this period, with the exception of the points that relax.

The same rule should be observed for reflex zones: carefully avoid zones corresponding to the genital organs and pelvis. To have top security avoid all stimulation of the face, except in cases of real need.

### High and Low Blood Pressure

Dien' Cham' is very effective in treating both high and low blood pressure. When the points and zones are well-chosen, one or two minutes of massage can raise or drop the blood pressure by three or four points!

Quite evidently it follows that in case of an error, there is the risk of seeing a patient with high blood pressure redden and perspire, if the points that raise the blood pressure are stimulated. Or, on the other hand, you may see a young woman with low blood pressure rapidly go pale or feel faint, if the points tending to drop the blood pressure are stimulated!

It is important in both cases to always check chapter 5 for relevant warnings before beginning a massage. Since a mistake is always possible, a precaution has been introduced in the massage techniques for points related to blood pressure: the systematic and frequent stimulation of the zone around point 0, with sweeping movements along the line situated in front of the ears, from the base of the earlobe to its upper connection with the face. You will notice that all sessions end with stimulation of this entire zone, sometimes just called point 0 for short, and it is often stimulated during sessions too. This reflex zone with many properties regulates excesses and shortcomings that can happen during a session. The habit of always returning to and ending with this zone will protect you from committing errors, including those concerning cases of high and low blood pressure.

If you see a patient suddenly redden or go pale, please do not panic. Strongly stimulate the zone around point 0 and all will be well.

## THE STANDARD SESSION

After you have become quite comfortable with performing the Basic Session, the next step is to elaborate it by adding the reflex zones and points that are suitable for the problem you wish to treat. First I would like to suggest a short Standard Session that you can use as a model and which will help you to answer questions like:

- Where shall I start?
- In what order do I stimulate the points and zones?

During your apprenticeship, start by memorizing and then massaging the reflex points given in the Basic Session and in this model session. It is important to be able to do this so that you can use them in any circumstances in case of need.

**Several pieces of practical advice**

Before going further, contemplate the following guidelines that indicate the way to proceed:

- Use the first part of the session to make a general tour and locate sensitive points.
- Never stimulate insensitive points for long. If you over-stimulate a point that is not painful you may reverse the effect. With this in mind, go rapidly over any insensitive points and spend more time on

those that are sensitive. There is such a big choice of zones and points with the same function or the same organ. One may well be sensitive and the other not. This fact will guide you to the correct practice! Have confidence in the body!

- Spend five to ten seconds on each point (around twelve to fifteen sweeping movements), longer on those that are painful.
- It is not advisable to make a diagnosis based on the sensitivity of certain points. Things are not so simple and this can lead you into error. For example, sensitivity of point 37, which corresponds to the spleen, does not necessarily imply a problem with blood composition or natural defenses. It could just be that you are suffering from heavy legs at the end of an exhausting day!

## Points in Proximity

As you already know, each point has several correspondences. Please remember the following rule:

### Basic Rule 8
Each point acts primarily on the closest organ.
Then it acts on the sick organ.

Let us go back to an example already used. When you discover that you have forgotten to water your houseplant and you find it wilting, what do you do? You should bring it water in small quantities to begin with, so as not to stress it further. Where is this water going to go? To the leaves that are all yellow? To the stalk that is bending over? To the roots? What is the point of thinking about that? You know it needs water and the plant itself is going to make sure that the best use possible is made of the water in order to survive.

It is exactly the same with your body. It needs energy and you free it up. That is all you have to do because your body will look after the rest!

In practice it means that the points located around the eyes, for example, first have an effect on eyesight and only subsequently on other areas. Hence stimulation of point **73** under the eye will treat troubles with vision before acting on corresponding organs like the breasts and the chest and so on. It will also have a selective action on the sickness and will not affect the functions other than that. Please be reassured and have confidence in the innate wisdom of your own body and the "computer keyboard" hidden in your face!

## Practicing a Standard Session

Let us now take a look at the Standard Session and the basic points. Here I will give only the main indications, which will be enough for the time being. When these are familiar it will be time to turn to the following chapter where you will find all useful indications and various correspondences, enabling you to tailor your sessions to specific health problems.

It is preferable to stimulate these points in the order given below. The order is logical and takes proximity into account. Please refer to **Diagram 1**. Remain at each point for a few seconds, just long enough to perform twelve or so rubbing movements, then continue. Performing a session will take you less time than to read the description!

### Basic Rule 9
When points are aligned or in the same zone they can be stimulated together in the same sweeping movement. How it saves time!

Start with the Basic Session (to relax and tone up). Then begin your Standard Session on the cheeks, first on the right, then on the left:

### Point 50
Located just under the cheekbone on the right side of the face only.

Liver, problems of digestion, flatulence, constipation, stops hemorrhage.

*Rub with sweeping horizontal motions below the cheekbone.*

## Point 41

Also located under the cheekbone on the right, near point 50.

Gall bladder (even after surgical removal), cholesterol, digestion, migraines.

*Points 50 and 41 can be stimulated together with the same sweeping motion.*

## Point 37

Located under the cheekbone on the left side of the face.

Spleen, blood and energy circulation, problems of digestion, immune response, depression, and heavy legs.

*Rub toward the ear with a sweeping horizontal motion below the cheekbone.*

## Point 39

Located just below point 37 on the left cheek.

Stomach, digestive troubles and gastritis.

*Stimulate with a horizontal sweeping motion toward the ear. Points 37 and 39 can also be stimulated together with a vertical motion.*

## Point 73

Located at the top of the hard bone just below the eye, in line with the center of the eye.

Eyes, lungs (coughs), breasts (mastosis), ovaries.

*Stimulate gently by making small circles on this delicate point.*

## Point 3

Located on the cheekbones just below point 73.

Lungs, heart (only on the left).

*Massage horizontally toward the ear.*

Now descend to the creases at the sides of the nostrils and work up to the nose:

## Point 61

Located in the creases next to the curve of the nose.

Lungs, liver, stomach, spleen/sinusitis, blocked nose, stops hemorrhage, deadens pain. This point supplies natural endorphins (analgesic and anti-inflammatory qualities), produces warmth, stops the nose from running (head cold).

*Rub back and forth in line with the curve of the nose.*

## Point 8

Located on the bridge of the nose between the eyes.

Heart, cervical or neck vertebrae, throat and thyroid gland, slows the heartbeat (tachycardia), lowers blood pressure, frees up cervical vertebrae, calms sore throats.

*Steady your fingers on the nose and stimulate in small circles.*

You have now reached the forehead. Do not be surprised that this involves further stimulation of points that have already been treated! They are important enough for it to be worthwhile coming back to them:

## Point 34

Located just above inner corner of each eyebrow.

Shoulders and arms (moving along the eyebrows from point 34), eyes, and the sinuses. Relaxes the nervous system and combats insomnia (can be stimulated along with point 124, which is located above it and toward the outer edge of the forehead).

*Rub along the eyebrow in the direction that the hair grows or in a sweeping diagonal motion including point 124.*

**Point 26**

Located between the eyebrows.

Cervical vertebrae, throat, sinuses, pituitary gland, third eye. Calms the mind (which is useful for hyperactive children); can also wake one up; acts on mental balance (do not over stimulate); reduces pain of headaches.

*Stimulate using repeated small movements, from the top down or with small counterclockwise circles.*

**Point 106**

Located on the first quarter of the line between point 26 and the hairline.

Spinal column, cervical vertebrae, throat, eyes, and sinuses.

*To stimulate point 106 (and all points located on the forehead) tap with the ends of your fingers or perform downward sweeping movements from the top downward.*

**Point 103**

Located at the center of the forehead, halfway up the vertical line between point 26 and the hairline.

The crown of the head, pituitary gland, spinal column, memory, stimulates chakras.

*See point 106 for stimulation directions.*

**Point 126**

Located at the midpoint of the hairline, with influence extending in a line along the hairline.

Spinal column, lumbar vertebrae, coccyx, anus (piles).

*Tap the forehead along the hairline.*

**Point 342**

Located three-quarters of the way up the vertical line between point 26 and the hairline.

Spinal column, lumbar vertebrae (lumbago). (Remember that the dorsal vertebrae correspond to the bridge of the nose and the cervical vertebrae correspond to point 26).

*See point 106 for stimulation directions. Then return to . . .*

**Point 126**

*Stimulate top to bottom using short movements then go back to . . .*

**Point 342**

*Tap descending the forehead and nose, go back up again and finish on point 0, found on a vertical line in front of each ear.*

The following points should be given additional attention according to specific spinal problems:

- For problems with the cervical vertebrae: Make sweeping movements over the zone between points 8–106. These points should be massaged vertically, either together or separately.
- In case of problems with shoulders and arms: Work along the eyebrows.
- In cases of sciatica: Massage the nostrils (buttocks), around the nostrils (groin) and the nasogenian crease.

Now you are going to leave the forehead via the temples and work on the lower part of the face:

**Point 124**

Located toward the outer edges of the forehead on a horizontal line with point 103.

Relaxes the nervous system.

*Perform horizontal sweeping movements of half an inch to an inch over this point.*

**Point 180**

Located near the temples.

Solar plexus, migraines; can provoke perspiration (the hands sometimes slightly damp).

*Massage point moving toward the ears.*

Now you are on the upper lip, which has many points related to the hormonal system:

*You can stimulate the following five points above the upper lip together, using small vertical or horizontal sweeping movements. Points located under the nose must be stimulated vertically.*

## Point 19
Located directly below the nose above the upper lip.

Nose, liver, stomach, colon, lower abdomen. Boosts the heart at the same time as toning it up: stimulate this point in the case of dizziness or faintness. Increases blood pressure; increases energy available. Stomachache; constipation, stops hiccups, stops vomiting, provokes contractions of the womb (**prohibited for pregnant women**).

## Point 63
Located below point **19**, just above upper lip.

Colon, pancreas, and womb. Constipation, indigestion, pains, dizziness. For childbirth provokes contractions of the womb, stops uterine hemorrhage.

## Point 17
Located above the outside corners of the mouth.

Adrenal glands, frees natural corticoids (anti-inflammatory action).

## Point 113
Located toward the outer corners of the upper lip.

Pancreas (diabetes), ovaries, prostate gland, sexual problems, womb (helps with menstrual difficulties), cystitis, indigestion.

## Point 7
Located above the upper lip on either side of point **63**.

Has similar properties to **113**.

## Point 38
Located near point **17**, above and outside the corners of the mouth.

Knee (arthrosis), knee problems, infections (produces natural antibiotics).

*Stimulate both sides of the mouth vertically.*

Now you are going to stimulate points located on the chin:

## Point 127
Located in the center of the crease between the mouth and the chin.

Small intestine. Corresponds to the Yin Conception Vessel. Heel, menstrual pain, menopause, sexual problems generally. Spasmodic colitis, diarrhea (in cases of diarrhea, stimulate the point early on).

*The points on the chin (127, 22, 87) must be stimulated with downward strokes.*

## Point 85
Located along the creases at the sides of the mouth.

Ureters, kidneys, elimination, water retention.

*The massage should usually be performed by associating this point with the kidney zones using a vertical movement, up and down, on either side of the mouth.*

## Point 87
Located on the midline of the chin below points **127** and **87**.

Bladder, womb.

*See point **127** for stimulation directions.*

## Point 22
Located on the midline of the chin between point **127** and point **87**.

Bladder.

*See point **127** for stimulation directions.*

### Point 51

Located on either side of the chin on a horizontal line with point 87.

Feet, toes (along the chin), big toes (on the edge of the chin, at the center). In the case of a headache, it is generally yang energy that has moved into the head. Stimulating this point induces this energy to descend.

*Push the tip of your sharper instrument in and stimulate upward. You can also perform sweeping movements to reach all of the points.*

### Point 365

Located at the bottom tip of the chin.

Toes, anus, feet, and large intestine.

*This point's area of influence stretches along the lower jawbone on both sides in the same way that point 126 influenced the entire hairline. Remember that the big toe is closer to the center with the smallest furthest away.*

Now finish up on the ear zones:

### Point 16

Located at the point where the upper ear joins the head.

Ears. Stops all excess loss of body fluids: internal or external hemorrhage, menstrual flow caused by fibroids, excessive perspiration, runny nose, tears, and so on.

*Stimulate this point by massaging in small circles, with a finger or end of a ballpoint pen.*

### Point 14

Located in front of the earlobe at the junction of the earlobe and the face.

Ears, throat, parotid and thyroid glands (hypothyroidism), deafness, earache, salivation. Unblocks the jaw.

*Massage horizontally just under the lobe, then rub again vertically.*

### Point 15

Located in the hollow behind the earlobes.

Ears and jaws. Decreases the blood pressure by three or four points. Helps with hypothyroidism.

*Massage by rubbing horizontally, then vertically.*

Terminate as always on point 0:

### Point 0

The 0 zone is a vertical zone located just in front of each ear, the actual zero point lies at the midpoint of this vertical line on either side of the face.

Kidneys, ears, eyes, mouth, nose, spinal column. Please note that point 0 (if taken separately) corresponds to the solar plexus. This point—which you will always use to end the session—regulates the blood pressure, whether too high or too low, and stimulates the life force. In the case of a weak individual, always start with point 0.

*Massage the whole zone vertically from top to bottom to relax everything and make everything peaceful.*

This Standard Session is useable in all situations as all organ functions are treated. In addition, even if you do not have a particular health problem, you can use it once or twice a week to boost and maintain all of your vital functions. Once you are comfortable with the Standard Session, you will be ready to tailor it to create a massage to treat a specific condition.

> **Vital energy has three sources**
> • Life force or sexual energy
> • Food
> • The breath
> To preserve your health you need to care for the quality of these three sources!

# THE CHOICE OF REFLEX POINTS

How do you plan a massage, especially when you are a beginner? You may well feel a little apprehensive about the apparent complexity of the various diagrams of the reflex points and zones, asking yourself how it is possible to choose from them the ones that will be effective in a given case.

It is true that due to the numerous correspondences between points, reflex zones, organs, parts of the body, and functions, there is an infinite number of possibilities of stimulation. In addition each point of the face can be in correspondence with several organs and functions. Be reassured right away that the action will only have an effect on the malfunctioning organ or depressed body function. You have to have confidence in your body's own wisdom!

There are several different ways of determining zones to be massaged to guide your practice of Dien' Cham'. In all cases, you should refer to basic **Diagrams 1, 2, 3, 9, and 10** (given in chapter 2), unless you have a medical qualification. The seven ways to plan your massage are:

## 1. Following skeleton and organ projection diagrams

This is the possibility that is the easiest for beginners. By using skeleton and organ projection diagrams, such as **Diagrams 2 and 3,** you can determine which facial reflex zone corresponds to the part of the body or internal organ in need of healing. You can stimulate the zone in question as a function of the problem, without having to know the reflex points. This allows effective treatment of complex chronic complaints, as each point has dozens of functions and can act on several organs, even though it will primarily act on the affected organ.

Furthermore, when you stimulate a reflex zone you go over several points while doing so.

Remember there are nearly 600 points on the face, even if I have only mentioned 57 in this work!

Take the case of someone affected by a blockage of the cervical or neck vertebrae. The relevant zone is located between the eyes and the eyebrows. It is usually enough to stimulate this whole zone to relieve a stiff neck! Knowledge of reflex zones allows treatment of sicknesses with a simple and recent origin, especially those with obvious symptoms like aches, blockages, headaches, migraines, and so on.

## 2. Following the "live" reflex points

It is possible to base a massage on the points that have symptoms and are particularly painful, which you will find by exploring the face with your fingers or an instrument of some description (ballpoint pen, steel or glass point, roller, flexible hammer, rubber hammer, and so on). Such sensitive points, called "live points" only appear following trouble in an organ. The most common are those indicated on the diagram of the reflex points but there are others.

> The same thing is seen in acupuncture with painful points, which show an ongoing disturbance, an affected organ, an energy deficiency, or an inflammation.

In practice this means that if you detect a painful spot outside those specified in **Diagram 1**, it is certainly in relation with one or other of your problems and there is nothing stopping you from stimulating it.

## 3. Following points known for their action

You can choose points known for their effects and their correspondences with organs, in accordance with a particular symptom or illness, without it being necessary to seek for a sensitive spot. For this, you will want to refer to the Practical Dictionary of Therapeutic Sessions in chapter 4. Sometimes it is just a question of stimulating one or two points to solve a problem. For example, in the case of a cervical vertebrae pain, the relevant points are **26, 8, 106, 34, 65**. Correct stimulation of these points can free up the cervical vertebrae in just a few seconds without requiring manipulation of the spinal column. This is a dream come true for osteopaths, chiropractors, and physiotherapists, who will be able to treat their patients effectively without running any risks, in just a few seconds, without fatigue. (A gain in time is a gain in energy!)

## 4. Following a formula proposed in the Practical Dictionary of Therapeutic Sessions

A fairly simple and effective stimulation sometimes necessitates a special technique. These techniques are described in more detail in the Practical Dictionary of Therapeutic Sessions given in chapter 4. Chapter 4 not only shows the correspondence between various conditions and the pertinent zones and points, but also offers formulas for treatment that have been established by experimentation concerning the types of cases already healed by Dien' Cham'. It is advisable to use them to begin with, until enough experience has been gained and until each reflex point is sufficiently known. These formulas are generally effective but not always so, because causes are often multiple, and it may be necessary in this case to adapt the treatment by using the following method.

## 5. By applying the method of choosing points explained in the personalized method

A whole chapter (chapter 6) is devoted to this advanced Dien' Cham' technique, which you can use as soon as you have acquired a certain experience. It will allow you to test each point to determine which will be the most effective at the time (which can vary from day-to-day, or week-to-week). Proceeding like this will optimize your ses-

sions. Therapists will be able to establish personal records, which they can pass on to their patients, allowing them to perform their own daily sessions. As this advanced technique is applicable to oneself as well as to others, it will be of great use.

## 6. According to Chinese acupuncture and energy system

This choice of reflex points is reserved to acupuncturists and therapists who have specialized in the Chinese energy system. It is interesting to note that all the yang meridians pass through the face, which is the area of the body that resists cold the best! It is the same thing for the two main channels: the Governing Vessel (GV), called Tu Mo, which rises alongside the spinal column and descends via the forehead and the bridge of the nose, ending under the upper lip at the gums; and the Conception Vessel (CV) called Jen Mo, which starts above the pubis and ends below the lower lip, above the chin. As certain Dien' Cham' reflex points are also acupuncture points, knowledge of the Chinese energy system allows treatment of problems as a function of Chinese pulse, knowledge of meridians, and related points.

Warning:
The use of needles on the face is certainly very effective but it can be dangerous and even fatal for inexperienced persons. This technique must absolutely be reserved for therapists who have followed a long training course with Professor Bui Quoc Chau. On the other hand stimulation using a finger or other suitable instrument such as the rounded end of a ballpoint or a roller is without danger.

## 7. Following classical medicine

This must be reserved for doctors only. As a function of their diagnosis they can choose reflex points known for their properties, according to each particular case. The results will depend on their knowledge of reflex points and experience in this area.

## LENGTH OF SESSIONS

There is no general rule about how long a session should last. A dozen strokes of a pencil can be enough, but sometimes more are needed. It is also possible for a session to last a lot longer, even though my experience inclines me to practice repeated short sessions, rather than one long one. It all depends on the case and the speed with which relief is felt. Let us just say that in a majority of cases two to three minutes is quite ample, sometimes even less.

Lumbago is the only common case where sessions last for more than two or three minutes! If one day you find yourself stuck in your bed without being able to get up because you are in so much pain, Dien' Cham' will be of great help . . . but only after ten or so minutes of forehead massage! Stimulate according to the zones indicated in the Lumbago section of the Practical Dictionary of Therapeutic Sessions given in chapter 4 or the zone colored grey in Figure 3.6 and have a few moments' patience. Strange as it may seem, you will suddenly realize that you can get up with little or no pain. Generally just one session is sufficient, if the treatment is given with adequate pressure. It

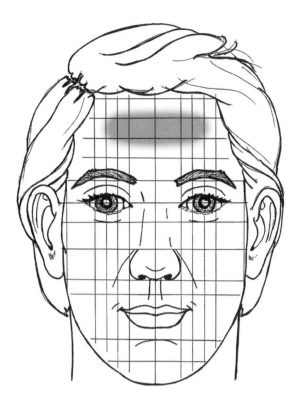

Figure 3.6. Reflex zone for Lumbago

will be for you to choose between your back and your forehead!

When you have no particular sickness, it is quite enough to practice the Basic Session to maintain a good circulation of energy. This will only take around thirty seconds! The same session can be repeated during the day, or in case of tiredness, or after having been under tension. Everything is quickly put back into place and your peace of mind is restored.

## SESSION FREQUENCY

In the case of someone in good health, who has no sickness and feels in shape, just two or three sessions of Dien' Cham' per week can maintain good energy circulation. It is easier to prevent sickness than to cure it! When you are relaxed and your energy or chi is moving well, you will never fall sick. Therefore it is a shame to wait for the situation to deteriorate to intervene.

### When You Rise

Start the day with the short Basic Session lasting about one minute. This is much better than a cup of coffee. It puts you in shape and allows you to start the day with great vitality. You will feel relaxed and well within yourself.

### When You Go to Bed

The effect of relaxing your nervous system and dissipating tiredness after the day's work or various activities is generally enough to prevent sickness from arising, so why not give yourself a Dien' Cham' session every evening in the way you would have a shower? It is a favorable way to practice hygiene with respect to your health, as well as your human contacts in general: as you recuperate a good level of energy, you will also recover interest in spending a pleasant evening with family, or with friends, which could be spoilt by untimely tiredness.

### Prior to Skin Care

I advise women to practice their session before looking after their skin in the morning and the evening. The massage comfortably stimulates the peripheral circulation in the face allowing the skin to better absorb creams, lotions, and other products. Dien' Cham' is also an excellent natural anti-wrinkle treatment!

### Every Time You Feel the Need

In fact the Dien' Cham' reflex should be acquired so that it is thought of at the first, even minimal, sign of pain or disturbance. Can you feel a headache coming on? Thirty seconds are enough to rid yourself of it before it becomes established.

Do you have backache after several hours spent in front of your computer? Do you have stinging eyes and are the documents on your desk becoming blurred? If you stimulate several points discretely with your pen things will get better. Can you feel a cold coming on? Thirty seconds of massage as soon as the first signs are noticed, without waiting for the nose to run abundantly, will solve the problem.

In addition, as I am sure you have understood, this massage can be practiced just about anywhere, discretely and with anything at hand. Even at the office, no one is stopping you from shutting your door to do it!

The important thing to understand is that the quicker a correct level of circulating energy is re-established after the first symptoms appear, the better the result is and the less you have to perform sessions! To take an example, chronic bronchitis can be treated and the symptoms completely suppressed in two or three sessions, sometimes four, depending on the state of the person. In-depth treatment can necessitate several supplementary sessions aimed at improving energy circulation and warming up the body.

In the case of acute problems, you can start with two or three sessions or even more during the same day. Then it will be up to the person to see how often the sessions are to be.

### Example: Common Cold

Let us have another look at the simple example of the common cold. If you are a little attentive to what is going on in your body, you will know the

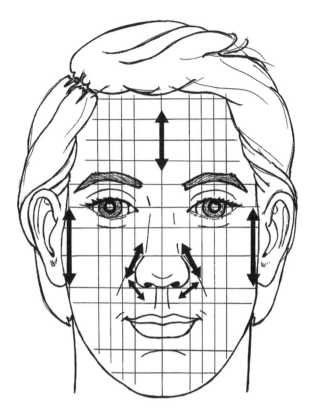

Figure 3.7. Treatment for the onset of a cold

thumb, vigorously massage the center of the forehead at the level of points **106**, **103**, and **342**. Finish up with the **0** zones in front of the ears. Just the trick! In such cases one session is enough. Do you know a better way of ridding yourself of a cold?

I remember one particular day when I suddenly felt the first symptoms of a cold. It was a warm day in the fall and I had been driving my automobile with the windows wide open from the start of the trip. I was on my way to an exhibition of natural medicine in Geneva where I was to spend several days giving conferences and signing books. You can see the problem if I had come with a red nose and all blocked up! I stopped at the next service area on the turnpike and performed the short stimulation for a head cold, which only requires use of the fingers. In less than a minute every sign had disappeared and I continued my drive with a calm mind.

### Another Example: Sciatica

In certain cases it is necessary to practice several sessions per day. The important thing is to listen to your body. When the body needs a little help it knows how to attract your attention! Let us take the example of a sciatica, which as you probably know is a burning and shooting pain descending from the right or left buttock to the lower leg. A bout of sciatica is quickly relieved by Dien' Cham' even if it is often necessary to do repeat sessions. In this case in particular the corresponding reflex zones (as shown on **Diagrams 2 and 9**) are especially painful and you will hardly be able to stand twenty seconds of massage during the early sessions. On the other hand, it is quite possible to repeat a brief stimulation several times over in the first half an hour, until you obtain real relief, which lasts for four hours on average. As soon as the pain returns, begin to massage the zones again. This time it is likely that you will be better able to stand your massage and that only a minute will be necessary for a big improvement to be felt.

Start over again every four hours or according

preliminary signs of one: haziness in the head, the beginnings of a sore throat, a dry and tickly nose, and the feeling that you cannot breathe so easily. Ideally you should act as soon as you recognize these signs without waiting to arrive back home. That might be too late! Please do not use excuses such as: I do not have my favorite instrument! I would prefer to have my book handy to be sure. I am going to wait until I get home this evening.

It is very likely that by then your nose will already have started running and in this case nothing will stop it, even though you may be able to procure some relief. If you had just given yourself thirty seconds at the outset, you would have saved yourself several days of misery!

Right at the start you need to reactivate your energy. To do this there is a simple movement that will only take you a few seconds. With the index fingers vigorously massage the ends of the nostrils as indicated in Figure 3.7. With the knuckle of the to the demands of your body until the problem disappears completely. Of course this does not mean that you should not go to visit your osteopath! But at least you will be able to go without having to resort to anti-inflammatory drugs and you will be better able to stand the manipulations. In certain cases Dien' Cham' has solved the problem of a sciatica without other intervention being necessary.

## A FEW SPECIAL MASSAGES

A fairly simple and effective stimulation sometimes necessitates a special technique. These are described in more detail in the Practical Dictionary of Dien' Cham' given in chapter 4.

### Constipation

This problem can be improved speedily by stimulating around the mouth as shown in Figure 3.8. This simple movement gives excellent results, even in the case of serious blockage having lasted several days. Using the index and middle fingers and the thumb as support under the chin, move around the mouth from right to left as shown in the diagram. Then, when you reach the center of the chin, purge using a brisk downward movement. Repeat this about fifty times without stopping.

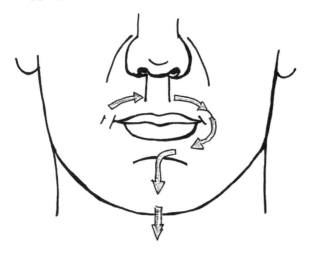

Figure 3.8. Direction of massage in case of constipation

It is of course possible to repeat this during the day as necessary.

To help you to remember the direction of this massage you can again use analogy. Consider your abdomen; the ascending colon rises on the right, turns behind the liver, then crosses the upper part of your belly toward the left. Then the descending colon descends on the left side of the abdomen.

Remember what your mother or grandmother probably told you when you were a child and were unable to go to the bathroom. Massage the stomach pressing down with your right hand flat, making wide circles, from the lower right abdomen upward toward the ribs, crossing the abdomen toward the left, descending and repeating over again!

On your face, the intestine rises in the same way on the right of the mouth, makes the right turn over the upper lip where it becomes the transverse colon, then descends toward the lower face, going around the left of the mouth, so you should stimulate the zones on the face in the same sequence. If you take account of this analogy you will never make a mistake.

Additionally, when you get up and before breakfast, drink a large cup of hot, slightly salty water (preferably using Himalayan crystal salt).

### Diarrhea

In case of diarrhea, use the same massage, but reverse the direction: starting at the zone corresponding to the lower abdomen on the left side of the face, using adequate pressure and the three fingers as above, massage up, across toward the right, and then descending to the right of the mouth.

Here the aim is to try to slow down evacuation rather than stimulate it. Although the result will only be temporary, it will allow you to gain a little precious time!

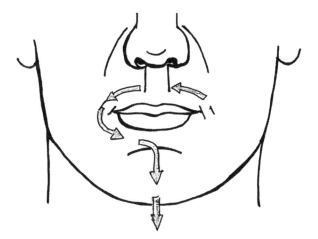

Figure 3.9. Direction of massage in case of diarrhea

## Typical Feminine Problems: Contraception, Menstrual Pain, Frigidity, Dryness of the Vagina, Consequences of Rape, and so on

This movement consists in stimulation of the area around the lips and the tip of the nose; its effect is further reaching than its primary action, which is contraception. (In chapter 4, you will find it described in detail under this heading.) It relieves menstrual pain and solves difficulties related to vaginal dryness after menopause.

This massage can also be useful following a case of forced intercourse. I have had the opportunity to check the effectiveness of this technique several times in cases where young women have been raped. Most often they later have great difficulty in their love life and a disabling dyspareunia: intense pain that sometimes prevents all sexual intercourse due to a physical obstruction or contraction of the whole region causing vaginal dryness, and so on.

In this case I advise using this massage technique in the minutes before sexual relations. Generally speaking, on the first attempt things improve perceptibly. Usually three or four massages are enough for the situation to revert to normal! It is much more effective than a long course of psychotherapy—and much less expensive!

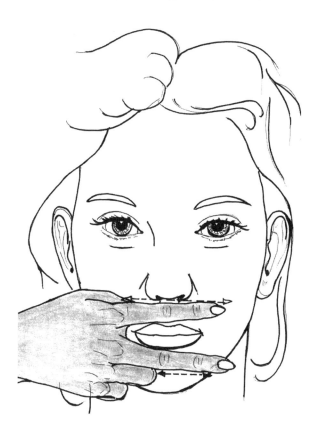

Figure 3.10. Feminine problems (first part)

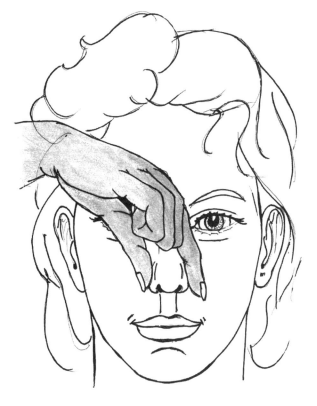

Figure 3.11. Feminine problems (second part)

*Method*[1]

For ten or so minutes before each sexual intercourse and also afterward, friction around your mouth with the index and middle fingers of, preferably, your right hand. This is to be done about 200 times, not too hard (so as not to hurt yourself), nor too lightly, which would render the massage ineffective. Then massage your nostrils by pinching them lightly between the thumb and index finger. This should also be done about 200 times but takes only two or three minutes. Pinch at the base of the nose and move toward the bridge of the nose in a brisk movement.

Zones stimulated in this way should warm up. This facial massage should procure a feeling of warmth in the pelvic region accompanied by agreeable sexual arousal. With respect to vaginal dryness: it will be a thing of the past! These signs validate the stimulation's effectiveness and guarantee a good result. Lack of them shows that the technique has not been correctly used: perhaps you did not massage the points long enough or with sufficient pressure. Sometimes a case of frigidity can be evidenced by an absence of signs, which can be treated using the same method used daily over a long period until the required result is obtained.

### Warning

This massage provokes a strong contraction of the womb and so must not be used in cases of pregnancy because of the risk of miscarriage or premature birth.

## DIAGNOSIS AND DIEN' CHAM'

In oriental medicine, the art of diagnosis is not just a classification of various symptoms from which one can deduce a possible pathology. In reality it represents a holistic way of considering the past, present, and even the future health and life of an individual. This kind of detection is above all based on the study of the face. Everything that can be read in it—such as lines, forms, and peculiarities—represents an exterior manifestation of the state of the blood, body fluids, organs, nervous system, bones, and the totality, all resulting from our heredity, our diet, our activities, and environmental conditions. The essence of the art is to apprehend in the face these slight modifications that announce problems to come, before they develop into an identifiable, declared illness.

Several centuries ago this traditional art of diagnosis was rediscovered and developed by Nanboku Mizuno. More recently George Ohsawa, founder of macrobiotics, decided to spread these ideas to benefit the West. Later, Michio Kushi further developed this technique, following his own observations. He is author of several books on health and macrobiotics, including an extremely interesting book—*Oriental Diagnosis*—to which you can refer if you wish to learn more about this method.[2]

However, diagnosis is certainly not necessary to practice Dien' Cham'. A good result can be obtained in a majority of cases simply by stimulating all the sensitive points you can find. Even though each pressure point of the face corresponds to several organs or functions, only the perturbed organ or function will react to stimulation!

As a general rule, when a patient goes to see a physician or therapist a diagnosis is made before any treatment is offered. It is the same thing with facial reflexology. An experienced therapist is capable of making a diagnosis in the very process of looking for painful, sensitive points and noting "silent," that is to say insensitive, ones. A silent point is generally found within a painful zone. This is the point where action is optimized and which corresponds to the Dien' Cham' saying:

Within the zone or point where pain is felt,
there is a painless point.

Specialists in facytherapy mainly look for these silent, painless points, for the purpose of both diagnosis and treatment, as they are considered the most active of all the possible corresponding points.

However, it must be remembered that each point of the face corresponds to several organs and functions and so diagnosis is sometimes difficult. If a diagnosis is based entirely on sensitive points an error is possible. Unqualified practitioners are advised not to fall into this trap. It is better to leave diagnosis to physicians using their usual methods. In fact, French law reserves the right to diagnose for physicians only.

A good result can be obtained in a majority of cases simply by stimulating all the sensitive points you can find. Even though each pressure point of the face corresponds to several organs or functions, only the perturbed organ or function will react to stimulation!

## Signs Revealing a Change in State of Health

Knowledge of facial reflexology can also allow you to take effective prevention measures, by drawing your attention to certain signs possibly manifesting on the face, which usually indicate a disturbance. It is therefore interesting to note any changes and to treat them as soon as possible. Generally disappearance of the change coincides with return to normal of the disturbed function.

There are three possibilities of recognizing these signs, the last being reserved for professionals:

### Signs Found on Examination
Spots, warts, wrinkles, alterations in the color and hue of the skin, dry or greasy skin, dilated pores, skin temperature relative to surrounding areas, changes in texture or elasticity of the skin at a specific location, swelling or depression, changes in bone or muscle shape, muscle cramps, obvious states of congestion, blotchiness, vitiligo, abnormal pilosity, sweating, and so on.

### Signs Noticed by the Patient
Feeling "out of sorts," aches, sharp pains, dryness of skin, paresthesia or local loss of sensitivity, burning, bites or spasms, whether the symptoms are felt on or under the skin.

### Signs Detected Using Instruments
Localized temperature abnormalities, electrical resistance of the skin, electromagnetic measurement of reflex points or zones, Kirlian photos, and so on. Any process that demonstrates an anomaly, whether it is a question of an excess or a lack with respect to surrounding zones. An interesting sign is the determination of a "soft" point, that is to say one that lacks firmness with respect to the skin around it. When you stimulate such a point there is an impression of sinking into the skin without finding the usual resistance. Even if it is not painful you must stimulate it. The degree of loss of resistance of the skin is in relation to the seriousness of the problem. When the problem is treated the sign disappears. Please note that this observation holds true above all in cases of acute problems, and not always with respect to chronic conditions.

All of these signs can reveal changes of a pathological nature. They can appear as forerunners of a problem which allow effective preventive measures, or as indicators of a developing sickness or an organ that is becoming fragile. Whatever the case, they should be taken into account. Often these signs present analogies with a specific pathology and can give indications on its gravity or site.

## BOTOX, BODY PIERCING, PEELING, AND TATTOOS

For esthetic reasons procedures such as botox injections, body piercing, peeling, and tattoos are used more and more often in modern society, but in truth they are not as harmless as they are often portrayed, as you have no doubt already thought to yourself! Their use on the face presents a significant risk of interference with your health because of the many correspondence points that can be affected.

### Botox

This is the famous botulinus toxin, which I should remind you is classified among the weapons of mass destruction! This says much about its so-called innocuousness! Its action is to paralyze, with the effect of preventing lines of facial expression. After receiving these injections you are no longer capable of wrinkling the area around the corners of your eyes when you laugh, which is so charming!

At present it is in fashion to inject a few drops of this botulinus toxin into the areas around the face that give rise to facial expression, several times per year:

- In the zone between the eyebrows at the root of the nose—point **26** and around it.
- Around the eyes—points **60, 130, 100, 180,** and so on.
- Around the mouth and the upper lip—not only points **38, 17, 113, 7, 63,** but **85, 6, 61, 39, 38,** and **50** as well.

These are zones of high sensitivity and conducive to stimulation. Besides their correspondences with organs and bones, there are multiple correspondences with the nervous and hormone systems. It is really to be asked what is likely to happen over the next years. Perhaps there will be various pathological consequences that no one will link with the presence of this toxin!

### Body Piercing

Over the years many therapists have warned parents against having the ears of their daughters pierced, so as not to disturb the fragile energy balance in the important reflex zones located on the earlobe, which are mainly linked to the head and nervous system.

At present, however, the simple earring seems to be quite modest! We now see studs and rings flourish in quantity on the ears, on lips—which is a very delicate zone with correspondences with the digestive and hormone systems—and also at the end of the nose. You are invited to refer to the listing of points in chapter 5 to see what points **19** and **143** correspond to. They also appear on the nostrils—points **64, 74,** and **61**—as well as at the corner of the eyes—points **60, 100, 130, 180,** and so on. Sometimes they are seen on the tongue itself, which is also an important reflex zone.

Before they make an appointment to have a few holes pierced and rings inserted, you could suggest that your adolescents take a look at the correspondences of the zones they are thinking about decorating in this way! You never know, common sense might carry the day.

### Peeling

Here I am referring to the deep peeling designed to rub out the small wrinkles acquired with age and certainly not the simple natural peeling that all women and now some men practice with the aim of removing dead cells from the surface of the skin.

Think about the extraordinary richness of the surface of the face in reflex zones, its highly complex blood circulation, and its abundance of ultra-sensitive nerve endings, directly connected to the brain. When you take account of the effect obtained in just a few seconds of gentle stimulation of the points and zones located on the face, it is difficult not to conclude that there must be considerable damage to the health and vital energy of a person who undergoes a procedure as destructive as this deep peeling while under anesthetic. Yet, in case of sickness, who will think about establishing a link?

Would it not be preferable to keep a few wrinkles, rather than risk spoiling one's health? They tell the story of the joys and pains of a whole life! Furthermore, the regular practice of Dien' Cham' will greatly contribute to the prevention of wrinkles, and keep you looking healthy, with no danger!

### Tattoos and Collagen Injections

Above all the concern here is tattooing around the lips and the eyes, sometimes called "permanent make-up." It might seem practical to be able to count on having made-up eyes and mouth when leaving the swimming pool, but is the risk really worth taking?

Remember that a tattoo is created by injecting inks with high proportions of heavy metals and colorings. That is the aim! It takes no account of the lesions inflicted on these zones, which are suddenly going to be submitted to hyper-stimulation by the multiple injections necessary!

There is also a modern trend to inject collagens into the lips in order to swell those considered too thin. Effects on the intestines and digestive system as a whole seem likely.

# 4

# Using Dien' Cham' for Prevention and Treatment of Health Problems
## A Practical Dictionary of Therapeutic Sessions

**Warning**

Let us first reaffirm here that in the case of serious illness or severe cases of fainting or loss of consciousness it is not advisable to attempt treatment with Dien' Cham' alone. In an emergency it is essential TO CALL FOR PROFESSIONAL HELP.

However, while you are waiting for the doctor, you may be able to use facial reflexology to effectively ease the person's suffering without any risk of making matters worse—it is better than just standing there doing nothing! So please do not hesitate to use this method as a complement to professional medical treatment.

## GETTING STARTED

This Practical Dictionary of Therapeutic Sessions was designed for beginners, to enable you to start using Dien' Cham' techniques after simply reading the basics of the method. Later—when you are more familiar with the practice and you know the various diagrams well—you will be ready to use chapter 6 where you will learn how to create a personalized session, either for yourself or for any other person. For the moment, be happy to follow the advice given and this will allow you to obtain your first results!

In each of the cases presented here, you will find the main pressure points indicated. The locations of the points are clearly shown in the accompanying figure, making it unnecessary for you to refer back to the main diagrams in chapter 2. You will be able to memorize the reflex points to be stimulated just by glancing at the figures given here.

Each case also includes a second figure with gray-shaded areas, which indicates the main reflex zones concerned, or at least some of the correspondences. These zones must be stimulated in the same way as the points. This will serve you as an example that you can put into practice and use generally on all kinds of troubles and sicknesses.

Please remember that one of the great advantages of Dien' Cham' over other reflexology techniques remains its ease of execution. Please do not say that you have forgotten your special ballpoint, or roller, because you can always use your fingers, or any other instrument with a rounded end, and this will usually be sufficient.

It is now time to get started!

## Acne, pimples, blackheads
**37, 38, 39, 63, 124, 127, 0**

### As well as
**60, 61, 3, 156, 143, 0**

In addition to the points indicated, stimulate the nasogenian creases (the small creases that link the nostrils to the corners of the mouth), as well as points along the upper lip. Where you find it appropriate, also treat for Constipation (see below).

If you suffer from chronic acne, think about changing your diet by adding vegetable fibers from fruit and vegetables and decreasing your intake of refined sugar, dairy products, and meat, especially pork-based products.

The zones to stimulate are mainly those corresponding to the digestive tract: the liver, gallbladder, pancreas, large intestine, and colon. Do not forget the hormonal correspondence zones, above all those on the upper lip, in girls and in boys.

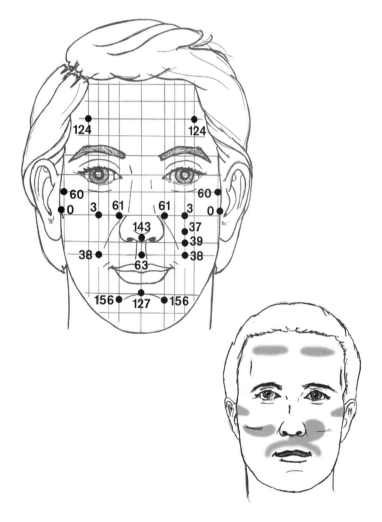

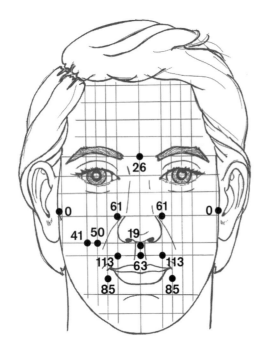

## Alcohol, Immediate Effects of Drinking
**19, 61, 26, 41, 50, 63, 85, 113, 0**

It is possible to reduce the effects of a meal during which too much alcohol was ingested just by massaging a few points for two or three minutes. This will allow your liver and pancreas to better perform the extra activity forced upon them and you will recuperate better by removing some of the effects of the alcohol. All will quite naturally depend on the amount drunk and your metabolic rate.

In any case improvement of the situation will rapidly become obvious. Please do not use this technique as an excuse to drink in excess. The alcohol test for drivers will only show negative when all of the alcohol has been eliminated from your body, even if this is speeded up somewhat by stimulation of the points given, either during or at the end of a meal!

### Hangover
**19, 61, 26, 0**

If you have abused the liquor bottle the evening before and forgotten to practice the stimulation given above, simple massage will reduce that hangover the following morning by suppressing the effects of alcohol.

In addition, soothe the liver and gallbladder by stimulating the reflex zones corresponding to these organs.

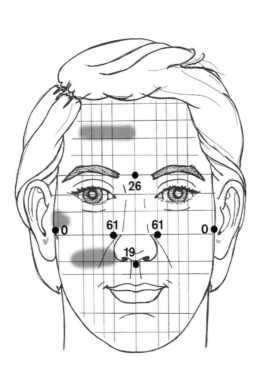

# Alcoholism

## 26, 74, 85, 127, 50, 41, 113, 0

Points 0 and 26 in particular favor elimination of alcohol. Of course it is generally necessary to treat for anxiety or worry and work out an overall program for fitness. Stimulation alone will never induce someone to stop drinking alcohol. If someone has made the decision to stop, however, these pressure points can come in handy by assisting detoxification of the body and calming the withdrawal symptoms that will inevitably arise, especially at the beginning.

Here it is advised to stimulate the reflex zones corresponding to the emunctories—the liver, gallbladder, intestines, and kidneys—as well as the pancreas and the nervous system.

**Important:** Contrary to the usual advice, it is better to give up all the various kinds of sugar and, if possible, even coffee. On the other hand vitamin B and C supplements are recommended.

# Allergies, Food

## 61, 50, 3, 26, 60, 74, 17, 0

These reflex points and zones promote digestion and reduce the risk of food allergies, which have become so frequent these days. One of the causes is that our food contains more additives of all kinds and the result is disorders of the immune system. It is interesting to attempt to discover the allergy agent in question and try to avoid ingesting it but this is sometimes difficult to accomplish. If this is the case, then use Dien' Cham', which will usually give satisfactory results.

The most pertinent reflex zones are obviously those dealing with the digestive system: stomach, liver, pancreas, intestines and kidneys. It is also beneficial to stimulate the immune system and the spinal column.

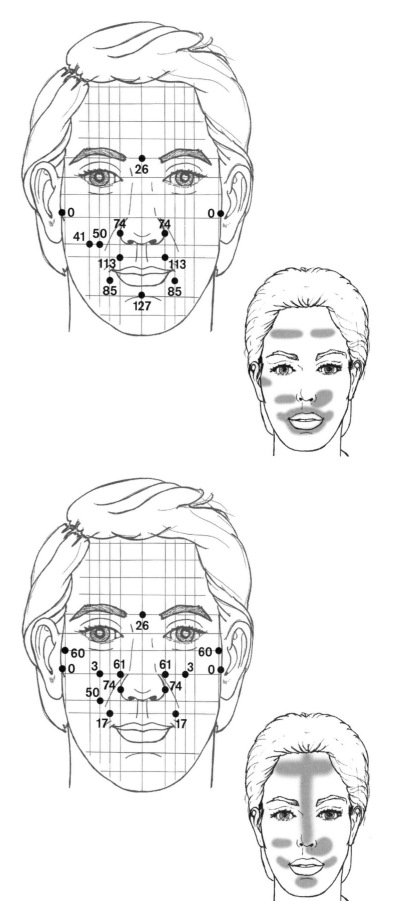

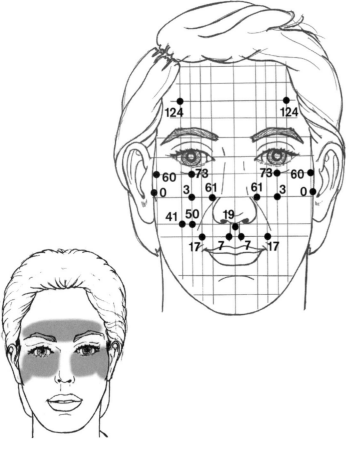

## Allergies, Respiratory
**3, 7, 17, 19, 41, 50, 60, 61, 73, 124, 0**

Numerous points on the face favor regulation of the body's natural defenses or immune system and boost them. The points above correspond particularly to sicknesses linked to respiratory allergies such as asthma, bronchial asthma, chronic bronchitis, sinusitis, and allergy-provoked runny nose (hay fever). Perform this stimulation daily or several times a day as soon as you detect the presence of the allergic agent (pollen, grains, dust, animal fur, feathers, and so on). If you are allergic to pollen or grasses, try to start your treatment before they appear, at the beginning of the spring!

Widely stimulate the upper respiratory tract and lung, nose, and sinus reflex zones, following the indications given here.

Remember to perform a nose and forehead massage as soon as symptoms appear (see the sections entitled "Example: Common Cold" and "A Few Special Massages" in chapter 3).

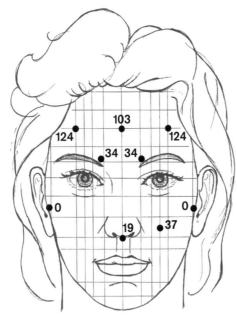

## Anemia
**37, 124, 103, 34, 19, 0**

This disorder of the blood—which shows up as a deficit or small size of the red blood cells, giving a low rate of hemoglobin—is generally linked to a lack of iron. Women are generally affected more than men, in part because of the loss of iron during menstruation, but men can suffer from this as well. It provokes a whole series of troubles, including chronic tiredness, reduced resistance, paleness, irritability, dizziness, even palpitations, headaches, stomachaches, and itching over the entire body. Remember to monitor your food intake and enrich it with iron and also vitamins C and B.

## Anorexia

**14, 37, 39, 41, 50, 19, 0**

When you are treating for this, it is a good idea to also stimulate the points associated with Relaxation and Toning Up, as well as those concerning Anxiety. Sometimes it can be necessary to treat for endocrine problems too (using points relating to the ovaries and uterus for example), and digestive disorders. Very often the appetite as well as the capacity to digest return at the same time, as these disturbed functions are reactivated.

This wide-ranging treatment must be practiced regularly, twice per day if possible, until a clear improvement is felt. It is then possible to make do with a single daily session until the problem is totally cured. Before and after meals it is helpful to stimulate points and zones corresponding to Indigestion.

## Anxiety

**124, 34, 103, 106, 26, 8, 60, 0**

Numerous points regulate and stimulate the nervous system. A regular or occasional stimulation of them will help considerably, without any of the secondary effects usually experienced when strong medicines or drugs are taken!

If you are subject to nocturnal anxiety that stops you from getting to sleep, stimulate these points before going to bed. The very same points will help if you have to confront a stressful or worrisome situation during the day, such as an examination, important interview, or being asked to speak in public.

Remember to check on your liver function because that can often be the cause in certain cases of illogical worry or anxiety, especially if worry becomes acute between one and three in the morning!

Please also remember to regularly practice the Basic Session, as it can be of immediate use at any time of the day!

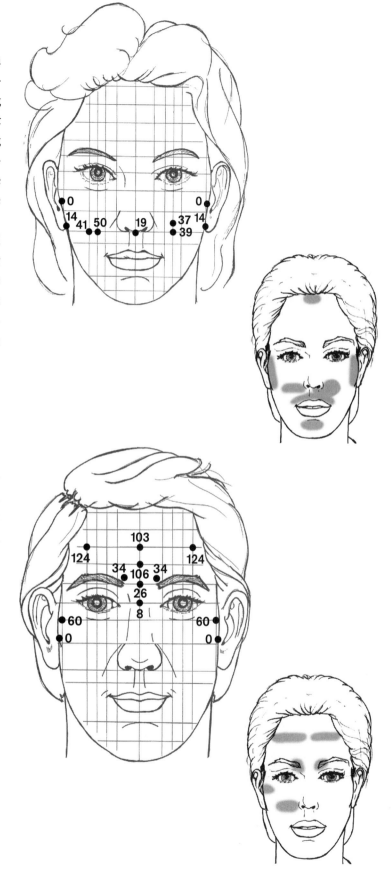

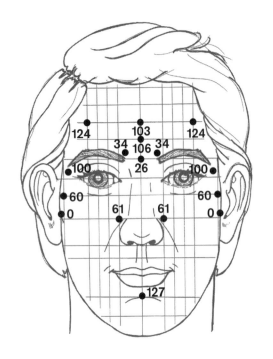

## Anxiety, Child
### 34, 60, 61, 26, 100, 103, 106, 124, 127, 0

We live in a strange age where it is necessary to give tranquilizers or sedatives even to babies! In this regard, France has the dubious distinction of holding the world record. It is however quite possible to treat nervousness and anxiety in our children purely using natural and harmless methods, which give good results. These include stimulation of the points given here, using short sessions.

For a very young child, just delicately stimulate the relevant zone with the end of a finger. Your massage will feel like a caress and you will see the little one relax quite naturally.

## Aphonia
### (see Laryngitis)

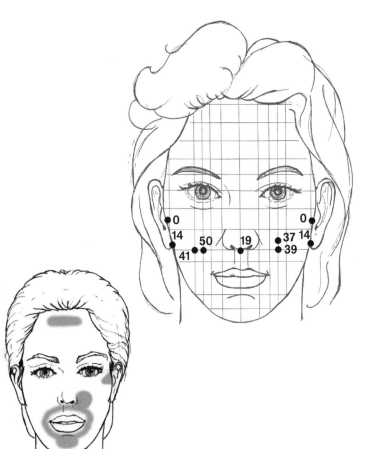

## Appetite, Loss of
### 14, 41, 50, 19, 37, 39, 0

A loss of appetite results in a lack of dynamism and often a liver or intestinal malfunction, especially in children and older or fragile persons. This can cause deficiencies, which will cause other problems like demineralization, spasmophilia, and so on. To prevent all of the above, stimulate the points indicated before meals.

Also stimulate zones assisting the digestive function to promote assimilation of food and elimination of waste matter.

# Arrhythmia of the Heart
## 1, 8, 19, 34, 61, 100, 106, 60, 0

These points regulate the heartbeat. Here again we find point 0 with a regulating effect, calming excess. If your heart is beating too fast, or too slow, point 0 will help to establish equilibrium again (see Tachycardia).

Massage corresponding reflex zones as well.

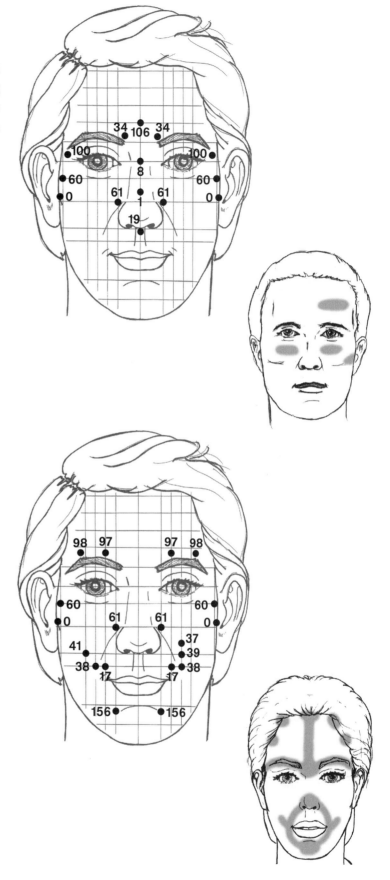

# Arthritis
## 17, 41, 60, 97, 98, 156, 0

### Always add the following points
### 37, 38, 39, 61

These points will treat arthritis as a whole with its related inflammatory pain syndrome. Work out your own program relative to the specific troubles being experienced.

According to the case you may add the following points:

| | |
|---|---|
| 34, 51, 65 | for arms and shoulders |
| 130, 100 | for hands and wrists |
| 130, 51 | for legs and feet |
| 197 | for knees |
| 98 | for elbows |

Remember that all joints correspond to each other! So, in some cases, it may be a good idea to stimulate all of the joint-related zones (shown in **Diagram 11,** chapter 2).

Here is a new chart. You can experiment with it as you see fit.

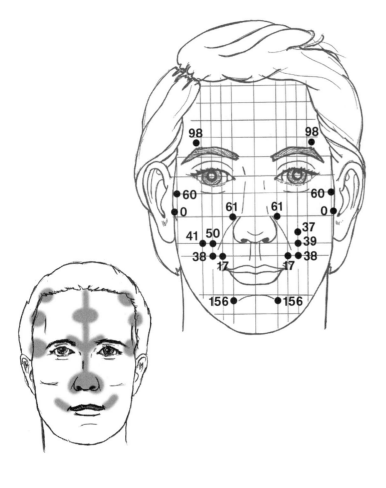

## Arthrosis
### 17, 41, 50, 60, 98, 156, 0

You can adapt your session to your specific troubles, following the pertinent entries for arthrosis seen below.

This degenerative sickness could reach all of us sooner or later. It is remarkable, however, to see how quickly it is spreading in young people, whereas previously only older people were susceptible. It is evident that our intake of artificial foods is in question here (with its accompanying additives and sugar abuse), which acidifies the body,* along with the sheer pace of modern life, also acidifying, and a lack of physical exercise, which is always harmful. The points indicated will help you to soothe the pain and improve your health generally. Take up some physical exercise again and change your diet, increasing the proportion of fresh uncooked vegetables like carrots and celery.

Take advantage of this session to stimulate the whole of your joint-related zones as well as those corresponding to your spinal column. Do not limit yourself to the areas affected, but go over all of the zones systematically and insist a little on the areas that are most painful.

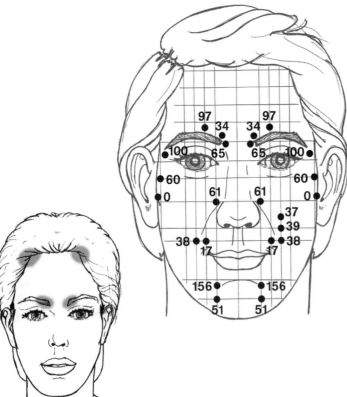

## Arthrosis of the Arm and Shoulder
### 65, 34, 51, 17, 60, 156, 0

### If necessary, add the following
### 61, 37, 38, 39

If your arthrosis only affects your arms and shoulders, you can limit yourself to the first sequence of points listed here. If not, add the second sequence.

Please do not forget that a Dien' Cham' session combines reflex points and zones! Add those that correspond the best!

---

*For a good explanation of acidification and why to avoid it see *The Acid-Alkaline Diet for Optimum Health: Restoring Your Health by Creating Balance in Your Diet* by Christopher Vasey, N.D. (Rochester, Vt.: Healing Arts Press, 2003).

# Arthrosis of the Hands and Fingers
## 130, 17, 100, 156, 191, 0

### If necessary, add the following
#### 61, 37, 38, 39

To the points indicated above, you can add the points corresponding to the fingers particularly affected (see Fingers). Refer also to the other entries for Arthrosis.

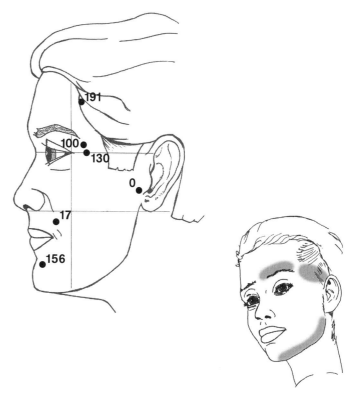

# Arthrosis of the Hip
## 63, 17, 41, 156, 0

### If necessary, add the following
#### 61, 37, 38, 39

It is important to treat this very serious kind of arthrosis, which is a degenerative condition, as quickly as possible, to avoid the necessity of corrective surgery. This is possible, as long as the condition has not reached an irreversible stage. Refer to the advice given above (see Arthrosis) and do not hesitate to add points given for arthrosis in general. In any case, relief will be rapidly forthcoming.

To these points, add stimulation of the nostrils. Rub the fleshy part of both nostrils energetically with the fingers or the ballpoint pen.

You can also stimulate corresponding areas of the forehead.

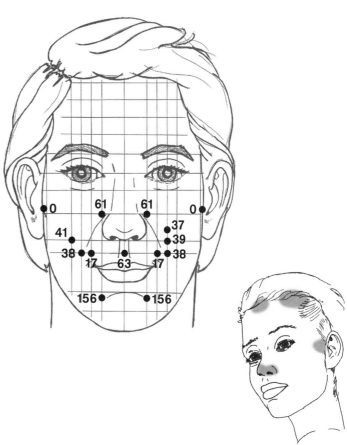

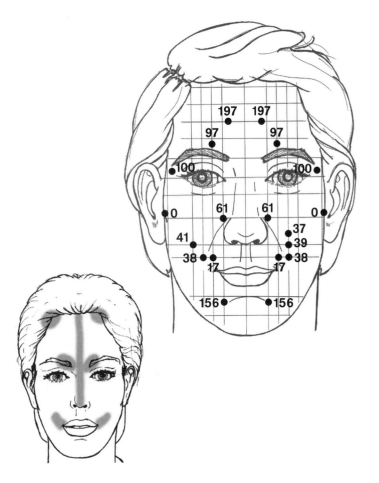

## Arthrosis of the Joints
### 97, 156, 100, 17, 41, 197, 61, 37, 38, 39, 0

All of these points can be stimulated in association with the basic arthrosis session or otherwise according to your judgment. Do not hesitate to perform two or three sessions per day until a lasting improvement is felt.

Regular and frequent massages of the joints affected using St. John's Wort oil will soothe painful and inflamed joints. It is also advised to drink a decoction of harpagophytum (Devil's Claw) or take this plant in the form of capsules or extract.

In addition to the above points, stimulate the joint zones affected, concentrating on the side of the body in question, going quickly over painless or slightly painful reflex zones.

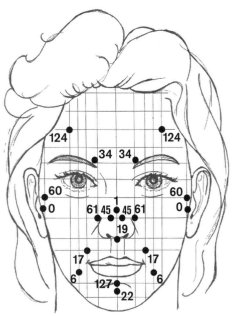

## Asthenia, Chronic Tiredness
### 124, 34, 1, 45, 60, 61, 19, 17, 127, 22, 6, 0

Asthenia corresponds to a state of habitual tiredness, which is both physical and nervous. Stimulation of these points wakes up energy and promotes its circulation throughout the body, dynamizing the function of the brain and boosting natural defenses. It is advised to make sure that you stimulate all of the points shown, as this will ensure you treat simultaneously troubles that are likely to be at the origin of the asthenia. In addition, a rapid result is encouraging and helps one persevere.

Regularly practice the Basic Session, as well as the Standard Session detailed in chapter 3, which will allow you to stimulate all of the body in just a few seconds.

# Asthma
## 26, 19, 3, 61, 17, 37, 60, 0

This sequence and the two others shown below can be practiced alternately and as frequently as necessary. After a few attempts, use the one that suits you the best. Another idea is to design a personal program based on the points indicated, by choosing the most sensitive ones, and then practice it at least once per day. As soon as the first symptoms of breathlessness or dyspnea occur, stimulate the points and you will be surprised to see that your attacks become less severe, rarer, and then disappear all together.

It is advised to remember the reflex zones too. And as soon as a cold starts, practice the special massage for this (see Cold).

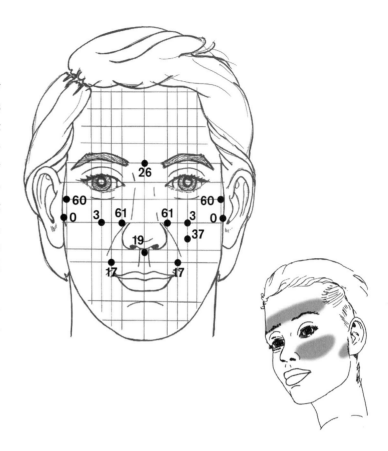

## Alternative Sequence
### 14, 37, 39, 50, 3, 61, 0

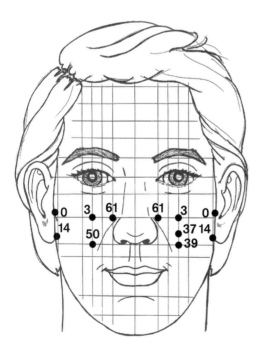

## Alternative Sequence
### 60, 85, 87, 51, 113, 19, 0

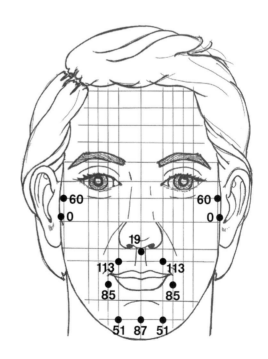

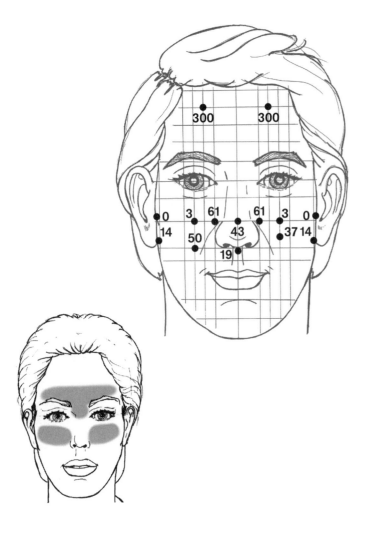

## Asthma Attack
### 19, 61, 3, 14, 37, 50, 43, 300, 0

Never neglect an asthma attack. Besides the serious suffering an attack causes, it can also have serious consequences if intervention is not done in time. Start by strongly stimulating point **19**, if possible at the beginning of the attack, and then the other points indicated here. It could well be that the attack will stop. If not then the usual treatment should be used. Relief of asthma will come progressively, by treating it every day.

Add these reflex zones.

> **Please Note:**
>
> It should be repeated that you must not stop your medical treatment. Dien' Cham' is complementary and absolutely not a substitute! However you will find that you need your usual treatment less and less.

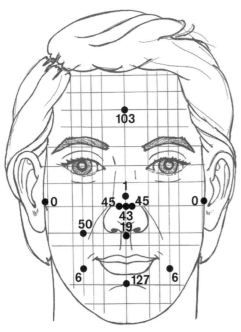

## Athletic Conditioning
### 19, 1, 45, 50, 43, 6, 103, 127, 0

All of these points are aimed at reinforcing the natural defenses and toning up the body, which sportsmen and women often overwork during their training. Of course these are points that can also be used in case of simple tiredness. Preferably this sequence should be practiced in the morning or during the day.

# Back Problems
**19, 26, 38, 43, 63, 103, 106, 0**

**As well as**
**124, 126, 143, 300, 342, 0**

**(see also Cervical Vertebrae, Coccyx, Lumbago, Lumbar Vertebrae, Neck, Spinal Column)**

The following points relieve specific areas as follows:

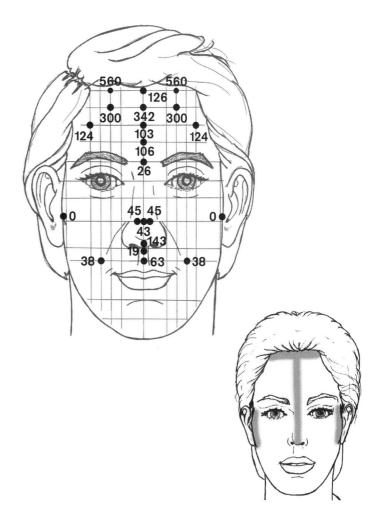

- dorsal vertebrae:  106, 103, 342
- lumbar vertebrae:  300, 560, 126, 43, 45, 0

The points given on the figure provide stimulation of the whole of the spinal column. Whatever the specific location of the problem, it is always better to start by stimulating all of them, and then concentrate on the zone concerned or where the pain is present. You can, if necessary, select a few of the points to make the session shorter if required, at your workplace for example. In this case you will concentrate on applying the massage as soon as the pain starts, rather than waiting for the pain to become entrenched and then trying to do something.

Stimulation of these points and zones is advised even when there is no back pain, especially in subjects suffering from tiredness or who have sedentary sitting or standing occupations.

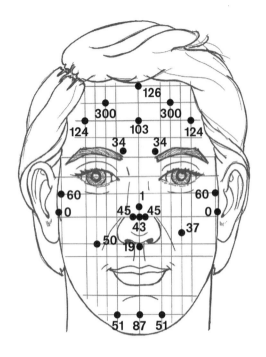

## Bedwetting, Enuresis
**124, 34, 87, 19, 43, 45, 37, 300, 0**

**Or**

**126, 103, 1, 50, 37, 87, 60, 0**

Contrary to received wisdom, this problem is mainly due to an allergic reaction. The psychological processes usually identified as the cause of this are merely the result of the allergy and the child is helpless in dealing with the consequent humiliating circumstances. Scientific studies have put the ingestion of cow's milk, eggs, chocolate, and citrus fruit into question and indicate these foods may well have a role in causing enuresis. (For more details please refer to work by J. C. Breneman of the American College of Allergists). Besides stimulation of these pressure points, try to find the cause of the allergy and eliminate the specific food-type. Regular consumption of quail eggs in the form of capsules sold in specialist shops often solves this disorder quickly.

**Simplified procedure**
**87, 51, 0**

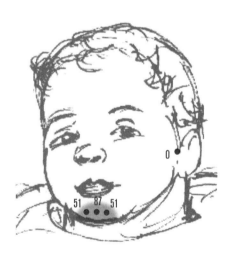

# Bladder Problems

85, 87, 22, 26, 3, 60, 0

### (see also Incontinence and Cystitis)

These points favor a return to normal in all problems affecting the bladder. They improve cases of weakness leading to incontinence, prolapse or sinking of the bladder, and infection or inflammation caused by various agents (cystitis). It can be usefully noted here that cranberry juice is beneficial in chronic cases of cystitis. It is also advisable to drink water abundantly.

During the same session also stimulate the corresponding reflex zones. The massage can be performed several times per day until pain and discomfort subside.

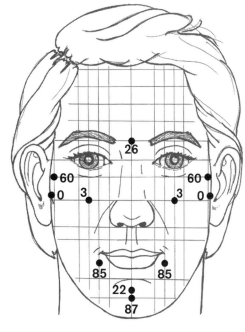
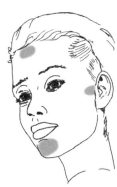

# Blood Circulation

7, 37, 50, 60, 73, 74, 156, 0

### (see also Legs)

Do you suffer from varicose veins or have the feeling of heavy legs at the end of the day? These troubles indicate a lack of tonicity of the vein walls. These reflex points and zones are here for you.

Use them several times every day if you are obliged to spend many hours in front of your desk, or on the contrary have to run around behind a shop counter all day. In both cases your blood circulation is placed in stressful circumstances. Never forget that the best remedy for this is regular physical exercise!

**Please note:** In this case point 0 tones up the veins, by promoting their contraction.

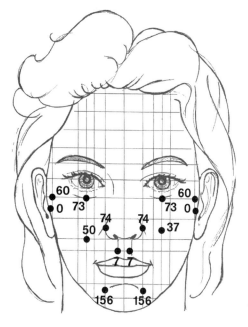
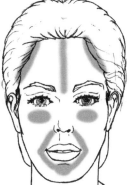

## Breastfeeding

**73, 39, 60, 87, 0**

Stimulation of these points promotes the production of milk. You should practice this straight after the birth and continue daily or even several times a day, just before giving the breast and as needed.

At the same time, it is also good to stimulate the hormonal correspondence zones on the upper lip, along the chin, and the hairline.

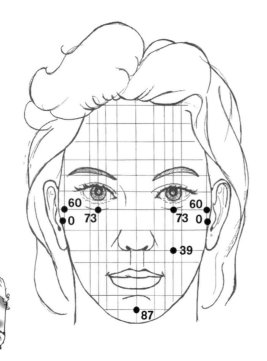

## Breasts

**73, 7, 113, 39, 60, 0**

**(see also Mastosis)**

These points correspond to the breasts and you can therefore stimulate them whatever the problem: nodules or nodes, cysts, mastosis, overdevelopment, or underdevelopment.

Add these corresponding reflex zones.

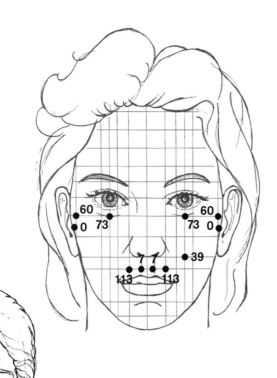

# Breathlessness

## 34, 8, 0

These points will help any person short of breath, whether it is in the case of walking up steps or during a run. When these points are stimulated the heartbeat is slowed, which is particularly useful for those practicing a sport. As these points are readily accessible, you can even use them during a competition, in particular the whole of the zone in front of the ear.

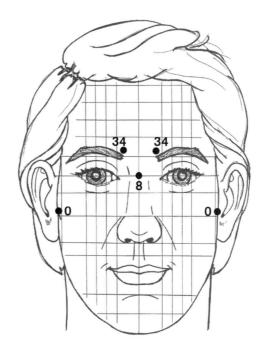

# Bronchitis

## 3, 17, 26, 8, 61, 37, 51, 73, 38, 14, 0

Whether it is a case of simple bronchitis (after catching a chill in the winter), or chronic bronchitis linked to an allergy or smoking, these points will allow a rapid improvement in the situation. As in other ailments, they can be stimulated while the patient is undergoing other forms of treatment, if this seems appropriate. If you stimulate these points at the onset of symptoms such as a sore throat or cold, you may not get to the coughing stage.

Always remember to take magnesium chloride,[1] as for all cases of infectious sickness.

The reflex zones to be stimulated are, above all, the lung and bronchial zones, but you can include the liver, kidney, intestinal, and spinal column zones, which will have the effect of toning up the emunctories and life energy.

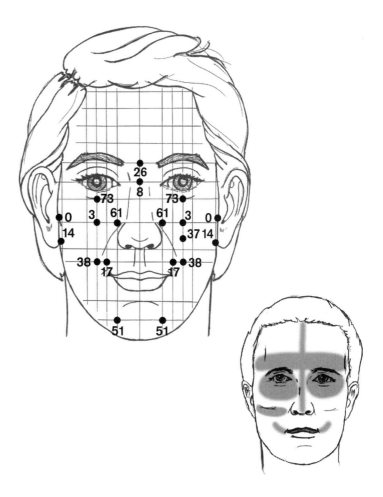

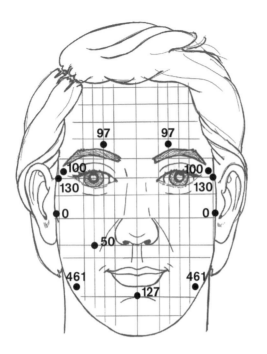

## Bruising, Dislocations, Sprains
### 50, 461, 130, 127, 100, 97, 0

It can be beneficial to learn these few points well because in the case of a sprain or twisted ankle it is far preferable to perform the stimulation as soon as possible. You can avoid pain and the situation worsening. Also think of cooling the lesion by running cold water over it for a few minutes. Please note that point **100** corresponds particularly to the wrist, and points **97** and **127** to the ankle.

To these points it is a good idea to add the reflex zones that correspond to the location of a specific lesion. For this see **Diagrams 2, 4, 6,** and 8 in chapter 2.

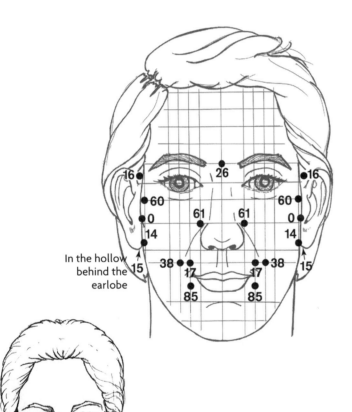

## Burns
### 17, 26, 38, 85, 60, 61, 14, 15, 16, 0

These points procure relief from pain. You can also add points that correspond to the affected area. Also remember that application of a clay[2] or mud pack soothes effectively and promotes rapid renewal of skin tissue.

The reflex zones to stimulate are the ones that correspond to the parts of the body concerned. The figure here has no zones indicated on it. This will allow you to adapt it for different areas affected by burns.

# Burping Babies

## 126, 19, 0

To provoke a burp, simple and gentle stimulation of these points with the end of a finger should be enough. Mother and child will then be fully satisfied!

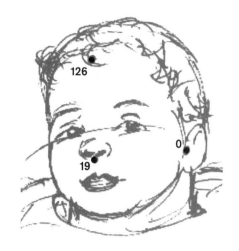

# Cellulitis

## 26, 3, 85, 87, 50, 37, 39, 74, 143, 0

### As well as
### 85, 87, 22, 0

These points help to fight against your body's natural tendency to stock water. Regular stimulation acts against the notorious cellulitis that all women abhor. It is necessary, however, to persevere to obtain a lasting result. In addition, in certain cases it is preferable to stimulate the points relative to the endocrine system (see Contraception), the thyroid gland (points **8, 14, 15**), the pancreas (points **7, 113, 63**) and sometimes the heart (**3, 9**).

At the same time, it is advisable to stimulate reflex zones corresponding to the endocrine system, the thyroid glands, the pancreas, the heart, and the kidneys.

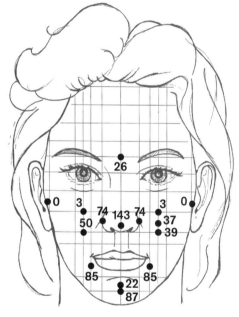

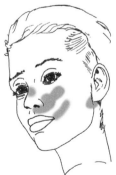

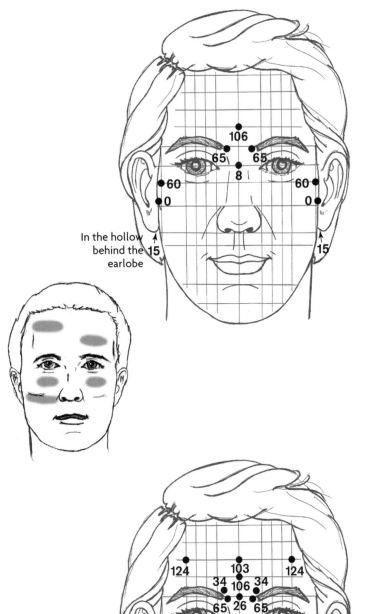

## Cerebral Blood Circulation
### 106, 65, 60, 8, 15, 0

Good circulation of blood around the brain is important to maintain. Many conditions in modern life tend to reduce this, such as dietary habits that cause stress, lack of exercise, lack of sleep and relaxation, to say nothing of the abuse of certain drugs including tobacco and alcohol. Aging is also an important factor. To preserve this circulation as far as possible, remember to use these points in case of troubles. A strong stimulation of point **15** with a pointed instrument will have an immediate effect on irrigation of the brain.

Add the reflex zones corresponding to the liver, the gallbladder, and the heart as well as those concerning the head in general.

## Cerebral Functions
### 124, 103, 106, 60, 34, 26, 65, 0

The reflex points and zones given here improve cerebral functions such as memory, concentration, and attention, in cases where a deficit has been noticed due to aging, overwork, lack of sleep, or sickness. According to the individual, these points can be stimulated when the need is felt, such as to complete a piece of work, an examination, and so on, or daily when a long-term result is sought. Remember to include the basic points for Relaxation and Toning Up.

## Cervical Vertebrae

### 8, 34, 26, 65, 106, 16, 0

If you suffer from cervical vertebrae pain, arthrosis, headaches, or shoulder or arm pain, perform sweeping movements in the area between **8** and **106** and then stimulate the zone along the eyebrows, which corresponds to the shoulder and arm: right arm/right eyebrow; left arm/left eyebrow. Remember that the spinal column is also represented by the entire zone that is vertically aligned with point **0** situated in front of the ear. Therefore it is important to stimulate it carefully in cases of back or neck problems. (See **Diagrams 8** and **12**, chapter 2.)

Cervical vertebrae pain, as well as stiff neck, is rapidly relieved by simple stimulation, for a few seconds, of the zone located between the eyebrows, at the root of the nose.

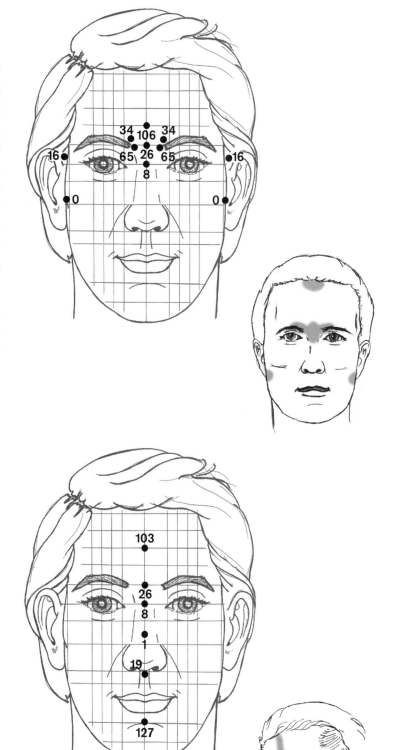

## Chakras

### 365, 127, 19, 1, 8, 26, 103

The reflex points corresponding to each of the seven chakras are distributed between the chin and the forehead in the following ascending order:

| 1st chakra | or sacral plexus: | 365 |
| 2nd chakra | or umbilical plexus: | 127 |
| 3rd chakra | or solar plexus: | 19 |
| 4th chakra | or heart plexus: | 1 |
| 5th chakra | or throat plexus: | 8 |
| 6th chakra | or forehead plexus: | 26 |
| 7th chakra | or crown plexus: | 103 |

Point **103** corresponds to the forehead chakra or third eye, and stimulates all of the other chakras as well as the pituitary gland, which is the corresponding endocrine gland, which has a regulatory function on the whole endocrine system.

It is also possible to find a projection of the chakras on the line in front of the ear. Point **0** corresponds to the solar plexus.

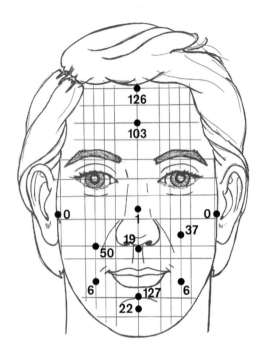

## Chi (to provoke its ascent)
### 126, 103, 1, 19, 127, 22, 6, 37, 50, 0

Those of you who practice one of the martial arts will know about Chi (Ki in Japanese), as practitioners learn to use this energy and direct it. It is synonymous with the life force but is more than that. In cases of sickness, this energy can be excessive or lacking and become blocked in one part of the body or another. The goal of all energy therapy is to restore balance by stimulating energy where it is blocked and directing it to places where it is lacking. There are cases where it is advisable to cause the Chi to ascend, which corresponds to a movement upward.

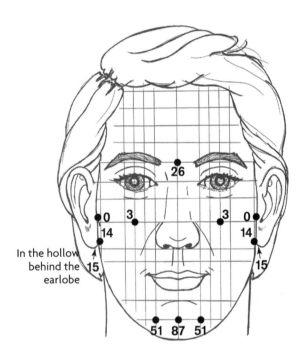

## Chi (to provoke its descent)
### 26, 3, 51, 87, 14, 15, 0

There are other situations where it is necessary to allow the Chi to flow downward. One example is when there is excess Chi in the head, which is the origin of many headaches!

# Chills

## 50, 127, 19, 3, 61, 34, 124, 0

Here we are talking about catching a chill, which often happens when the seasons change. It does not necessarily transform into a cold or rhinopharyngitis, but it is an indication of weak natural defenses. In Chinese medicine, it is considered to be a normal and natural reaction of the body against the invasion of a perverse form of energy, which is the cold energy. The main symptoms are eyes watering, a dry throat, a tickly nose, and fever. The stimulation of points indicated will underpin the body's attempts to adapt to changed circumstances and get rid of the problem.

Rub the ears vigorously, as well as the spinal column zones, in order to boost your natural defenses and life energy.

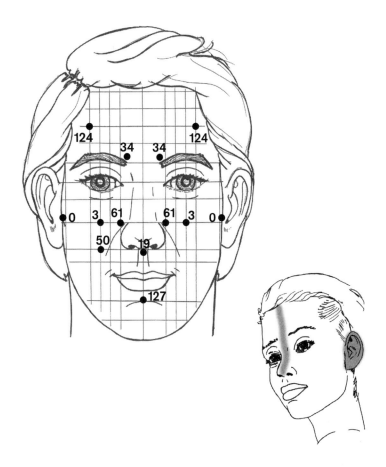

# Choking or Inhalation of a Foreign Body

## 19, 63, 7, 14, 0

This kind of mishap has probably already happened to you. Babies and children are often victims of this. Tapping the victim on the back is generally sufficient to dislodge the foreign body, but some cases are more serious. The following short sequence will be of great help in such a circumstance. Strongly stimulate point **19** with a ballpoint pen, the rounded end of a roller, or whatever else falls to hand. Rub the zone between the base of the nose and the upper lip. Generally simple stimulation of point **19** is enough to expel the undesired object.

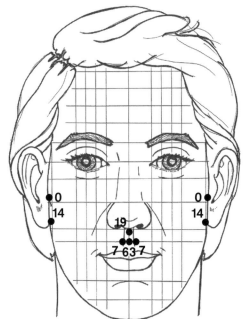

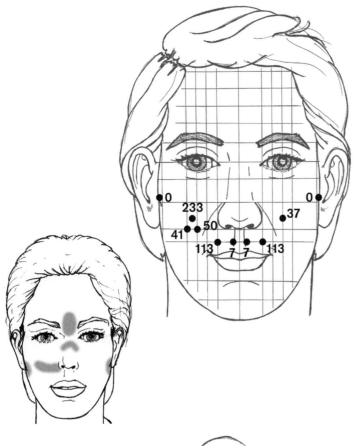

## Cholesterol Reduction
### 41, 50, 37, 113, 7, 233, 0

The link between a high level of cholesterol and cardiovascular disease is well known. If your level of cholesterol is too high, especially if you have high LDL and triglycerides, supplement your modified diet with stimulation of the points shown. If, in addition, you suffer from hypothyroidism and, in spite of your efforts with your diet, your LDL or triglyceride level does not drop, stimulate the following as well: points **8**, **15**, and **14**.

Excess cholesterol is also linked to a poor liver function and sometimes to hypothyroidism as well. In this case it is advised to stimulate the correspondence zones of these organs.

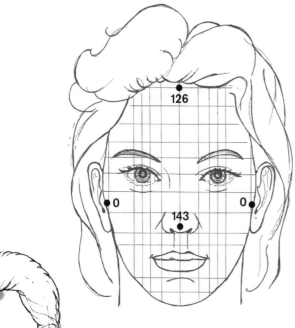

## Coccyx
### 126, 143, 0

If you suffer from pain in the coccyx, such as following a fall or after long periods spent sitting, stimulate these points for as long as it takes to obtain total relief from the pain.

You can also stimulate these reflex zones.

# Cold, the Common

## 50, 19, 3, 61, 26, 124, 106, 103, 342, 0

A Japanese saying has it that a cold that is neglected can open the doors to all kinds of sicknesses. Even if a cold usually leaves without a trace, we must remain alert to the possibility of complications, especially in children and older people, whose natural defenses are weaker. It is advisable to remember this and the fact that over two hundred viruses can come into play! So keep stimulating these pressure points with your instruments! Most people catch two or three colds a year, with all of the usual complications: mucus, sometimes sinusitis, runny nose, watery and irritated eyes.

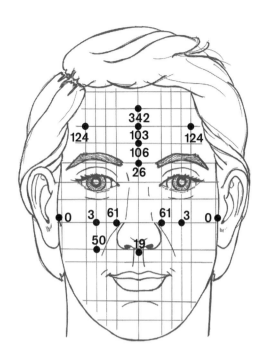

The stimulation of the points indicated will bring rapid relief—to your great surprise, because of the poor results usually obtained with other therapies proposed. Try to remember to repeat this stimulation, if you are again obliged to go out into the cold!

### The Beginnings of a Cold

It is only necessary for you to be a little tired for a chill to penetrate. A while later the head cold starts with its usual first symptoms of a runny nose, itchy throat, and sneezing. You must boost your energy right away.

Using your index fingers rub around the nostrils up and down vigorously, as shown on the figure, as well as in front of the ears.

Using the knuckle of the thumb, energetically rub the center of the forehead at the level of points **106**, **103**, and **342**. It is advised to consume only warm liquids!

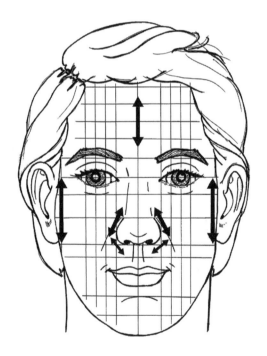

You can also warm the points indicated using a joss or incense stick as a moxa (i.e., by burning a compressed herbal stick—most commonly artemesia—and holding it close to the skin to warm an acupuncture point). Just bring the red hot end close enough to the chosen point so that you can feel the heat, but not touching. Above all do not burn yourself!

You can also warm up your face using your hair dryer! Strange, but it works!

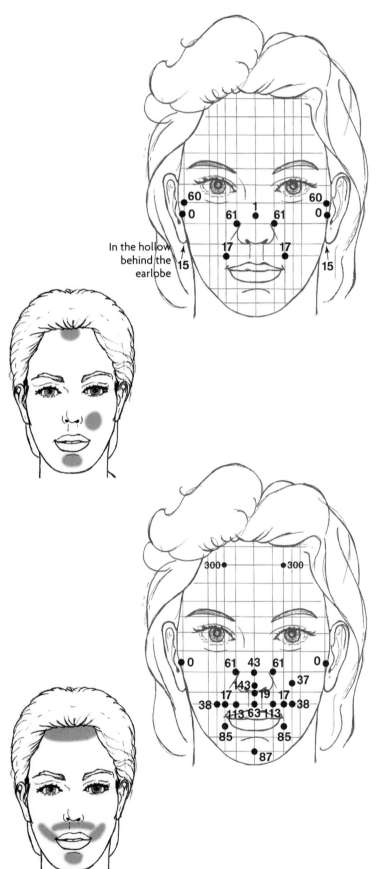

## Cold Sensitivity
**15, 17, 60, 61, 1, 0**

**(see also Numbness at Extremities)**

This refers to the regular feeling of being cold that is not linked to a fever during sickness. It is sometimes linked to a case of anemia that must be treated as well. All of the points given here warm the body up. If you often have cold feet, also stimulate points 87 and 342.

Remember to stimulate the chin and the center of the hairline as well.

## Colibacillosis
**19, 17, 38, 43, 143, 113, 61, 63, 37, 300, 85, 87, 0**

All of these points have a beneficial effect on this intestinal infection, which is often painful. It is often also the cause of urinary infections with accompanying cystitis. You can also stimulate all of the points located on your upper lip and the chin.

Also stimulate reflex zones corresponding to the intestines, kidneys, and bladder to prevent cystitis from returning.

# Colitis, Functional Colopathy

**127, 63, 19, 61, 0**

## Or

**342, 98, 19, 17, 38, 0**

Colitis is linked to an inflammation of the large intestine and is often the cause of recurring abdominal pain, sometimes accompanied by spurious trips to the toilet. Colitis can be associated with a chill or a functional anomaly of the intestine and is sometimes accompanied by diarrhea. It is usually provoked by an unbalanced diet, too rich in meat and meat products and too low in vegetable fibers. The points indicated should be stimulated in the absence of diarrhea and the pain will quickly disappear in the two or three minutes following the treatment.

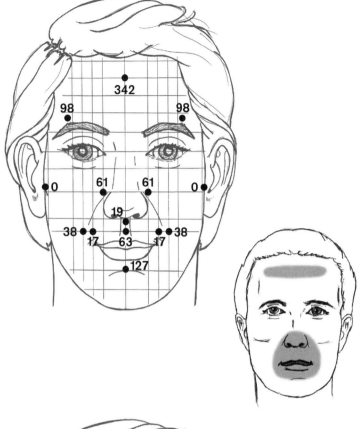

# Colitis with Spasms

**127**

For this painful condition, point 127 is the single most important point to remember.

### Stress-Related

Here is another sequence, useful above all in cases of colitis related to stress: first points **124, 34,** and **8** for relaxation, then **61**, following the nasogenian crease, then back to point **61** again, horizontally over to point **3**, which you rub well, and finish using point **0** as usual.

### With Diarrhea

If the colitis has provoked diarrhea you can try the following points: **103, 50, 37, 63, 127, 22, 365, 19, 0,** or see Diarrhea.

You may also try the reflex zones shown here.

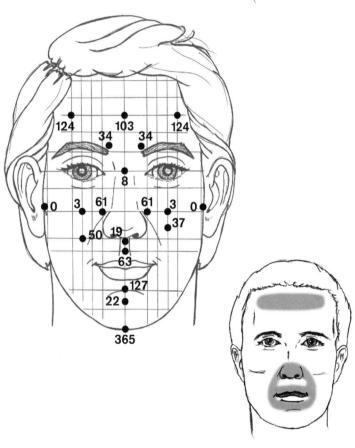

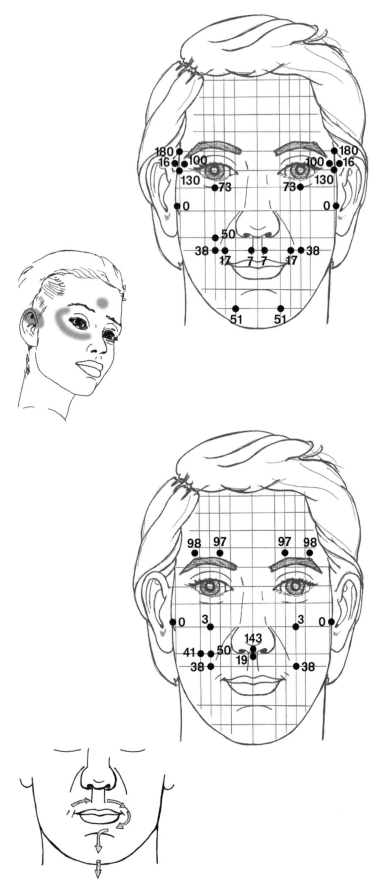

## Conjunctivitis
### 73, 180, 130, 100, 16, 51, 50, 38, 17, 7, 0

This painful inflammation affects the eyes and makes them look red and teary. Conjunctivitis can be the result of an allergy or provoked by dust particles in the air. It is important to resist the temptation to rub the eyes; rather you should stimulate the points and zones given here for as long as is necessary to obtain relief.

## Constipation
### 50, 19, 3, 143, 41, 97, 98, 38, 0

This can be provoked by delays in visiting the toilet to evacuate fecal or waste matter or simply because its volume is insufficient. The possible underlying causes are several. There could be an obstacle, such as a stricture or narrowing of the intestine at one point, or it could be a malfunction like a decrease in muscle tone or even an excess of this, resulting in painful spasms. The latter is very frequent in subjects with high blood pressure who often eat large quantities of meat and pork-based products, as well as those who eat insufficient quantities of the vegetable fibers present in fresh fruit and vegetables. The effect is compounded by drinking too little water and a lack of physical exercise.

In addition to the sequence shown above, there is another simple form of treatment that gives excellent results, even in the case of a serious blockage having lasted several days. In the morning before breakfast, drink a big cup of warm, lightly salted water. With the right thumb placed firmly under the chin, use two or three fingers of your right hand—the index and middle finger, possibly accompanied by the ring finger—to move round the mouth from right to left as shown in the figure. Then, when you reach the chin, make a brisk gesture downward. Repeat the above massage fifty times without stopping.

It is of course quite possible to repeat this during the day if necessary.

# Contraception

Although this method may sound very strange, it is used with success by thousands of women in southeast Asia. I will relay this to you accompanied by the customary message of caution. Several of my readers have attempted to use this method and it seems that it has been an effective means of contraception for them; however, I have also been told of one failure. It is important to keep in mind the cultural dimension of a tradition or a belief, and, in this area, particularly, we have to be circumspect. It is quite possible for the psychological aspect to play a determining role in the likelihood of conceiving a child or not. We only have to consider how many women become pregnant right after having adopted a child, following years of having been considered sterile!

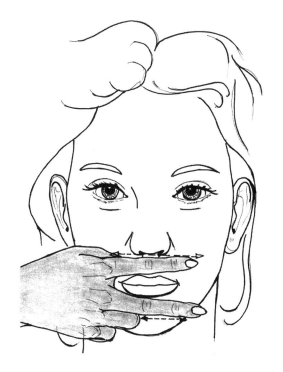

According to the principles of facytherapy, the nose reflex zones are in close relationship with the uterus, in the same way as the points located above the upper lip and below the lower lip are linked to the ovaries and the uterus. Stimulation of these reflex zones—which can be performed by pressing, rubbing, or tapping—induces hormonal, muscular, and biological type modifications at the level of these organs.

This particular technique is not confined to contraception; it has many other interesting and beneficial results, being particularly effective in cases of vaginal dryness, dyspareunia or pain during sexual intercourse, frigidity, period pain, giving birth, and vaginal tightness, which are all generally linked to trauma of a sexual nature.

## Method[3]

- For about ten minutes before sexual intercourse and straight after, rub the area surrounding your mouth back and forth 200 times with the index and middle fingers of preferably your right hand. Do not rub so hard as to cause injury but strongly enough to make the massage work.
- Then massage your nostrils, pinching them lightly between the thumb and index finger

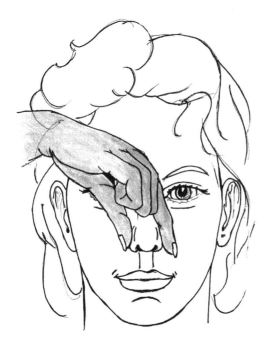

about 200 times. It should only take two or three minutes! Pinch from the base on each side and move toward the bridge of the nose in a brisk upward movement.

- This facial massage should cause a sense of warmth in the pelvic region together with a pleasant sexual feeling. As for the common symptom of vaginal dryness: it should be a thing of the past! These signs show that the stimulation has been effective and are the guarantee of good contraception. Absence of them indicates that the technique has been badly performed, either due to the stimulation being too short or the pressure inadequate.

- The two hundred strokes only represent an average. In the case of a young sensitive woman in good health, fifty strokes can be enough for the warmth and other sensations to be felt. On the other hand, a mature woman or one with less vitality may have to practice this massage for longer to feel the effects.

- Whatever the case, the important thing is to feel warmth in the face and pelvic region, along with sexual arousal, including lubrication of the vagina and sometimes even toning up, which is when you feel the vaginal muscles move. When these indications are experienced, contraception should be effective. To obtain a good contraceptive effect it is sufficient to practice this technique during the fertile period. Instruments are now available in pharmacies that allow this period to be determined with precision.

Sometimes the lack of signs evidences a form of frigidity that is easy to treat using the same method, but practiced daily over a long period until a satisfactory result is obtained.

### Warning

This massage provokes strong contraction of the womb, preventing nidation or implantation. It is to be avoided in cases of pregnancy because of the risk of a miscarriage. On the other hand, it can be practiced at the time of birth, when it soothes pain and relaxes.

# Cough

## 73, 26, 8, 61, 51, 3, 14, 0

Bouts of coughing are more frequent at night and make life unpleasant. They are caused by slightly more alkaline blood due to the predominance of the parasympathetic nervous system, or changes in the recurring secretion of hormones at night with respect to the daytime. It is also likely that mucus accumulates more easily at night when it is not naturally rejected, and obstructs the higher respiratory tract. This obliges the person to breathe the cold night air through the mouth causing further irritation. These points can be stimulated as often as necessary and this usually brings rapid soothing of the symptoms.

In addition to this sequence, also remember to stimulate the points that decrease or increase secretions:

- in case of a dry cough see Secretions (increasing)
- in case of a productive cough see Secretions (decreasing)

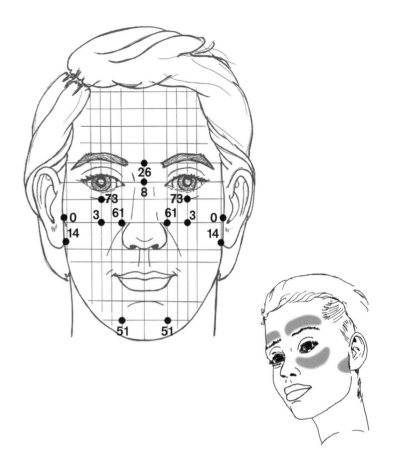

# Cystitis

## 61, 19, 87, 63, 50, 7, 17, 0

Cystitis is an inflammation of the bladder caused by bacteria often linked to colibacillosis. A symptom of this is a frequent need to urinate with painful passing of water. You will be very surprised to note the rapidity of the relief obtained using the stimulation of the points given here! Choose either this sequence or one of the sequences on the next page, according to your intuition, and repeat it until this annoying problem disappears. Drink plenty of warm lemon water and treat yourself for an intestinal infection. The use of clay and magnesium can also help.

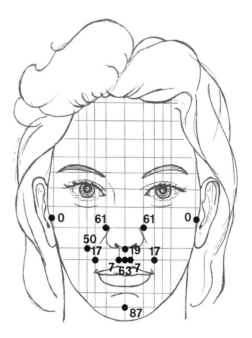

## Alternative Sequence (Cystitis)

**61, 63, 7, 113, 127, 51, 87, 73, 0**

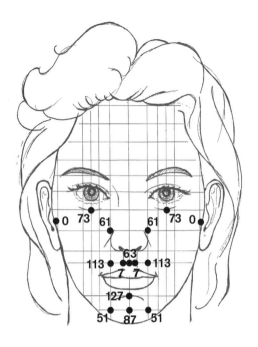

## Cystitis
### (simplified for emergencies)

**22, 17, 156, 0**

It is possible to add reflex zones corresponding to the bladder and intestines. Stimulate using broad sweeping movements around the chin and the upper part of the forehead.

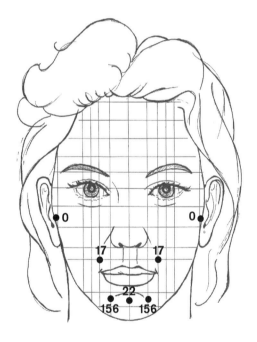

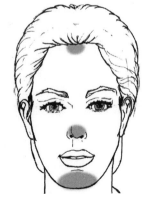
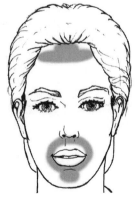

## Deafness

### 14, 15, 16, 45, 65, 74, 0

All of these points often allow total or partial hearing to be recovered, as long as the problem is not too entrenched or the lesion irreversible. Whatever the case you risk nothing by trying! Very often your efforts will be compensated for by a happy result! Try this session for a while. If you are not satisfied with the results, try the session below to see if it will be more effective. Or start with the second session, if you prefer, and move to this one if you are not satisfied.

Add these few reflex zones corresponding to the ears.

## Deafness, Hearing Difficulties

### 65, 3, 45, 300, 14, 15, 16, 0

Try these points whatever the degree of your hearing troubles. Results are rapid on a recent and moderate hearing loss. If your problem is an old one, do not expect a miracle but some improvement is usually experienced.

Treat these reflex zones as well.

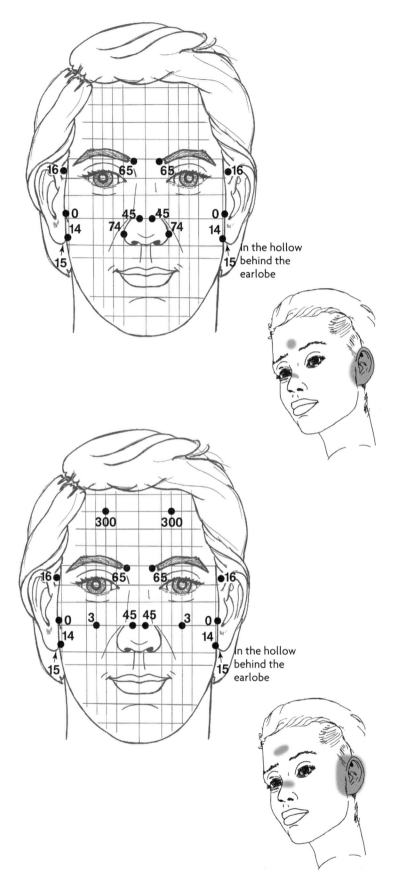

In the hollow behind the earlobe

In the hollow behind the earlobe

## Decalcification, Demineralization
### 85, 87, 43, 45, 20, 300, 0

These points facilitate the use of calcium and help fight against osteoporosis, which is a kind of decalcification common in postmenopausal women. Point **20** corresponds to the parathyroid glands, which are small endocrine glands located on either side of the thyroid gland that play a vital role in the metabolism of calcium. These points can help sustain growth in a child, especially during the growth spurt of puberty, and also assist the body in repairing a fracture!

In case of decalcification of the hip, add point **64** to the above sequence.

In addition, stimulate the reflex zones corresponding to the skeleton as a whole (as shown in **Diagram 2** in chapter 2), as well as the thyroid and parathyroid gland zones.

## Depression, Nervous
### 34, 124, 22, 127, 50, 1, 19, 103, 0

Nervous depression has become a common sickness, above all in women who are twice as likely to suffer from it as men. Sadness, discouragement, insomnia, chronic tiredness, headaches, incapacity to make decisions, problems with concentration, and negative views on everything mainly characterize this affliction, which spoils the lives of those who suffer from it, together with their friends and family.

Very often the cause is not psychological but physiological. The hormone system plays a part in this sickness, together with hypoglycemia or low blood sugar. Certain nutritional deficiencies are involved as well, such as tryptophan, vitamin B6, and folic acid. Stimulation of the points corresponding to these troubles allows the subject to fight against this serious and painful sickness.

## Detoxification, Drainage

**26, 3, 85, 87, 0**

**Or**

**7, 19, 26, 38, 50, 61, 85, 124, 87, 0**

Good health depends on maintaining a body free from excess toxins or toxic substances. Detoxification and drainage is the basis of all natural treatment and plain common sense. Awareness of this is important, since modern life obliges us to live in polluted environments, ingesting liquids and foods that contain all kinds of doubtful substances that can accumulate and become toxic over the years. There is also the danger of overworking the liver and kidneys by overeating or drinking, made worse by insufficient physical activity. This is why it is important to help the body to liberate these poisons.

You can stimulate these points and zones to give yourself a detoxification cure several days per month.

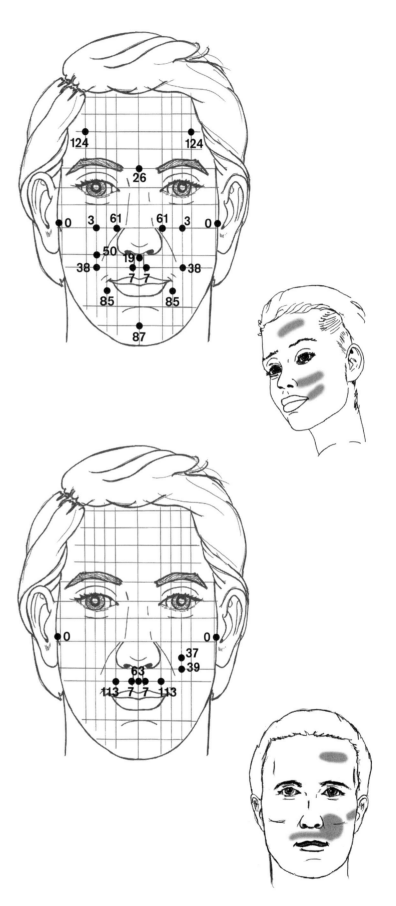

## Diabetes

**7, 63, 113, 37, 39, 0**

Diabetes comes from a disorder of the metabolism of carbohydrates. Insulin, which is a hormone secreted by the pancreas, is no longer sufficient to regulate the level of glucose in the blood. In serious cases of this sickness, insulin injections are necessary. The number of people suffering from diabetes as well as allied complications is growing constantly. Age and weight are important factors.

The points and zones given here stimulate and regulate the pancreatic function. In fact all of the points located on the upper lip have a regulatory effect on the pancreas. Regular stimulation of these points will help if you have a tendency to low blood sugar or diabetes. It is also a good idea to improvise a short Dien' Cham' session whenever you eat rich foods or drink too much alcohol!

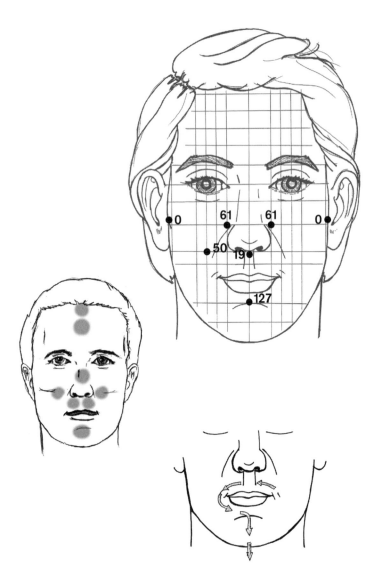

## Diarrhea
### 50, 127, 19, 61, 0

### (see also Colitis)

Bouts of diarrhea can be the sign of a poor intestinal function caused by colitis or the consequence of a chill. Sometimes it can also mean there is a more serious sickness if there is loss of mineral elements due to an infection like dysentery, amoebiasis, cholera, or simply gastroenteritis. There are two methods for treating diarrhea, in addition to the appropriate treatment for the case of infectious sickness.

The first consists in stimulating the points and zones shown here.

The second is illustrated in the second diagram and consists of a simple massage around the mouth. Be careful of the direction, as the opposite one cures constipation! With the thumb of the right hand steadying under the chin, two fingers—the index and middle fingers—move round the mouth from left to right pressing quite strongly, until they reach the reflex point for the anus, point **365**, at the center of the chin base, where you perform a brisk downward "evacuating" movement. Repeat this about fifty times.

This simple massage can come in very useful in case of a pressing need at a delicate moment or difficult place!

## Digestive Troubles
### (see Indigestion, Gastritis, Flatulence)

## Diuresis (facilitating)

### 26, 3, 85, 87, 0

These points promote the elimination of urine and tone up the kidney function. Use them in cases of water retention, whatever the cause, and kidney fatigue. After an infectious sickness, especially if it has necessitated the taking of drugs such as antibiotics, it is recommended to drink as much as possible and stimulate the kidney function to clear the body of toxins.

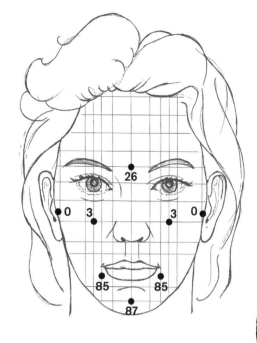

## Drug-induced Shock

### 19, 127, 0

These two points in particular can save someone's life in case of shock, whatever its cause, such as: ingestion of medicines that the body is reacting against, an allergic shock caused by local anesthetic or any other substance which is toxic for the body, various drugs, alcohol, household chemicals, and so on. This should in no way obviate the need to call a physician as quickly as possible. *Start by calling the emergency services,* and stimulate the pressure points while you are waiting.

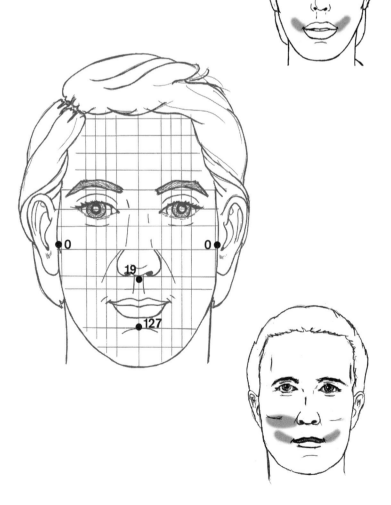

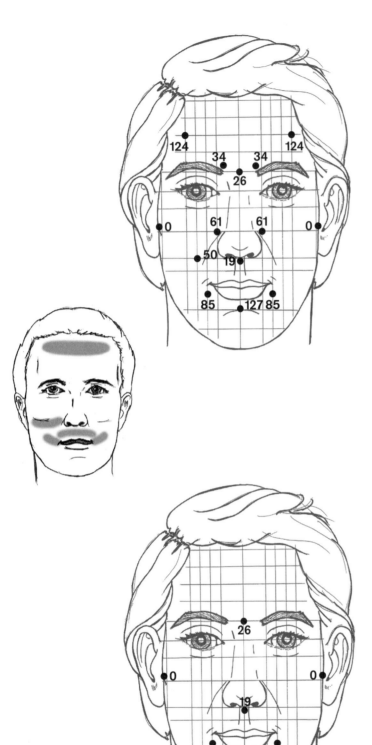

## Drug Problems
### 34, 26, 19, 50, 61, 85, 124, 127, 0

It is obviously impossible to treat this difficult problem simply by using Dien' Cham'. However it is possible to use it as an effective aid during the period of detoxification to accelerate body drainage, boost vital energy, and curb withdrawal symptoms. For this it is necessary for the patient to massage his or her face several times per day, as soon as the painful syndrome starts up. Points **61, 124,** and **127** attenuate withdrawal symptoms more specifically. Point **19** promotes the elimination of toxic substances. It is of course possible and recommended to treat the whole system by using the basic pressure points and points promoting drainage (see Drainage).

It is obviously better to associate this program with stimulation of the body's drainage zones, particularly those corresponding to the liver, gallbladder, kidneys, and intestines.

## Drunkenness
### 19, 26, 85, 0

### (see also Alcohol and Detoxification)

These points rapidly dissipate any effects brought on by the consumption of alcohol. To obtain an even better result, it is advisable to first apply an ice cube to these points for a few seconds. Then keep stimulating until the feeling of drunkenness dissipates.

## Dysmenorrhea
### (see Periods, Painful)

# Dyspnea

## 26, 19, 3, 38, 87, 0

These points rapidly relieve the trying feeling of not being able to breathe or suffocation that is generally linked to asthma, bronchial asthma, or tobacco smoking. It can also occur during a bout of spasms or during pectoral angina. Practice the stimulation for at least five minutes or more if necessary, remembering to treat the root of this acutely disturbing problem.

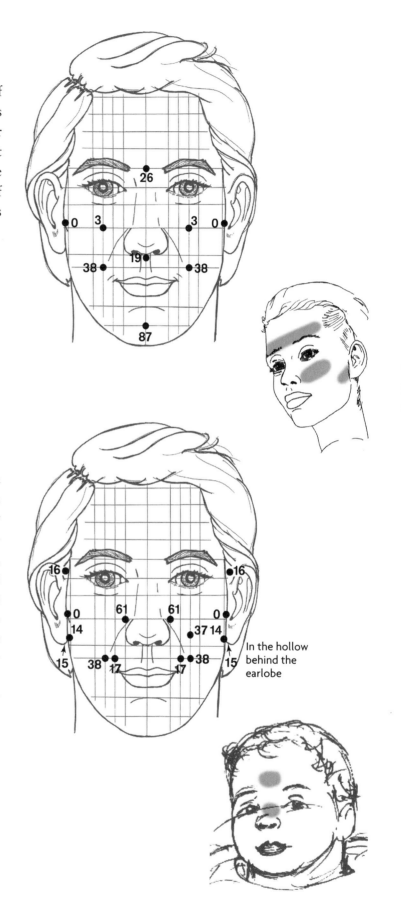

# Earache

## 17, 38, 37, 61, 14, 15, 16, 0

Children are often affected by a painful infection of the ear. Stimulation of these points will bring a rapid end to pain and inflammation. A mud or clay poultice or cataplasm, as well as taking magnesium chloride,[4] will rapidly remove the infection, as long as the treatment is undertaken as soon as possible. If in doubt, refer to your physician right away. It should be noted that the ingestion of too many dairy products and sweet foods is often the cause of repeated earaches. Make sure that your child is eating healthily.

You may also try these few reflex zones, away from the sensitive areas and therefore less painful.

# Ears

## (see Ears, Buzzing in; Earache; and Deafness)

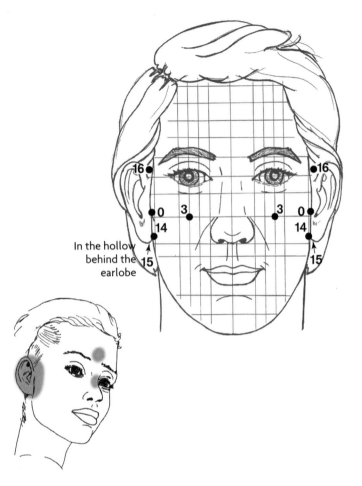

In the hollow behind the earlobe

## Ears, Buzzing in; Tinnitus
### 3, 14, 15, 16, 0

Disagreeable buzzing or whistling in the ears, sometimes reaching 70 to 80 decibels, can really spoil the lives of those who suffer from it, both at night and during the day. There are several possible causes and this should be determined before trying to treat the problem. A simple blockage due to wax can cause tinnitus and this can be removed quite simply. Other frequent causes include irritation of the auditory nerve, high blood pressure, in which case the noise is a whistling, arteriosclerosis, kidney or liver trouble, contraction of the cervical vertebral nerves, and so on. These few points will attenuate the problem and in certain cases stop it completely.

Please remember the rule that says that points and reflex zones are primarily active on the areas and organs close by. All of the area surrounding the ears is therefore considered a zone of proximity independently of the other possible therapeutic uses. Stimulate this region as soon as the buzzing is heard.

# Eczema
## 61, 50, 41, 7, 17, 87, 3, 60, 0

You can choose this sequence or one of the two alternates shown below. Experiment to find out which of them works the best in your case. You can also use them on alternate days. In acute periods do not hesitate to improvise a session several times per day until the situation improves. If at all possible avoid the application of various creams that are given to soothe itching. They generally only mask the problem and can ultimately provoke asthma.

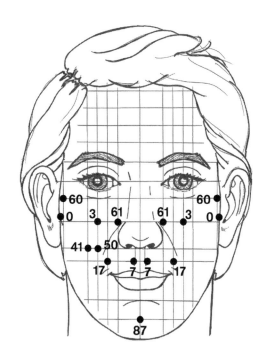

## Alternative Sequence
### 61, 37, 39, 63, 50, 41, 51, 0

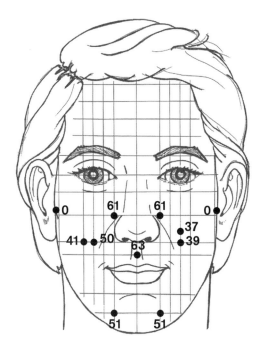

## Alternative Sequence
### 61, 41, 50, 124, 26, 0

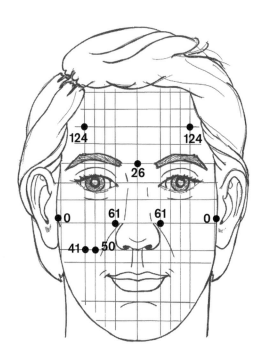

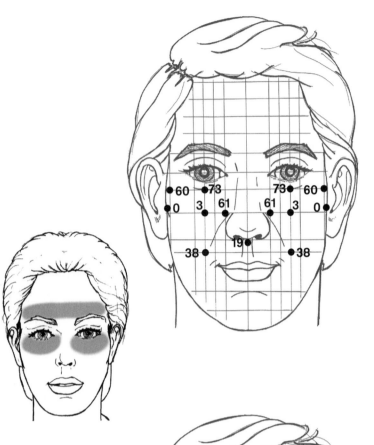

## Emphysema, Breathing Impairment
**19, 60, 3, 38, 73, 61, 0**

This pulmonary condition is characterized by a cough and a tiring inability to breathe, or oppression, accompanied by whistling noises. This sickness often starts with chronic bronchitis and the cause is usually tobacco smoking or atmospheric pollution. These points should be stimulated daily and every time that the need is felt.

Also stimulate these reflex zones when necessary, with the knuckle of a finger if you have nothing else handy.

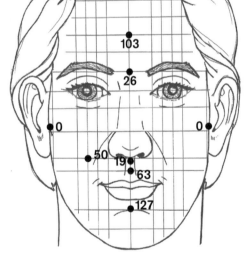

## Epilepsy
**19, 26, 50, 63, 103, 127, 0**

These points should be stimulated every day. The epileptic fits will become less frequent and decrease in intensity. It is essential to continue the prescribed medical treatment at the same time.

## Epileptic Fit
### 19, 127, 0

Start by pressing strongly on point **19**. If this does not work do the same on points **127** and **0**. Vigorously rub the ears of the patient.

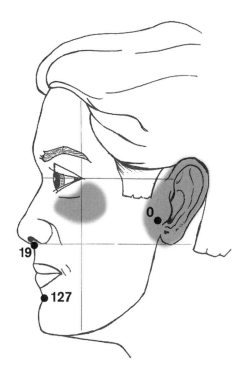

## Exhaustion, Nervous
### 19, 126, 103, 124, 106, 34, 1, 50, 127, 22, 0

This kind of tiredness is one of the characteristics of our way of life, where "better" always means "faster." A hectic lifestyle is often associated with a lack of peaceful exercise like golf, walking, or any other open-air sport, and it is the origin of troubles like pent-up nervous tension. It can be noted here that running from the office to the gym, and then running back home to perform a hundred and one domestic tasks, is not a way of dissipating nervous tension either. It is often better to take a short walk in the park or any other activity that helps you to really relax. Do not become hooked on hyperactivity, love yourself, and stimulate the following pressure points!

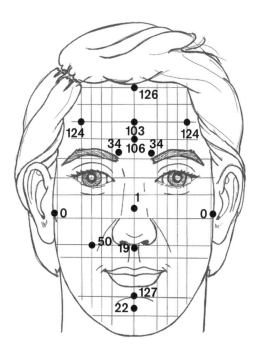

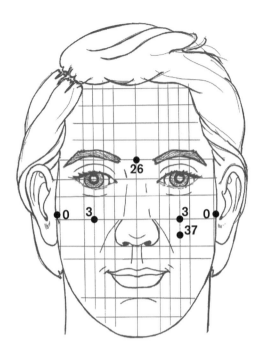

## Expectoration
### (clearing upper respiratory tract)
### 37, 3, 26, 0

### (for opposite effect see Secretions, decreasing)

Several kinds of breathing troubles are helped by expectorating, which is to say, eliminating excess mucus. This is the case with various types of bronchitis with dry coughing, asthma, tobacco smoking, and so on.

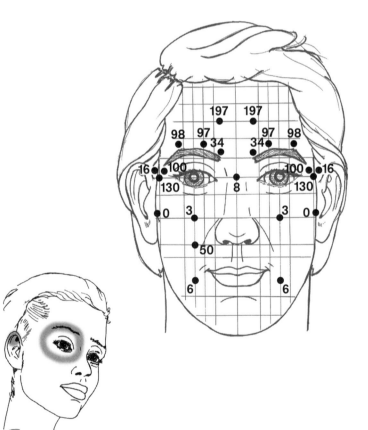

## Eyesight Troubles
### 3, 6, 8, 16, 34, 50, 97, 98, 130, 0

### Ocular Pain
### 130, 100, 0

To improve your eyesight stimulate these points and determine which ones suit you the best. They are generally the ones that are most sensitive. Work out your own program and try to be regular in your practice.

There is another method that can be used as an alternative or as a complement to the sequence described above: stimulate the area around the eye, on the edge of the orbit, as is shown on the figure here. These points will help you to treat a number of vision problems, whether you are shortsighted, or suffering from astigmatism or farsightedness. The more you stimulate them the quicker you will obtain a lasting result. It should be remarked, however, that an improvement is often felt during the first session.

**As well as**
**60, 177, 185, 191, 195, 197, 0**

Also shown are the eye reflex zones.

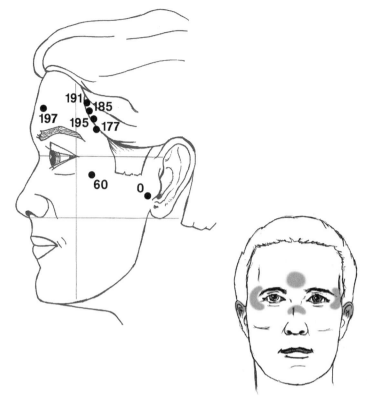

# Eye Tiredness or Fatigue
## 73, 3, 34, 103, 130, 0

It sometimes happens that after a lengthy period of concentration, particularly on a computer screen, one feels a dull pain behind the eyes, occasionally even a burning feeling when they are closed, together with the inability to concentrate properly and a dose of irritability. This phenomenon is called asthenopia. It should not be confused with conjunctivitis or a sequel to a shock involving the eye. In fact the origin is lack of sleep, overwork, and sometimes also bad lighting on the worktable or desk. In can be noted here that it is a problem typical of those who have to keep their eyes on their screens many hours every day. (I have had enough experience of this to tell of the extraordinary power of these few points, which I massage as soon as tiredness starts to impede my sight, and when a headache is on the horizon!)

You can also massage these reflex zones with a knuckle of a finger, when you do not have the time to do something more precise.

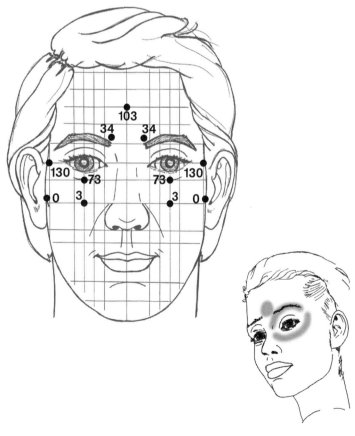

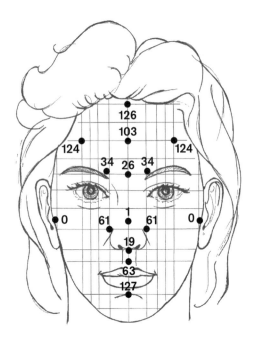

# Fainting
**19, 26, 63**

**Followed by points for Relaxation**
**124, 34, 26 and**
**Toning Up**
**127, 19, 103, 126**
**Or**
**19, 127, 61, 1, 124, 103, 34, 0**

It is always useful to know what to do if someone faints in your presence. There are a few sequences usable in these cases. If you are not sure of the exact points to use, at least be able to perform the Basic Session in addition to point **19**, the reanimation point.

## Simplified procedure

If you are unable to memorize all these points, this short sequence will come in very handy: **19, 127, 0.** Strongly press on point **19** until the person regains consciousness. If the faintness continues stimulate points **127** and **0**. Rub the ears vigorously.

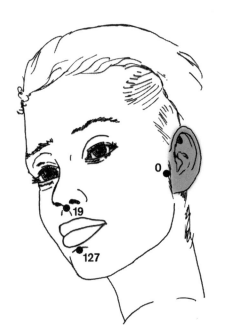

# Fatigue, Chronic or General
50, 127, 19, 26, 103, 0

**Or**

1, 6, 17, 22, 43, 60, 124, 106, 0

Tiredness, which can become chronic exhaustion, is the price we often pay for lives lived at a hundred miles an hour, even during the holidays. Overwork, poor dietary habits, lack of sleep, worry, or an exceptional physical effort can all provoke tiredness or exhaustion of energy. It is the same for the aftereffects of infectious sicknesses, as well as for those people suffering from fibromyalgia or spasmophilia, which is a complaint usually linked to a lack of either calcium or magnesium. All of the above can cause the body to become prematurely worn out. In such a case, correct, healthy conditions must be restored if the person wants to ward off more serious problems in the future! These points will allow you to boost your energy and tone up your body instantly.

Remember to perform the Basic Session several times per day. This will often be sufficient to restart body processes and cancel mental tiredness in just thirty seconds or so.

A short session of tapping the forehead can also work wonders, as well as massaging the ears.

# Fever, High Temperature
26, 3, 8, 38, 85, 60, 87, 180, 14, 16, 15, 0

All of these points act in the case of fever and you should not hesitate to use them. Choose those points that seem to work the best by testing their sensitivity, and taking account of their main indications. Of course this does not mean that you should not treat the condition at the origin of the high temperature, but this massage will provide relief and help the immune system to react effectively.

Also thoroughly massage the ears.

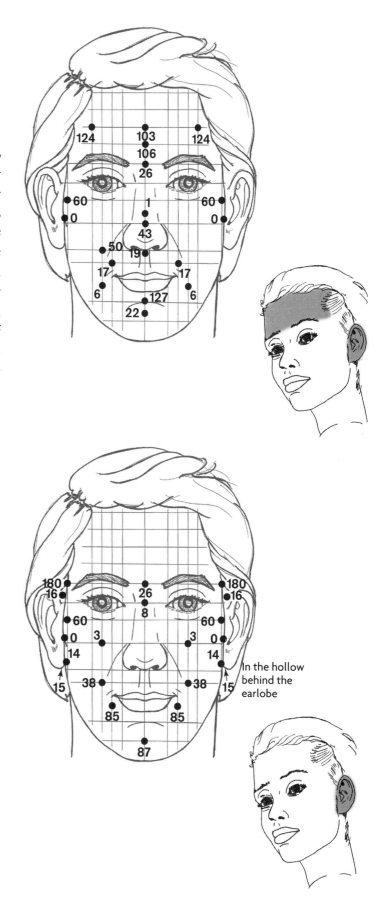

In the hollow behind the earlobe

# Fibromyalgia
## (see Spasmophilia)

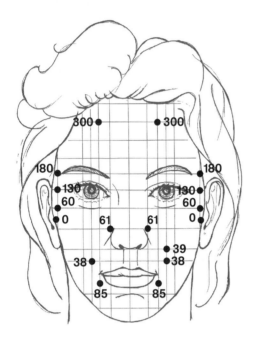

# Fingers
## (abscesses, whitlows, various other problems)
## 38, 39, 60, 61, 85, 130, 180, 300, 0

There are many correspondence points for the fingers. Do not hesitate to use them in case of a lesion whatever the cause: fracture, sprain, burn, cut, abscess, or whitlow, and so on. The energy released locally will facilitate healing and self-regeneration.

Here are the points more particularly related to each finger:

- thumb                61
- index finger         185
- middle finger        195
- ring finger          177
- little finger        191

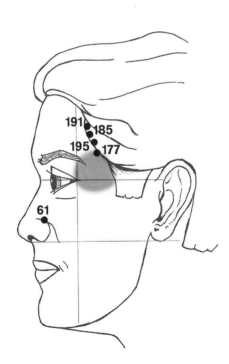

## Flatulence, Intestinal Gas
### 41, 50, 38, 127, 37, 0

Troubles linked to gas in the digestive system, whether in the stomach or in the intestines, are treated by using the same points. For a long time it was thought that flatulence was linked to excess swelling of a pocket of air located inside the stomach. This is not the case. Air cannot enter the stomach as it is rejected as soon as it reaches the lower part of the esophagus. Distension or flatulence are linked to nervous system factors and can also indicate the presence of a serious digestive disorder, such as gastritis, stomach or duodenal ulcers, hiatal hernia, gallstones, and sometimes intestinal colitis or worms.

Following surgery it is often difficult to evacuate intestinal gases. For this there is a simple remedy: the stimulation of points **38** and **19** from one to several minutes, until a result is forthcoming.

## Frigidity
### 7, 1, 19, 45, 63, 156, 87, 43, 287, 124, 34, 60, 0

There are multiple causes for this condition and several ways of treating it. It can just as well be caused by a hormonal problem as by the behavior of the partner! The psychology of the sufferer is often responsible and it is here that the solution lies. However if in general all seems well, stimulation of these points will be an effective measure.

You can also refer to the massage for the mouth zone indicated under Contraception.

The zones situated on the chin and the upper lip can also help. Stimulate them for several minutes before sexual intercourse.

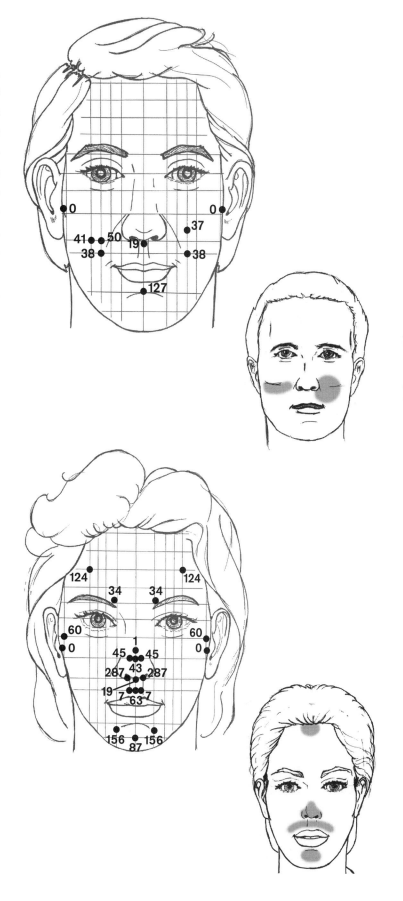

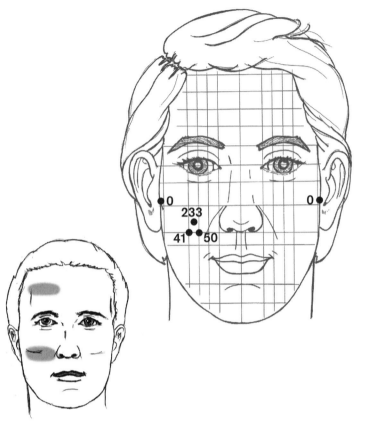

## Gallbladder
### 41, 50, 233, 0

**(see also Gallstones)**

This small organ is located below the ribcage, behind the liver, and its function is to secrete bile. The stimulation of these pressure points several times per day will have the effect of eliminating stones and biliary mud, which are the cause of pain. The effect of this massage will be to stimulate a lazy gallbladder, which is often the cause of insomnia between 1 and 3 AM. Of course this does not replace a change in your food intake. You would be further well advised to supplement your diet with a few spoonfuls of top quality olive oil taken regularly in the morning before breakfast, until the troubles disappear.

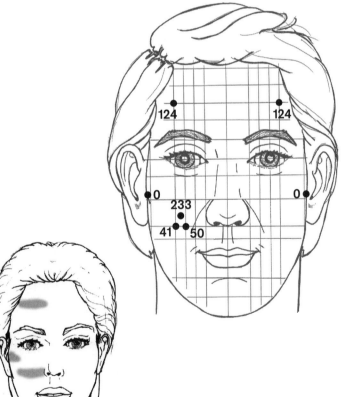

## Gallstones (Bile Lithiasis)
### 41, 50, 233, 124, 0

Of course it is possible to prevent the formation of these by changing to a diet that is low in animal fats and sugars, thereby avoiding gallbladder pain. However, when they are present, it is best to intervene as rapidly as possible to avoid surgery. In association with the absolutely vital changes in dietary habits and amount of physical exercise, stimulation of these reflex points and zones most often provokes evacuation of biliary mud and small stones together with relieving the pain and discomfort caused by the nausea, hot flashes, and so on. Larger gallstones will also often dissolve too, but if not it is vital to consult your physician. Every morning take several tablespoonfuls of high quality olive oil, followed by a cup of a beverage such as herbal tea, lemon in water, or something similar. Eat soy lecithin but, above all, take up a diet with less animal fat.

# Gastritis
**39, 37, 50, 61, 45, 63, 19, 127, 0**

**(see also Ulcer, Gastric)**

Gastritis is an inflammation of the stomach, generally resulting from overeating or the consumption of inappropriate foods, which irritate the stomach. This benign or minor problem is evidenced by heartburn or stomach acid flowing back into the esophagus. Excess acid can be soothed during eating, which can lead to overstepping the mark and eventually making the problem worse. Try to be reasonable and regulate your food intake. Stimulate these points before and after each meal. You will find digestion easier and see that your state of health is improving rapidly.

Choose the zones that are the most responsive from the ones given, and remember to practice your Basic Session regularly, as well as the points for relaxation. Your stomach will thank you for it!

Did you know that raw potato juice and cabbage juice—from a good supplier of organic foods of course—magically heal gastric and duodenal ulcers? A half a glass of either of these should be drunk before every meal.

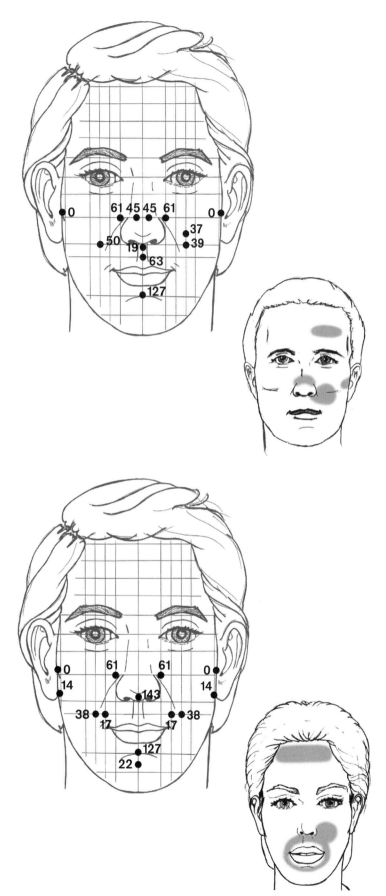

# Gastroenteritis
**14, 17, 22, 38, 61, 143, 127, 0**

This tiresome condition is generally caused by an amoebic infection or colibacillosis. It is usually contracted during vacations spent in tropical or subtropical climates but nowadays more cases are being reported in temperate zones. The main source of infections of this kind is food and drink. Water from piped domestic supplies and fruit and vegetables washed in unclean water are often sources! The main symptoms are diarrhea, vomiting, together with a high temperature. The points given here will help you to treat them . . .

. . . and these few reflex zones will too!

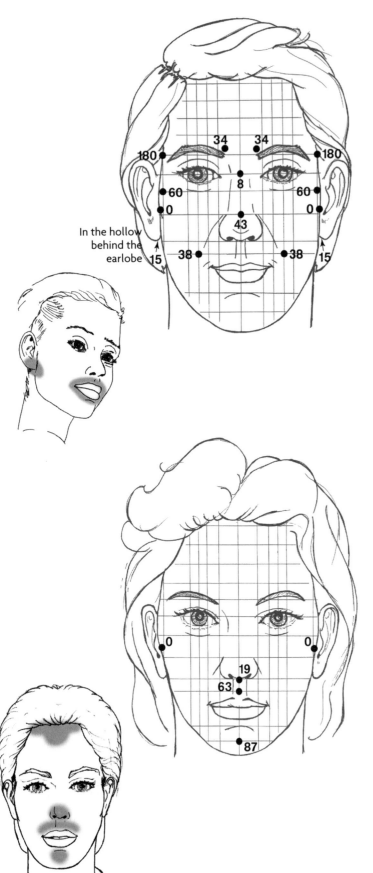

## Gingivitis
**8, 15, 38, 43, 34, 60, 180, 0**

Are your gums so fragile that they bleed when you start brushing your teeth or when you bite into an apple? You are probably suffering from gingivitis. Stimulate these points and use a soft-bristled toothbrush after meals. Great benefit can also be derived from performing a mouthwash every morning for ten minutes or so with top quality olive or peanut oil.

Please remember the basic rule to first massage the adjacent areas where possible. Also stimulate around the mouth as shown!

## Giving Birth
**19, 63, 87, 0**

Stimulation of these points and zones at the beginning of the delivery favors contractions. It should also be performed just after the birth. Stimulation of point 0 provokes contraction of the womb, which decreases the risk of bleeding or hemorrhage.

> **Warning:**
> Never stimulate these points during the pregnancy as there is a risk of causing premature delivery.

As soon as the delivery is under way, stimulate the nostrils and the region around the lips as is described under Contraception. This technique relaxes the pelvis and soothes pain.

In addition the whole of the chin should be massaged, and along the hairline.

# Glands, Swollen

## 37, 50, 0

These points allow drainage of the lymphatic glands and elimination of toxic substances released, the accumulation of which is responsible for the appearance of the well-known swelling below the ears, around the neck. Stimulation of these points should last several minutes.

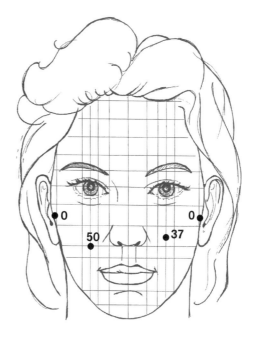

# Goiter, Basedow's Disease

## 7, 8, 14, 100, 106, 0

Goiter can be caused by an overactive or deficient thyroid function. You will need to check which is the case by referring to your physician. These points will contribute toward regulating your thyroid function and can be stimulated whichever your problem.

You can also massage the neck reflex zones, which cover the thyroid zones.

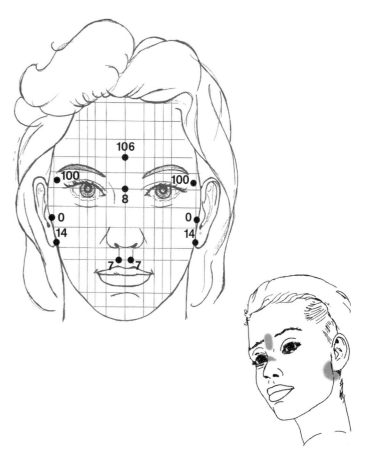

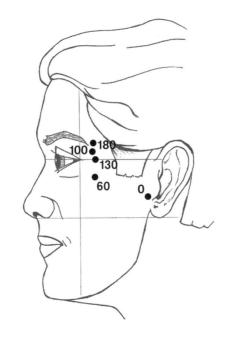

## Hands

### 60, 130, 100, 180, 0

Whatever the problem with your hand—sprain, fracture, wound of whatever kind, burn, and so on—the repeated stimulation of these points will bring relief, and promote healing and a return to normal.

Also stimulate the various reflex zones corresponding to the hands, concentrating mainly on areas where pain is felt.

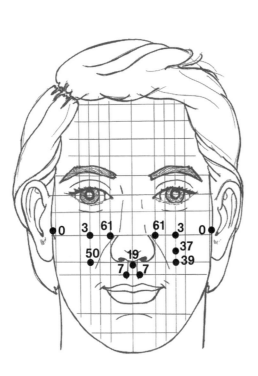

## Hay Fever

### 50, 19, 7, 3, 61, 37, 39, 0

The kind of spasmodic coryza that is usually called hay fever is a kind of allergy. Sometimes it lasts for a considerable time, at least until the pollens responsible for the problem disappear. It spoils the springtime for those who suffer from it and sometimes also a good part of the summer! The tedious symptoms include uncontrollable and continuous sneezing, runny nose, and watery eyes, but hay fever can also worsen leading to acute sinusitis or even asthma! It is often necessary to repeat the stimulation proposed daily, and according to the prevailing weather conditions.

Also perform the nose and forehead massage given for a cold. It brings rapid relief.

# Headaches
## 61, 26, 106, 34, 124, 0

Who has never had a headache at one time or another? On the other hand it is difficult to precisely determine their causes, as there are at least 140 explanations or reasons for them. However, it is easy to relieve headaches by stimulating these few points in the order given. Here Dien' Cham' advantageously replaces aspirin! In general headaches are related to tension. The muscular contraction created by the state of tension provokes spasms in the blood vessels irrigating the muscles. Energy circulation is reduced and the subject experiences a minor discomfort in that region of the brain. The tension can be caused by a busy lifestyle, noise, anxiety, stress, linked to overwork or a sustained effort. Using reflexology, immediate relief is obtained!

Headaches are often linked to poor liver function (see Headaches, Digestive Origin). Always remember to incorporate stimulation of the zones related to the liver and gallbladder into your session.

# Headaches, Crown of the Head
## 50, 51, 87, 61, 103, 0

This is another of those varieties of headache that is such a handicap! Always start with the general pressure points for headaches. If that is not enough to clear the pain completely, try these points, which may be more directly linked to your problem. The result in this case should be almost immediate!

The earlier that you practice this short session the better, more spectacular, and longer lasting will be the result. If at all possible the stimulation should take place at the very beginning. Do not get discouraged, however, if your particular problem is old. One of the specialties of Dien' Cham' is to soothe certain pains in just a few seconds, even when the pain has an origin in the distant past and has proved difficult to dislodge!

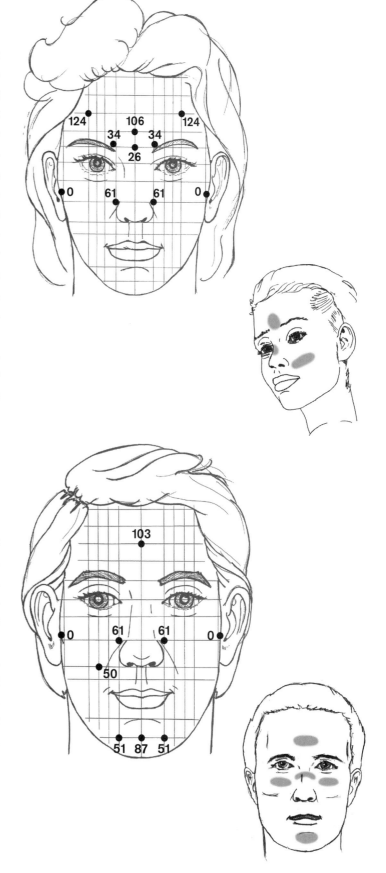

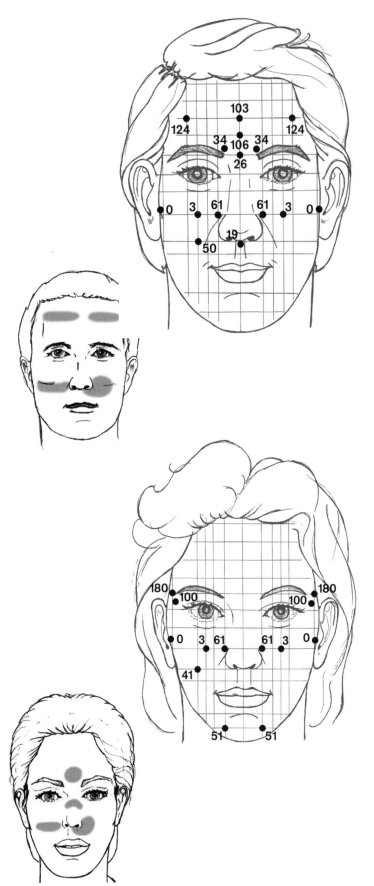

## Headaches, Digestive Origin
### 50, 19, 3, 61, 26, 106, 103, 34, 124, 0

As we have already mentioned, headaches can have many causes. Among these we can identify the common but seldom recognized phenomena of indigestion, caused by overeating, as well as being linked to poor liver function. These points should be stimulated as soon as the first symptoms appear to procure immediate relief. If the problem is a chronic one, get into the habit of performing this massage as a preventive measure after meals for a few days. Use the same simple routine in case of the occasional party dinner. Then you will feel quickly better and avoid spending the rest of the day or evening in pain!

Very often, there is a tendency to quickly put the blame on the stomach, when commonsense would tell you that it is caused by over consumption of alcohol! Some people feel the effect following ingestion of a tiny quantity of alcohol, whereas others who think that they can stand alcohol much better, sometimes pay for their excesses with a terrible headache.

## Headaches, One Side of the Head
### 41, 51, 61, 3, 100, 180, 0

Another variety of the many kinds of headaches! You can stimulate the points mentioned above concerning headaches in general. If that seems insufficient, add the points given here. Never hesitate to renew the stimulation as often as you think necessary. Headaches always give in to this kind of massage but sometimes return during the day. If you repeat this program of stimulation as soon as you feel the first pain, the headache will disappear in just a few seconds. It may come back attenuated, but finally it will stop.

Also stimulate zones corresponding to the head, at the center of the forehead, on the nose, and so on, and concentrate on those on the side of the headache.

In addition:

- if you have pain on the right side, stimulate liver and gallbladder zones
- if you are experiencing pain on the left, stimulate the stomach and pancreas zones

## Headaches, Temple
### 41, 61, 180, 3, 0

Pains, which can sometimes be acute, are felt at the temples. This symptom is often linked to gallbladder dysfunction. In the treatment of headaches that can be quite tricky to soothe, it is of major importance to know how to choose the pressure points, as a function of the probable origin of the trouble in the person suffering. This is the only way you can obtain an excellent result. These examples are given to allow you to establish your own program of points to be stimulated which you can adapt using your own intuition and experience.

To the above, add the liver and gallbladder reflex zones, above all if you are suffering at the right temple! If the pain is on the left side, stimulate the zones corresponding to the pancreas and stomach.

## Head Injury
### 87, 103, 127, 26, 124, 34, 0

These points can soothe troubles following a blow to the head, even if the incident was a long time ago. They can help dissipate dizziness, headaches, and feelings of nausea. Even if your child only has a small bump, stimulate them as soon as possible!

Also massage the reflex zones corresponding to the head, concentrating your efforts on the side affected.

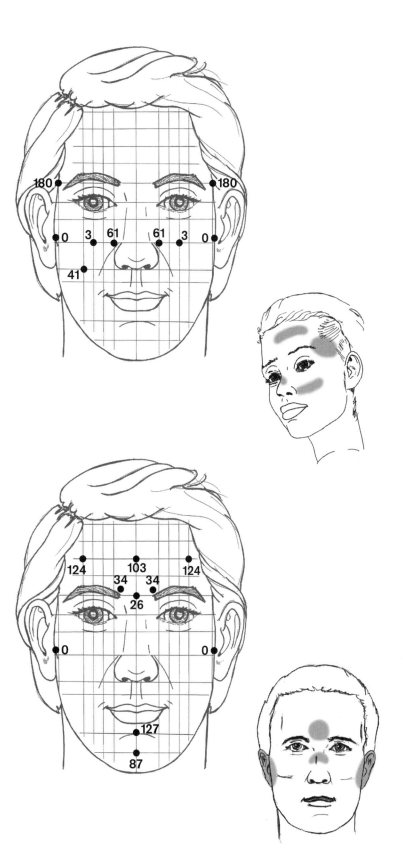

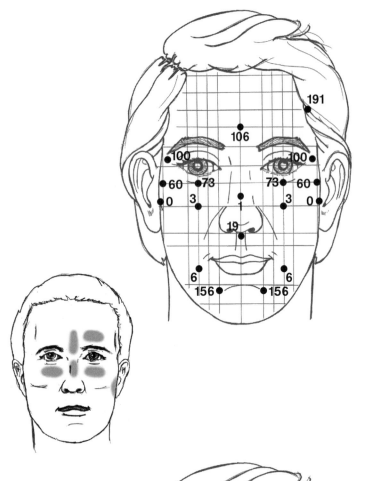

## Heart Insufficiency, Heart Failure

### 1, 3, 6, 19, 73, 100, 106, 156, 60, 191, 0

These points can be used in the case of pectoral angina, especially point **73**, as well as for all heart ailments. This is not a substitute for following the treatment prescribed by your physician, but you will undoubtedly experience some relief. Practice this stimulation several times per day if you feel the need.

Also stimulate the zones corresponding to the heart and the chest in general, as well as those to do with the spinal column, especially those dealing with the dorsal vertebrae.

## Heat Stroke

### 19, 26, 143, 85, 0

In a sensitive or fragile person, heatstroke can be caused by any of the following: falling asleep on the beach, even in the shade, working in the garden in the heat without taking the necessary precautions when you are tired, or spending hours in an automobile without air conditioning. Children can also fall victim to this. The points given act in urgent circumstances to cool the body down. Practice the stimulation for ten minutes or so. And to avoid this happening to yourself, remember to drink lots of lemon water during periods of great heat or take vitamin C. You can also spray yourself with cold water or rub your body down with a face cloth several times a day during the heat. The following session may be most appropriate if the heatstroke involves too much exposure to direct sunlight. You can decide which session is most appropriate by judging which points are most sensitive.

# Heat Stroke, Sunstroke
## 26, 103, 3, 85, 60, 87, 14, 15, 16, 0

Everyone knows that lengthy periods spent in full sunlight can have negative effects on the health. In spite of precautions however accidents can still happen. For example if you doze off lying on an airbed floating on the sea, rocked by the gentle movement of the waves, or perhaps heat stroke on a vacation caused by being blocked in an automobile in the sun during the hottest part of the summer! This is even more dangerous during long periods of very high temperatures. The risk of dehydration is further increased and someone's life can even be placed in danger. You must refresh yourself frequently, including the use of the points indicated here.

In the case of prolonged tiredness, a depression of natural defenses associated with dehydration is quite sufficient for this kind of problem to occur. Remember to drink plenty of water and do not try to eliminate salt from your diet. Children are particularly vulnerable to this kind of problem! The points should be stimulated for as long as necessary. Also apply cold compresses to the forehead, neck, and chest, and give plenty of water to drink.

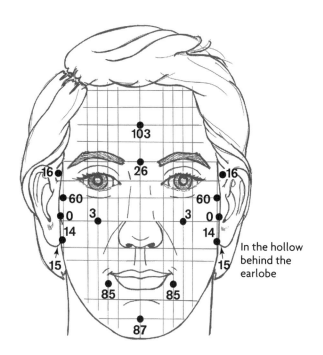

In the hollow behind the earlobe

# Hemorrhage, Bleeding
## (from the uterus or elsewhere)
## 16, 61, 17, 7, 50, 6, 37, 124, 34, 287, 0

All of these points tend to stop hemorrhage, except of course when it is caused by an accident: hemorrhage from the stomach, excess blood loss during periods, epistaxis or nosebleeds, bleeding from piles or from the gums, and so on. Points 0 and 287 in particular stop hemorrhage from the uterus (including that which occurs following childbirth), by provoking contraction of the uterus.

Remember to include stimulation of the reflex zones corresponding to the area affected by the hemorrhage: uterus, rectum, colon, and so on.

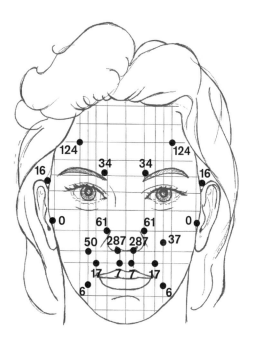

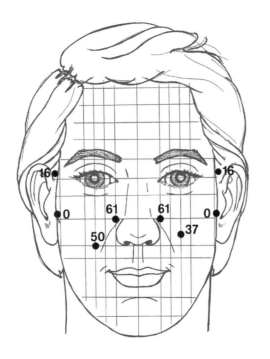

## Hemorrhage, Bleeding
### (from the stomach)
### 16, 37, 61, 50, 0

These points will stop bleeding from a gastric ulcer. Remember to treat the ulcer above all, but these points will avoid great loss of blood.

Stimulate reflex zones of the stomach too.

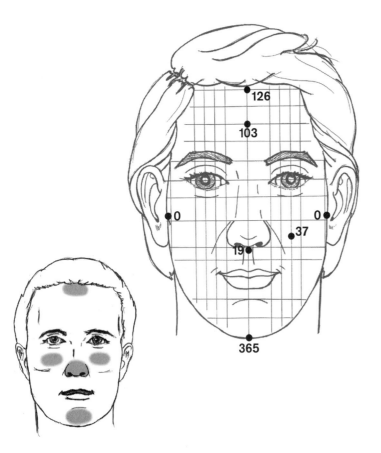

## Hemorrhoids or Piles
### 126, 19, 37, 365, 103, 0

These points will soothe pain due to the presence of hemorrhoids but will also help them to disappear by acting on the cause, which usually has to do with poor blood circulation and the liver. It should be noted that all of the points located on the line between points **126** and **365**, between the hairline and the base of the chin, have a beneficial effect on piles.

# Hepatitis, Viral

**17, 19, 38, 41, 61, 74, 50, 0**

An ever increasing number of people are affected by this disease. It is known that the majority of cases of hepatitis, types B and C, are contracted during blood transfusions. Type B can also be caught during sexual encounters, whereas type A (also called jaundice), which is more benign and the most common, comes from a dietary origin. Whatever the type of hepatitis you want to treat, stimulation of these points will be of great help. Certain plants (for example Desmodium and Chrysanthellum americanum), as well as high doses of vitamin C (4000 to 6000 U per day, if it has a natural source, sometimes more), will complete the treatment.

    Also stimulate the liver and kidneys reflex zones, as well as the points used for a general toning up as per the Basic Session.[5]

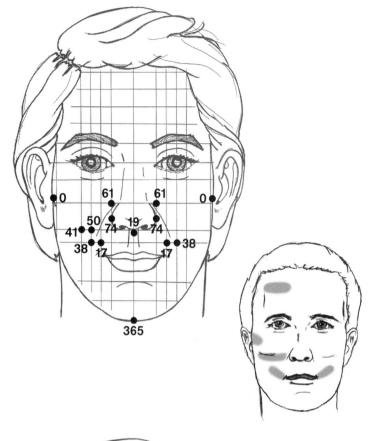

# Hernia, Hiatal

**61, 37, 39, 74, 0**

This minor problem is due to the upper part of the stomach passing through the hiatus, which is the orifice by which the esophagus reaches the stomach, followed by a shift upward into the thorax. This can provoke various symptoms, which can even make the sufferer think that he is soon going to have a heart attack! Very often just one Dien' Cham' session is enough to solve this problem.

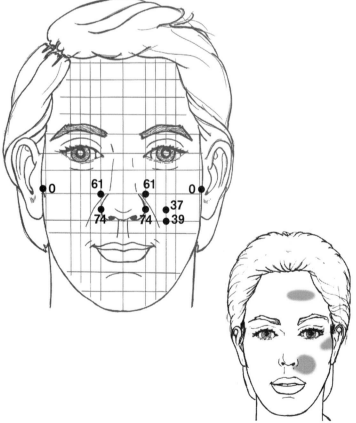

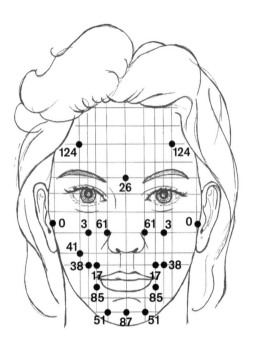

## Herpes
### 124, 61, 26, 3, 87, 51, 41, 17, 38, 85, 0

Here the subject is that cold sore or fever blister on or near the lip, which is common and tiresome! Herpes is caused by a virus caught by direct contact. It remains latent in the tissues most of the time and appears when the natural defenses are low, during a stressful period, overwork, or other sickness. Frequently stimulate points **61** and **124** and apply a little vitamin E locally.

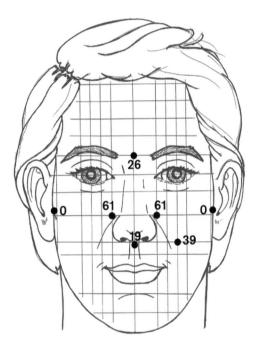

## Hiccups
### 19, 39, 61, 26, 0

Is there anyone who has never experienced this minor problem which can be tiresome, above all when one is in public? Sometimes there are cases where the bout can even last for several days, preventing the sufferer from eating, drinking, and sleeping. A bout of hiccups usually starts during a contraction while one is trying to eat or drink something. Something goes down the wrong hole or you laugh or speak while swallowing, which is of course something our grandmothers would reprimand! The problem can occur while the body is cooling down during a meal. This can cause a spasm of the diaphragm, which is called a hiccup. The best thing to do is to stimulate the points given as soon as possible, before the spasm and therefore the hiccup has time to take hold.

# High Blood Pressure
## 15, 61, 8, 26, 106, 3, 0

Most of the time high blood pressure is due to a diet which is too rich in animal protein, or the ingestion of excess alcohol, tobacco, or salt. The problem is often hereditary and, after the age of fifty, one out of ten people are affected. It provokes many symptoms such as headaches, above all in the occipital region, vertigo, insomnia, pounding of the heart, buzzing in the ears, dizziness, nocturnal oppression, chest pain, and constipation. Many disorders can follow: kidney complaints, thyroid problems, hormonal disorders, arteriosclerosis, nervous tension, and being overstressed. Point 8 is one that specifically treats high blood pressure. At the same time as the others, you can stimulate it each time you feel your blood pressure rise or your heartbeat accelerate.

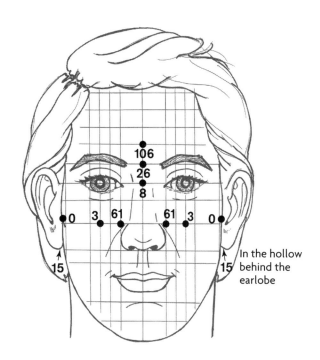

In the hollow behind the earlobe

# High Blood Pressure, Acute
## (simplified procedure)

When necessary, following stressful circumstances or any other cause, perform this simple massage which is easily memorized. (If you suffer from high blood pressure learn this straight away to be able to practice it easily, anywhere.) Using a roller or the tips of the fingers, rub the zones shown here pressing harder and harder. Do not worry about hurting yourself a little; these zones are sensitive precisely because of your problem. Rub your chin in the same way.

Finish the session by stimulating point **15**, until your blood pressure is normal. This can take five to ten minutes. This simple technique applied two or three times per day will allow you to obtain natural regulation of your blood pressure.

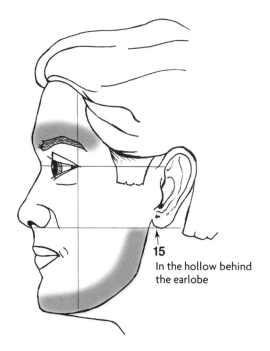

15
In the hollow behind the earlobe

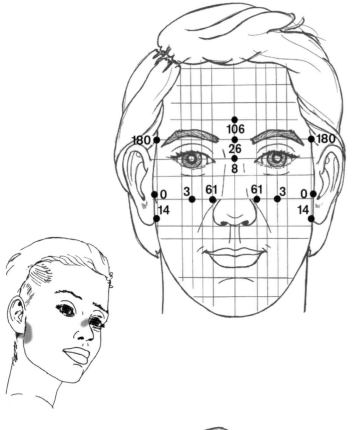

## Hoarseness
### 26, 3, 8, 61, 106, 180, 14, 0

There is little more annoying than becoming hoarse just before having to speak in public during a meeting or any other occasion. Teachers and lecturers know the problems that hoarseness can create in the classroom! Here is a simple method that gives good results with just a few minutes massage and can be repeated as often as necessary. Quite often, just one session is enough.

Even more simply, just massage these zones that correspond to the throat.

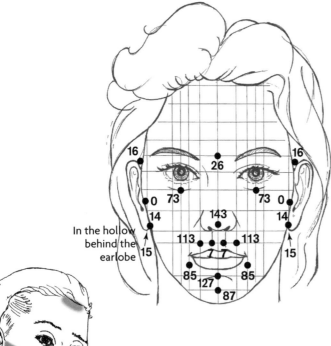

## Hot Flashes
### 7, 73, 85, 87, 127, 143, 0

### Or
### 7, 113, 26, 14, 15, 16, 0

This kind of disagreeable experience can follow menopause, total hysterectomy, or removal of the ovaries. Regular practice of Dien' Cham' will rapidly soothe this symptom. Make sure that you stimulate around the ears too. For this you can use your index fingers, which you use to rub all around the ears: in front, behind, at the base, and above. You should do this at any moment, as soon as a hot flash commences. Never forget to stimulate points relative to menopause every day!

You should also stimulate the hormone correspondence zones, which are in the center of the forehead at the hairline, at the end of the nose and nostrils, around the mouth and in particular the area between the base of the nose and the upper lip.

## Hyperactivity in Children
### 34, 8, 26, 106, 100, 124, 127, 61, 0

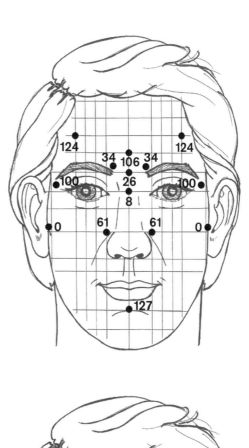

### (see also Anxiety, Child)

Stimulate these points in short sessions, twice per day if possible.

A hyperactive child is in permanent motion. This is mainly a problem in boys (90%) and constitutes a nightmare for the parents and teachers. The hyperactive child cannot stay still for more than a minute, is incapable of concentrating on a subject and, to complete the picture, manifests awkwardness and clumsiness. He is often aggressive, nothing seems to be able to stop him, and he listens to no one. In this way he becomes a very real danger to himself. Certain physicians accuse chemical food colorings and preservatives as well as salicylates. It is therefore advisable to correct the diet of the child in a radical way by avoiding all foods containing these substances. In any case a diet of healthy food, if possible organic, can only be beneficial to the whole family.

## Hypoglycemia, Abnormally Low Blood Sugar
### 7, 63, 113, 19, 0

Stimulate these points in case of faintness. This condition is not very well known and accounts for several varied symptoms, including hypersensitivity to noise, unexplained depressive states, crying fits, chronic tiredness, allergies, spasmophilia, difficulties concentrating, difficulties at school, irritability, and so on. The cause of the disorder is a lack of sugar in the blood (which is the opposite of diabetes). However do not jump to conclusions too rapidly and increase your sugar intake. In fact, refined sugar and carbohydrates are not advisable. Adopt a diet with plenty of natural non-refined products. Also take supplements containing zinc, chrome, and brewer's yeast.

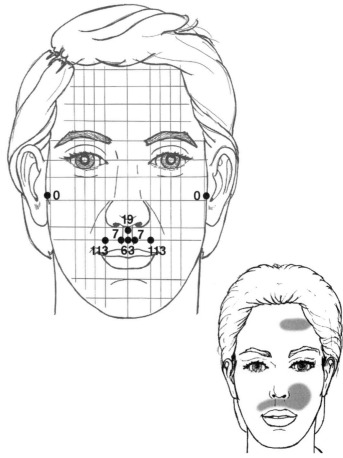

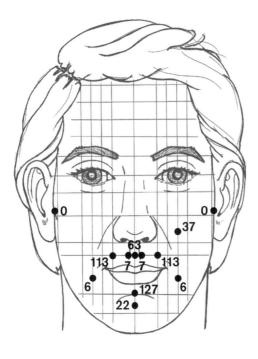

# Immune Deficiencies
**63, 7, 6, 22, 113, 127, 37, 0**

### As well as
**60, 61, 37, 50, 113, 127, 156, 17, 0**

Many people suffer from immune deficiencies, from the child who catches every passing ailment to the person suffering from cancer, an immunological disorder, or AIDS. In all of these cases regular and deep stimulation of these points will boost the body's effort to autoregulate. In the case of patients having undergone chemotherapy, it is advisable to stimulate the immune system at the beginning and at the end of every session. This will allow the treatment to have the best possible effect and, at the same time, preserve the natural defenses that are already diminished, as evidenced by the very presence of the sickness. It is essential to preserve the immune system because our health depends on this. Rather than go to war against countless so-called "enemies" of our body (which are often actually necessary to our survival), it is better to organize and back up our natural means of defense and autoregulation. Our body knows very well what is to be done and does it well as long as we assist it in its efforts and allow it to act beneficially!

These few points should be stimulated in case of tiredness, an epidemic of flu, for example, and in any other situation that is likely to interfere with our natural defenses such as overwork, stressful situations, and a generally poor state of health. In addition, vigorously rub above and below the mouth with your index and middle fingers.

Of course all of these points will usually be stimulated during the course of a single session. The two sequences given here are designed to allow memorization and thus be used in cases of urgency.

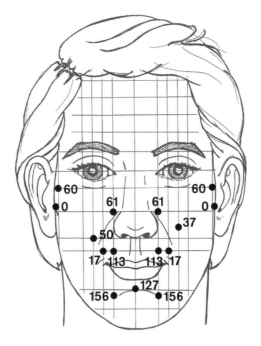

# Impotence

## 7, 1, 19, 45, 63, 156, 43, 0

Ever more men are suffering from this disorder of sexual function. The following diverse reasons are often given for this problem: stress, chronic tiredness, overwork, lack of self-confidence (the fear of not being up to expectations in today's society with its intense erotic climate), and hormonal problems, which some commentators think are linked to chemicals in foodstuffs. Regular practice of Dien' Cham' is usually sufficient to boost energy and solve this irritating problem. Remember that point 0 increases sexual energy and stimulates life energy. It also contributes to better sexual relations and avoids premature ejaculation.

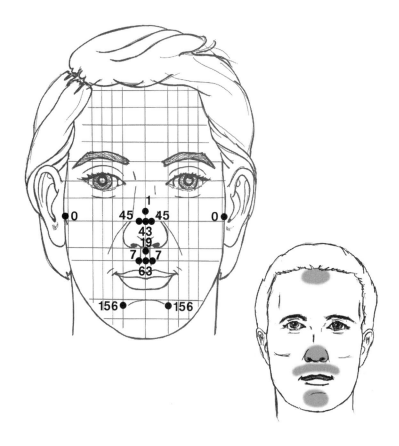

# Incontinence, Urinary

## 124, 34, 103, 37, 19, 1, 0

Whether the problem is due to aging, a serious sickness, a course of medical treatment, or a surgical operation, it can be progressively helped with reflexology. Of course the quicker you practice the stimulation, the better will be the result. It is not so easy to solve a case of years of incontinence, although it is quite possible to obtain an improvement.

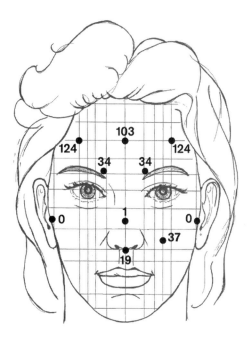

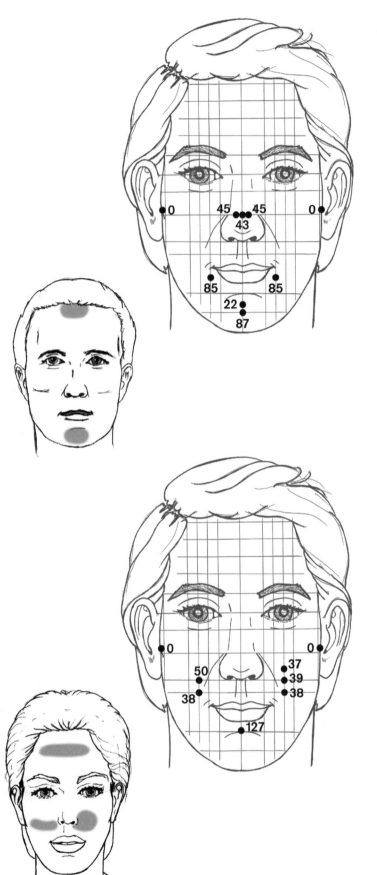

## Alternative sequence (Incontinence)
**85, 87, 22, 43, 45, 0**

Besides the stimulation of these points you can also use this simple method: Massage the zone around point **126** (at the top of the forehead, on the hairline) as well as the chin.

# Indigestion
### 50, 38, 127, 39, 37, 0

This problem is generally experienced either at the end of a big meal or one during which too much alcohol was consumed. However, it only manifests when the digestive function is otherwise disturbed. The liver, pancreas, stomach, gallbladder, duodenum, and intestine are closely linked to this dysfunction. Stimulate these points after a meal, or even beforehand if you have some warning in advance of the amount of food you are likely to eat.

Also stimulate these reflex zones.

# Inflammation

## 26, 3, 50, 17, 38, 14, 16, 61, 60, 0

It could be said that these are "natural anti-inflammatory points." In fact repeated stimulation of these for long enough procures a rapid and lasting relief of pain caused by inflammation. Duration has to be evaluated according to the relief felt by the patient, but stimulation should never exceed two or three minutes. It should be noted that the sedative effect is not just a passing one. Usually the improvement will last longer as the sessions continue. Quite often a single session is enough, however.

In all cases of inflammation, it is advisable to also stimulate the immune system, the emunctories, liver, kidneys, and intestines, as well as the zones corresponding to the spinal column.

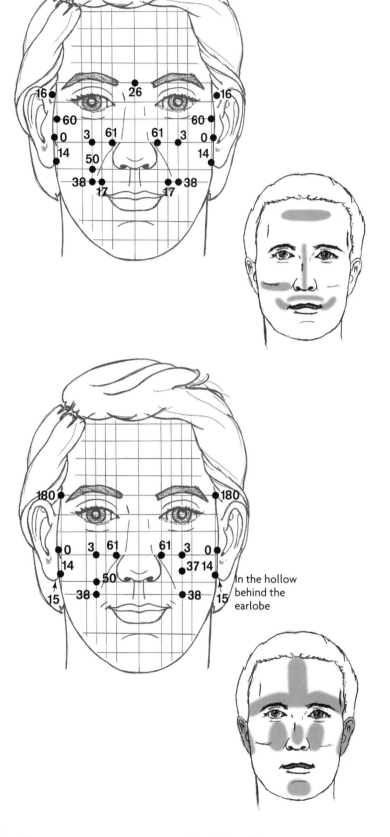

# Influenza, Flu

## 14, 15, 38, 61, 3, 37, 50, 0

### Also add the Relaxation and Toning Up points

Remember to take action as soon as the first symptoms appear without waiting for the flu to get established, otherwise it will be difficult to rid yourself of it. If your bout of flu does not provoke any perspiration, stimulate point **180** as well. You can use a roller, the end of a ballpoint pen, or just simply the ends of your fingers. Rub the ears thoroughly. Repeat this treatment several times during the day. It is also advised to use tiger balm on your neck, back, and shoulders (see Sore Throat).

On this figure you will also find the various components of a complete Dien' Cham' session as it is explained in chapter 6 in detail (Advanced Dien' Cham').

In the hollow behind the earlobe

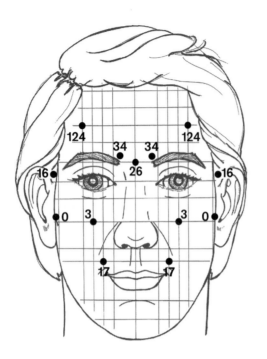

## Insect Bites
### 16, 17, 124, 34, 26, 3, 0

The stimulation of these points rapidly soothes the stinging or burning sensation following an insect bite. Stimulate them for two or three minutes until the pain disappears.

Also remember to apply vinegar as soon as possible, or rub the bite with some grass that you have bruised between your fingers.

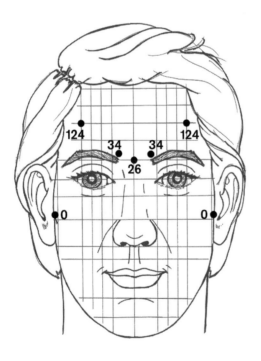

## Insomnia
### 124, 34, 26, 0

If you lack sleep often or have trouble recuperating fully when you sleep, you will have trouble waking up properly and your day will be spoiled. Your health will no doubt suffer in the long term. Indeed both your physical health and mental equilibrium depend largely on recovery during sleep. The impressive quantities of sleeping drugs sold in France and the rest of the industrial world prove the widespread nature of this problem. Sleep depends on a delicate balance, which is easily disturbed by several factors such as stress, overwork, worry, mental hyperactivity, and, sometimes, hormonal disorders. According to Chinese medicine, insomnia can also be linked to functional imbalance of the heart, liver, gallbladder, or kidneys. Try both sequences shown here to see which one suits you best. Stimulate the points before going to sleep and during the night if you wake up. In general a few sessions will be enough to recover a good night's sleep.

**A further sequence**
124, 34, 51, 16, 14, 0

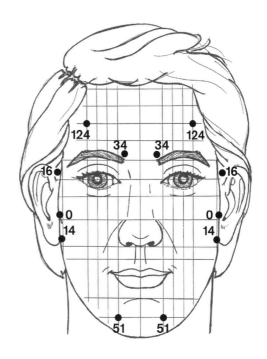

# Intestinal Gas
(see Flatulence)

# Itching and Scratching
26, 3, 17, 7, 50, 51, 61, 0

**(see also Pruritis)**

These points soothe pruritis and itching whatever the origin, including cases of insect stings (see Insect Bites also). Please remember here that itching could indicate a case of eczema or a circulatory disorder. Where necessary treat this too.

To the above add these reflex zones for the heart (and therefore circulation), liver, and intestines, which are often at the origin.

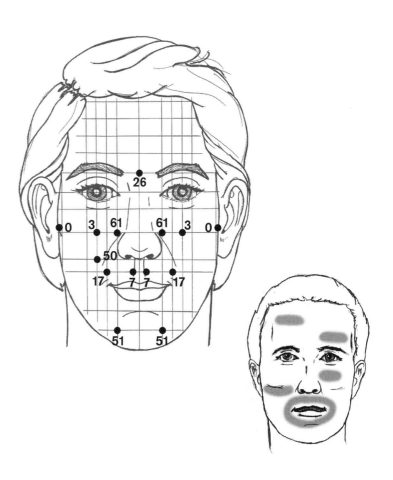

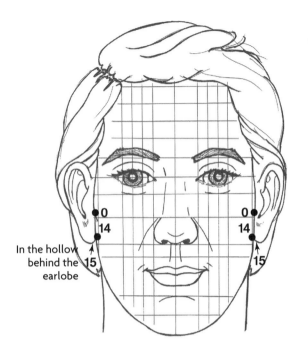

## Jaws
### (spasms and problems with articulation)
### 14, 15, 0

Does your dentist ever complain that you are not opening your jaws wide enough to enable him to work comfortably in your mouth? Does your jaw make a clicking noise when you yawn? Do you sometimes suffer from the "torture" of spasms of the jaw? Strong stimulation of these points will usually allow you to solve this kind of problem in a single session.

In the hollow behind the earlobe

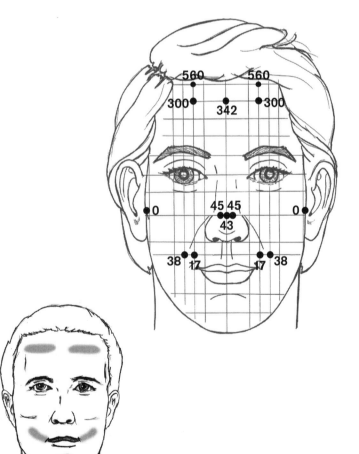

## Kidneys, Various Problems
### 17, 38, 300, 342, 43, 45, 560, 0

This sequence of points stimulates the renal function. It is therefore usable whatever the problem. In case of an infection, also use the points given for cystitis. Remember that it is advisable to stimulate the kidneys to promote elimination in numerous cases such as cellulitis, intoxication of different kinds, and where the body needs to be drained.

Also massage the various reflex zones corresponding to the kidneys and select the most sensitive.

# Kidney Stones (Renal Lithiasis)
## 38, 43, 45, 73, 300, 85, 0

Nothing is comparable to the very real torture that these tiny deposits lodged in the kidney can provoke. Here again it is easier to prevent them than to cure them, especially since these stones are almost impossible to dissolve. However if you only have small ones these points will help you to evacuate them with just a little pain. If you have already had kidney stones, you should regularly stimulate these points to keep them from returning. Also remember that regular taking of calcium and magnesium in sufficient quantity is an antidote to the formation of more kidney stones.

Contrary to common wisdom, some recent scientific work has proved that it is in fact a lack of easily-absorbed calcium that lies at the heart of the problem, and that dairy products are not a suitable source! On the other hand, we are not designed to eat rocks! If the water in your tap is too hard, filter it or consume water with just a few minerals. You can also take colloidal minerals which have a highly beneficial effect, such as: Hypertonic Marine Plasma, Quinton's Plasma, Himalayan Salts, or T. J. Clark's Phytogenic Mineral Formula, from the sea or from a vegetable source.[6]

# Knees
## 17, 38, 197, 300, 156, 1, 45, 37, 0

Whatever the problem with the knee—arthrosis, arthritis, accidental lesion, fracture, or sprain—you will be well advised to stimulate these points as soon as possible. A vigorous up and down massage of the zones close to the corners of the mouth will also provide relief.

Point 17 stretches an inch or two from the corners of the mouth, when you smile, toward the ears. Check which specific point is the most responsive. Also, stimulation of the chin is often very effective.

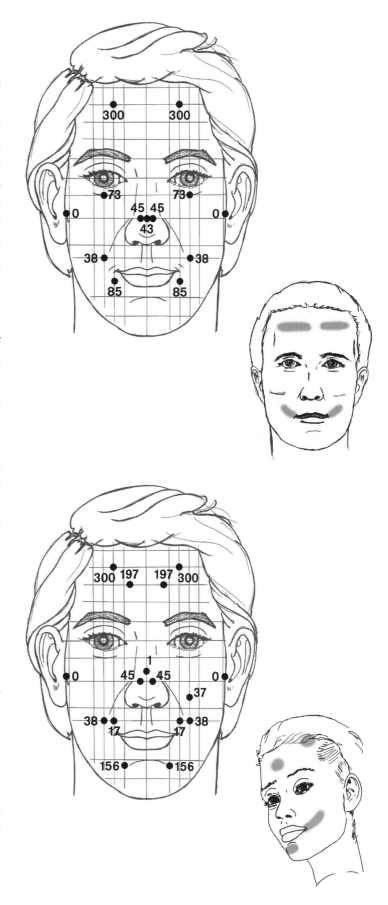

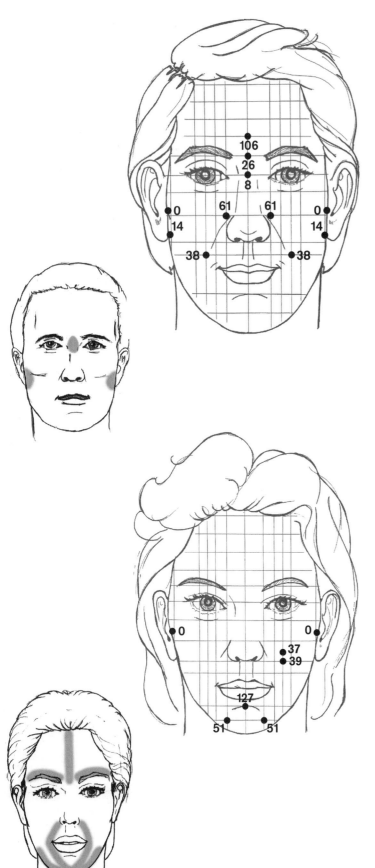

## Laryngitis, Loss of Voice
### 14, 8, 26, 106, 61, 38, 0

In cases of emergency, such as when you are due to speak at a meeting and you are unsure of all the points needed to treat your condition, just stimulate points **14** and **8** for a few minutes. Repeat this as necessary.

## Legs, Heavy Feeling
### 37, 39, 127, 51, 0

Sitting or standing for long periods, associated with lack of exercise, tends to accentuate blood circulation troubles. This is the most common reason for the unpleasant, heavy feeling in the legs that returns as soon as it is necessary to move a little (walk upstairs, go shopping, or just do housework).

Sedentary occupations are always associated with this condition and it can be further complicated by a decrease in the liver function or overwork of the gastrocnemian muscle ("calf spasm"). This is particularly the case if the professional activity of the subject involves long hours of shuffling around on the spot, like sales persons for example. Reflexology can be extremely useful in this kind of case by boosting the blood circulation locally and freeing up stasis. It should be practiced during the day and in the evening to eliminate tiredness and assist relaxation.

## Leucorrhea
### (see Vaginal Discharge)

# Lithiasis
## (see Gallstones, Kidney Stones)

# Liver Problems
## 50, 103, 233, 197, 0

All of the points given improve the liver function and promote drainage of this vitally important organ. These points will help you whether you just have a weak liver function or suffer from a more serious problem like hepatitis, cirrhosis, and so on. Always remember that it is possible and usually better to complement your medical treatment of whatever sort with this practice. The results can only be better. Also remember to lighten the load on your liver by eating a balanced diet, abstaining from the standard toxic substances: alcohol and tobacco, as well as all forms of drugs.

Try to find out which of the various liver reflex zones suit you the best, which is the most responsive!

# Low Blood Pressure
## 50, 19, 103, 0

Low blood pressure can be the source of weakness, problems with eyesight, fainting, and loss of consciousness. If you start to feel faint, lie down immediately and stimulate the points shown here.

Please note that point 0 has a regulating effect, which means that it can be used in cases of both high and low blood pressure. This is one of the reasons why it is advised to finish each session with point 0. If, for example, you make the mistake of stimulating a high blood pressure point in someone suffering from high blood pressure, you will, by ending at 0, regulate the whole of the massage and no harm will result.

Just to reassure you, remember that a habitually low blood pressure value is a factor for longevity, as long as it is not pathological!

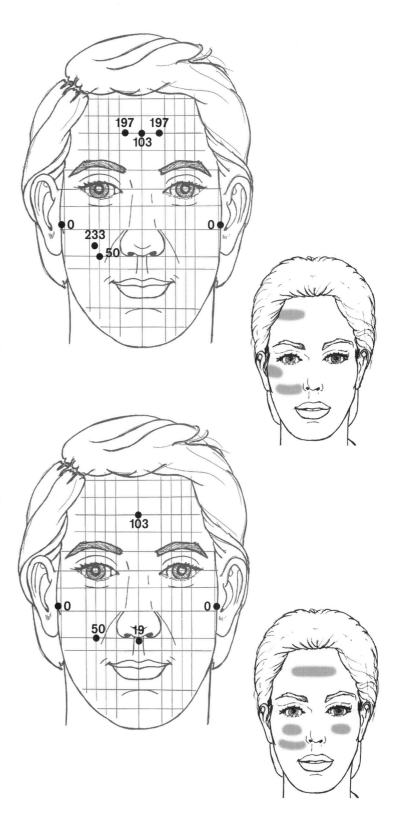

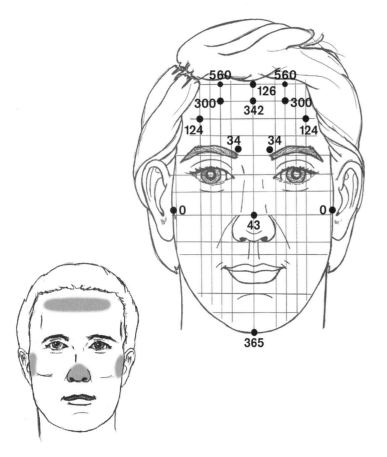

## Lumbago
### 124, 34, 43, 126, 342, 365, 300, 560, 0

Take your time to stimulate the points shown using a roller or ballpoint pen. At least ten minutes will be necessary. You can also work these points using your fingertips until relief is obtained. Repeat this session several times per day. If you perform this stimulation when you awake, it will usually allow you to get out of bed, which is quite a step as anyone having suffered from lumbago will know!

Besides the points indicated previously, there is one zone in particular that you should stimulate at length, for ten minutes or so. You will find it shaded in grey on the figure, in the middle of the forehead. As strange as it may seem, after doing this you will suddenly realize that you are able to get up with a minimum of difficulty. Generally the problem is solved in just one session!

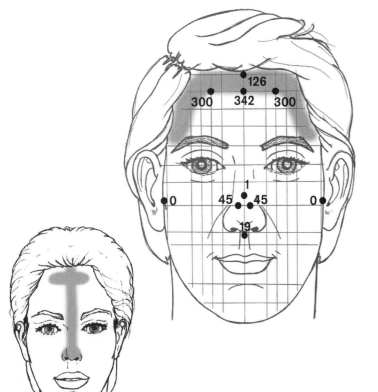

## Lumbar Vertebrae
### 19, 1, 45, 342, 126, 300, 0

In the case of lumbar pain, tap the forehead along the hairline as shown here, or make sweeping movements over the region using small up and down movements. All of the points between **126** and **19** unblock the spinal column and consequently you can stimulate all of this zone, sweeping downward or upward according to your intuition. In the first case you will cause energy to rise, and in the second to descend.

Also stimulate the other reflex zones corresponding to the spinal column, concentrating on painful areas.

# Lungs (all problems)
## 26, 3, 61, 73, 60, 0

### (see also Bronchitis, Cough)

These few points are easy to stimulate during the day and allow improvement of all respiratory problems, from allergies to asthma and chronic bronchitis, or just a simple cough caused by a cold. Do not hesitate to use the points as often as is necessary, in addition to the points more particularly indicated in your case.

Also massage the lung reflex zones on the cheeks and the forehead.

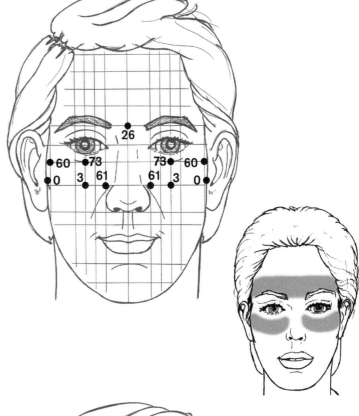

# Malaria
## 14, 15, 26, 34, 124, 0

It must be made clear that these few pressure points do not heal malaria, which is usually caught in the tropical or subtropical regions of the globe, following the bite of the anopheles mosquito. It is essential to treat this with standard medicines or drugs. On the other hand regular stimulation of the points indicated improves health generally. In case of a fever stimulate the points as soon as possible until an improvement is felt.

It is also recommended to add stimulation of the emunctories, as for all cases of infectious sickness. Practice the Basic Session several times per day to stimulate the natural defenses.

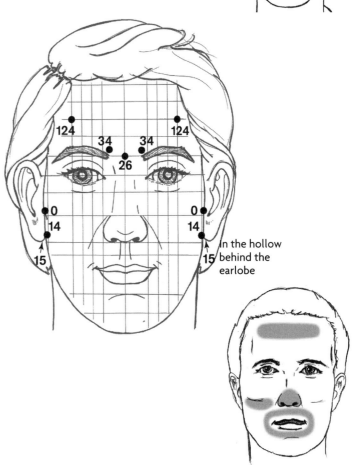

In the hollow behind the earlobe

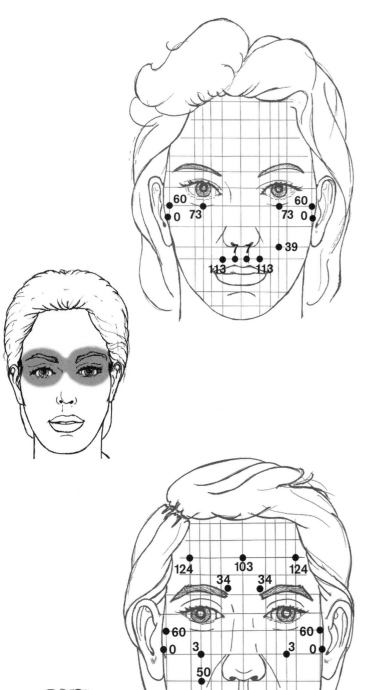

## Mastosis, Painful Breasts
**39, 73, 60, 7, 113, 0**

### (see also Breastfeeding and Breasts)

Regularly massage these points and add the points located around the eyes. Finger pressure will generally be enough.

With three fingers together exert medium pressure toward the nose root. Continue pressing round the orbit of the eyes starting under the eyebrows, moving along below the eye and finishing at the initial position.

## Memory
**103, 124, 34, 60, 50, 3, 0**

These points improve blood circulation and stimulate the cerebral function as a whole. They will be useful in cases of mental tiredness, overwork, and troubles with concentration and memory linked with aging. Stimulation of the points can help a student who has a block during an examination. In this case, it is enough to discreetly use the end of a ballpoint pen to obtain the desired result, which will be so appreciated!

You can also stimulate reflex zones corresponding to the head and located on the forehead and the nose.

# Ménière's Disease (or Syndrome)

## 63, 65, 34, 0

The symptoms of this disease are sudden bouts of dizziness or vertigo with buzzing in the ears and sometimes deafness that lasts for varying lengths of time. It is sometimes called labyrinthine syndrome or positional vertigo and is linked to a disturbance of the inner ear, which regulates balance of the body. It is due to vascular trouble together with high pressure in the labyrinthine fluid. In case of vertigo, stimulate these few points as quickly as possible. Renew this as soon as felt necessary and in any case daily.

To your session add these ear reflex zones.

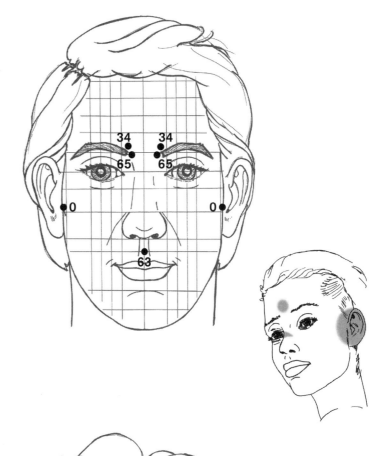

# Menopause

## 7, 85, 87, 127, 156, 0

Menopause arises when ovarian secretions diminish and this results in interruption of monthly periods. This period of hormonal change is sometimes troublesome but can easily be dealt with thanks to Dien' Cham'. Hot flashes, depression, irritability, headaches, and tiredness are just passing symptoms and certainly not a sickness. It should be noted that most women live through this transition with no bothersome problems.

Perform a general stimulation of the reflex zones located on the upper lip, chin, and toward the hairline.

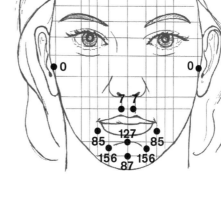

# Metritus
## (see Uterine Problems)

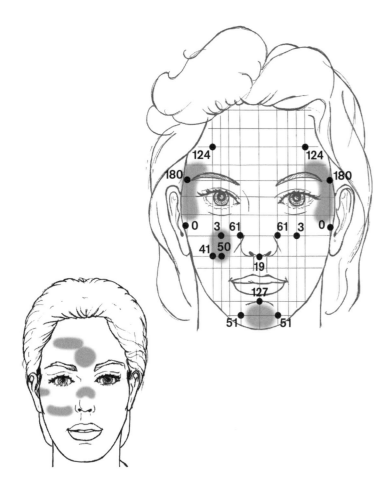

## Migraine
**50, 127, 19, 3, 61, 124, 180, 0**

### Or
**124, 41, 50, 61, 51, 180, 0**

Migraine is characterized by a dull pain in the head and throbbing, which is often just on one side. It can also be felt at the level of the temple and in the eye orbit. Migraines are often accompanied by autonomous nervous system disorders such as nausea, vomiting, general weakness or faintness, together with great tiredness. Most often digestive problems and stress are the causes, but other possible causes like high blood pressure and hormonal troubles should be considered.

When you want to tap your head against the wall (or preferably before that juncture), think Dien' Cham'! As a general rule the pain disappears in just one session. If it persists do not hesitate to consult a physician because the symptoms may correspond to something more serious. In the case of optical migraines, add points **100** and **180**. In Vietnam, one remedy is to apply fine slices of ginger root to the temples . . .

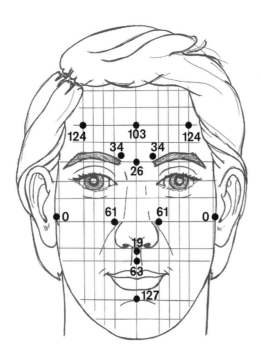

## Motion Sickness
**(automobiles, aircraft, boats)**
**127, 19, 26, 103, 0**

### Or more simply: 19 + Relaxing Points (124, 34, 26, 0)

### Seasickness
**63, 61, 26, 0**

Everyone must at some point in their lives have taken a child on a road trip and have him or her start vomiting or feeling sick. Sometimes even adults have this problem, which causes a considerable degree of unpleasantness for everyone! Not to mention the case of vacationers on a day cruise being afflicted by seasickness and who only really appreciate the view of the harbor at the end of the trip! Whatever the means of transport, travel sickness provokes powerful symptoms in sufferers, which can be cold sweating, nausea, vomiting, dizziness, and even fainting. In this case Dien' Cham' again comes to the rescue. You can stimulate the points indicated before leaving if you have apprehensions about the trip, or as soon as the first symptoms appear.

Tapping the forehead as described in the Forehead Massage in chapter 3 can also be effective as long as it is repeated whenever the need arises.

## Multiple Sclerosis
### 37, 60, 73, 74, 51, 63, 97, 98, 64, 0

All of these points treat the pins and needles, the paresthesia (loss of sensation), as well as the pain and paralysis in the limbs. This is why it is possible to use them to soothe this difficult sickness. It is sometimes a good idea to use the points given for facial paresthesia in addition to the points corresponding to dorsal back pain.

More specifically:

* point 51 treats pain in the arms and legs
* points 63 and 64 treat paralysis of the legs
* points 97 and 98 treat paralysis of the arms

Regularly practice general stimulation of the reflex zones of the skeleton, working particularly on sensitive areas or those corresponding to the parts of the body affected.

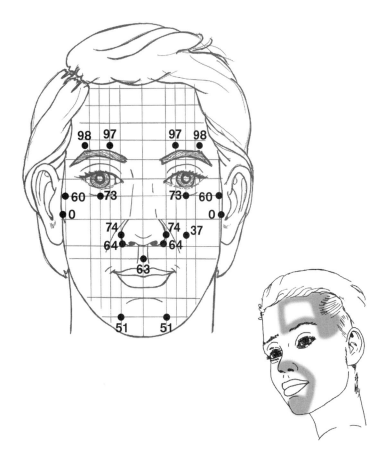

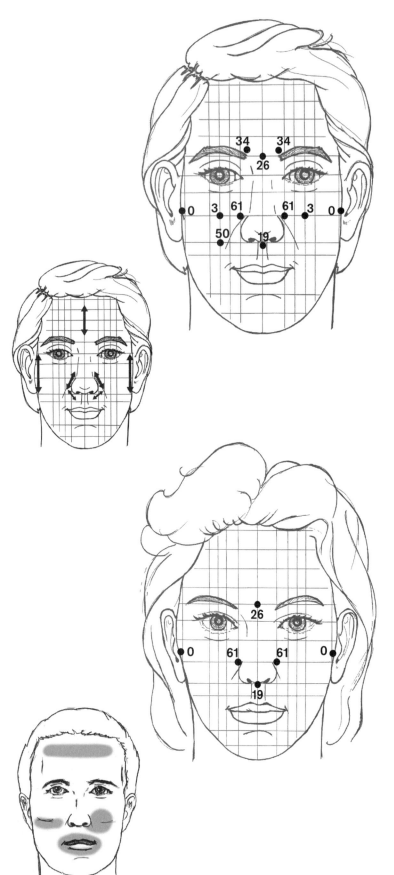

## Nasal Blockage
### 50, 19, 3, 61, 26, 34, 0

This is the first sign that affects us before the arrival of a cold or influenza. A blocked nose also limits our efficiency. It has been shown that breathing through the mouth gives free access to other ailments and decreases our intellectual capacity! It is just as well to act on this as soon as it appears. The stimulation of the points indicated produces an immediate and dramatic effect. The nasal blockage disappears during the first session.

Also use the common cold prevention stimulation technique described above. This will unblock the nose as soon as it is applied unless the cold is already entrenched.

## Nausea
### 19, 26, 61, 0

This symptom is very common and is generally not serious unless it persists and is accompanied by repeated vomiting, in which case a visit to a physician is necessary. Causes can include a problem with digestion, a migraine, an allergy, the beginning of a pregnancy, or a disorder of the inner ear, as is the case with motion sickness. In all these cases (except for pregnancy) stimulation of these points affords rapid relief.

It is also better to stimulate all of the zones corresponding to the digestive system: liver, gallbladder, stomach, pancreas, small and large intestine.

> **Warning**
>
> Do not stimulate in cases of pregnancy.

# Neck, Stiffness of
## 8, 26, 106, 34, 0

### (see also Cervical Vertebrae)

Whether it is a case of a twisted neck or the result of not moving for a long period, these points will rapidly remedy the problem. If you suffer from stiffness of the neck vertebrae, these same points will free them up effectively. Do not hesitate to stimulate them several times per day, above all if your employment obliges you to remain in the same position for long periods.

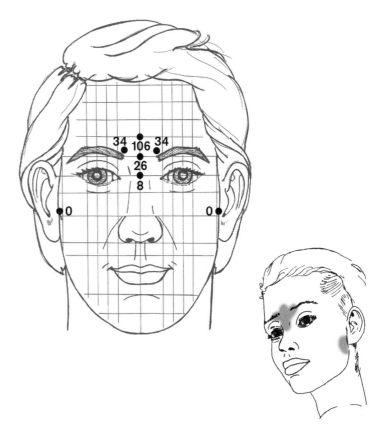

# Torticollis
## 34, 26, 106, 8, 50, 100, 87, 65, 0

A stiff neck is not just caused by a chill to the neck as is generally thought. It often stems from excess tension. In spite of the discomfort or even pain, a stiff neck is never serious and disappears after a few hours. However Dien' Cham' can usually get rid of one in just a few minutes! If you catch a stiff neck away from home and you cannot remember which points to stimulate, you just need to recall that the cervical vertebrae are represented between the eyebrows. Simple stimulation of this zone (around points **34, 65,** and **26**) should usually be quite sufficient to resolve the problem in less time than it takes to write this.

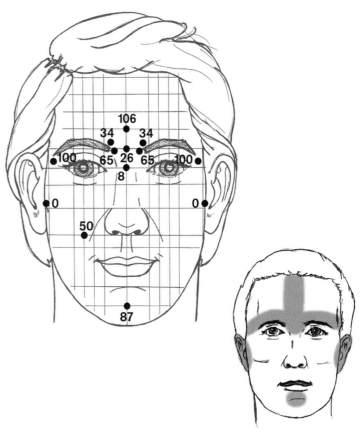

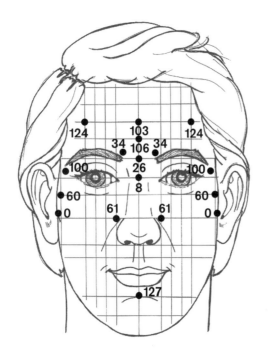

## Nervousness
### 8, 26, 34, 60, 61, 124, 127, 100, 106, 103, 0

Stress, overwork, worrying about problems, hormonal disorders, and so on can all contribute to a state of nervousness and hypersensitivity which can throw our lives out of balance. The same effect can also be the result of a lack of certain minerals and vitamins. Even if correction of the underlying causes must ideally be attempted, it is also necessary to try to rapidly remedy any clear manifestations or symptoms that could otherwise, at certain times, be detrimental to the sufferer's welfare in a broad sense. Stimulation of these points routinely twice per day is a good emergency measure. Of course these points can also help to calm a nervous child. It is also a good idea to give a vitamin and mineral supplement adapted to his or her age, above all colloidal mineral complexes,[7] which are available at health food stores.

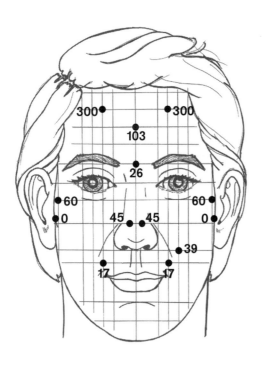

## Neuralgia
### 39, 60, 45, 17, 26, 103, 300, 0

Neuralgia is a pain that is situated on one of the nerve paths. It can be violent, tenacious, permanent, or intermittent, located in one particular place or moving along the whole nerve path. Whatever the exact location and cause, it is always a difficult pain to bear. These points suit all kinds of neuralgia but you can add other points and zones corresponding to the location. Stimulate until the pain disappears and again as soon as the pain returns.

# Nightmares

## 8, 50, 3, 37, 0

Pressure point 8 will enable you to go back to sleep after a nightmare. As a consequence it will be of great use to parents of children who remain worried and cannot sleep after having had a bad dream.

If you are subject to nightmares remember to stimulate relaxation points and zones assisting with the digestion before going to bed. This will promote peaceful and restorative sleep.

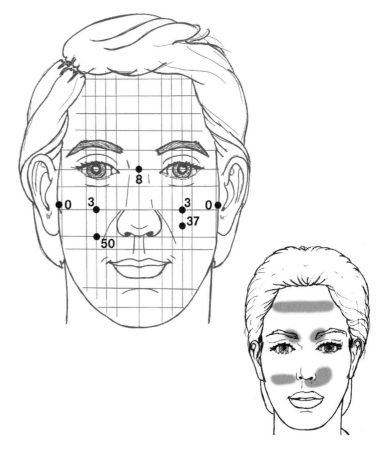

# Nosebleeds

## 16, 50, 61, 124, 17, 0

This problem is very common in children but it is not serious. It is often linked to a shock or the effect of blowing the nose too hard during colds. Try these points at the same time as pressing the bleeding nostril closed for a few minutes.

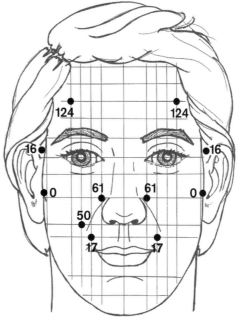

# Numbness

## (see Paresthesia)

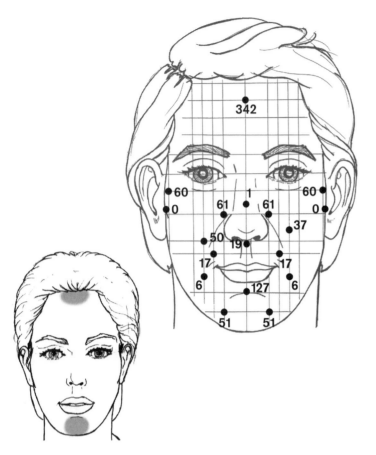

## Numbness at Extremities
### 1, 19, 17, 51, 127, 60, 50, 37, 6, 61, 342, 0

All of the indicated points provoke warmth. If you are one of the many people, mainly women, who always have cold hands and feet, stimulate these points daily. You can use all or just a selection of them. This will have the effect of improving your blood circulation and boosting your energy. As a consequence, you will suffer less from the usual ironic comments from your friends and family! Please note that point **342** has the special effect of warming the soles of the feet.

Quick procedure for relieving numbness in extremities: stimulate the zones shown on forehead and chin.

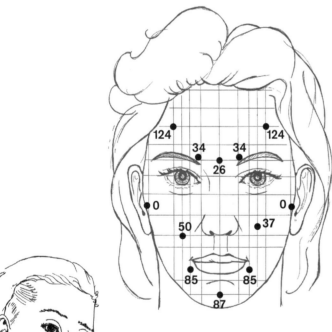

## Obesity
### 37, 85, 87, 50, 124, 34, 26, 0

These points can be effective during a slimming or weight-loss course, as they promote elimination and act against water retention. According to the case it can be useful to add the anti-stress pressure points and stimulate the glandular zones, above all in women.

In the latter case treatment of the zone above the upper lip by rubbing or massage of the points individually can be necessary. Also stimulate the thyroid using points **14** to **15**. The points which tone up the body can also be effective in boosting a weak metabolism (see Toning Up).

## Ocular Hypertension
### (high blood pressure in the eye)
### 16, 51, 0

This is a specific local problem that is dangerous for your sight and a common complication of high blood pressure. Above all remember the diagnosis from your physician. Follow his advice and stimulate the points given here.

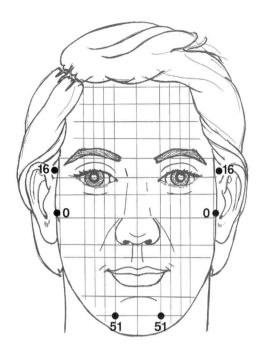

## Oppression, Feelings of
### 180, 73, 61, 3, 0

Stimulation of these points, which unblock the solar plexus, is usually enough to relieve the disagreeable feeling of oppression, whatever its origin. Never neglect this symptom however, and check with your physician that all is well elsewhere.

**Please Note:** These points often provoke perspiration.

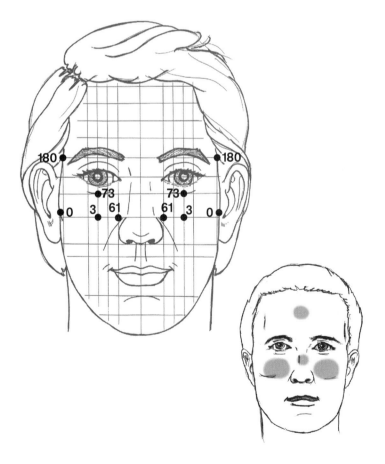

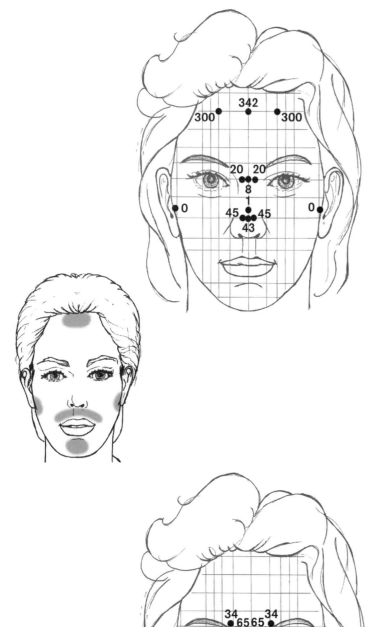

## Osteoporosis
**1, 8, 20, 43, 45, 300, 342, 0**

This is a generalized demineralization of the skeleton. The bones become brittle and fragile and this is the origin of numerous fractures, which sometimes occur spontaneously and are usually difficult to treat, such as in the pelvis and the thigh bone. This problem specifically affects women and takes place after menopause. The main causes are a drop in the level of estrogen occurring between the ages of fifty and sixty, linked to a lack of exercise and balance in the diet, but there can also be problems with the metabolism of proteins and digestive troubles, such as consequences of a gastrectomy, diabetes, cirrhosis of the liver, and so on.

Besides these pressure points, remember to stimulate those that treat hormonal problems, such as those for the thyroid glands and the ovaries. Also remember to take natural colloidal minerals that are easily assimilated by the body.[8]

## Ovarian Cysts
**34, 7, 113, 65, 73, 287, 0**

### (see also Ovaries)

Many women are subject to this benign problem, but such cysts are often the cause of painful periods or copious bleeding. They are caused by a hormonal disorder, stress, or—as is the case more and more often—linked to the consumption of dairy products, which are too rich in estrogen because of the treatment given to milking cows. Cysts often disappear spontaneously after a few months treatment if this massage is practiced regularly.

In addition, stimulate the reflex zones, above all those on the chin, toward the hairline, and on the upper lip.

# Ovaries

## 7, 22, 37, 63, 87, 113, 65, 73, 156, 0

## Or

## 34, 7, 113, 65, 73, 0

These pressure points soothe and also treat most of the problems related to the ovaries: cysts (see also Ovarian Cysts) of course, but malfunction and inflammation too. All of these points exert a regulatory effect on the endocrine system and this is usually enough to regulate ovulation and hormonal secretions.

Here are some reflex zones to try out as well.

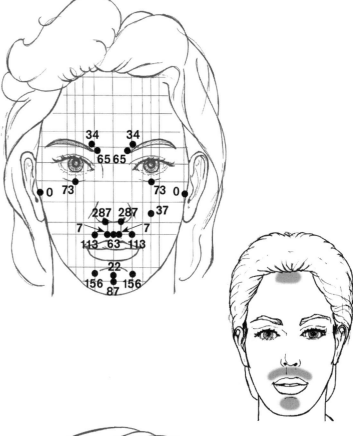

# Overwork

## 19, 124, 103, 34, 45, 127, 22, 0

If you have the habit of going beyond the feeling of tiredness during your activities, either physically or mentally, there is a risk that you could be overworking. Tiredness is an alarm signal that it would be better to follow in spite of the obligations of the modern world, but this is rarely the case. These days many children and adolescents also suffer from nervous exhaustion. They are overworked and habitually lack sleep, thanks mainly to watching the television too late at night, as well as going out in the evenings. It is of course necessary to address the causes of this situation, but stimulation of these points can be of great help nonetheless, to promote regeneration of a tired body.

Alternatively you can practice a short session using these reflex zones during the day.

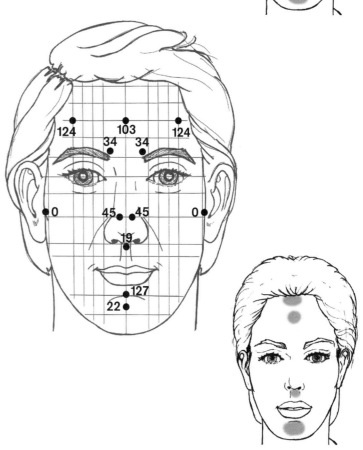

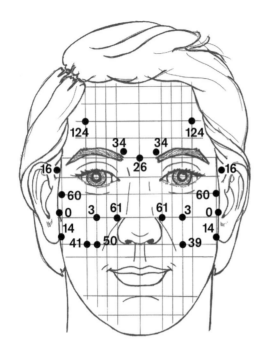

## Pain

**26, 124, 34, 61, 60, 39, 41, 50, 3, 14, 16, 0**

These points have a painkilling effect and afford rapid and natural relief from bouts of pain. In case of need use them freely. This can be enough to avoid having to ingest doubtful substances, which will end up upsetting your body or can even be toxic.

Never forget that pain is an alarm signal that your body is sending you to tell you that something is not quite right. Take this warning to heart and treat yourself in order to avoid more serious trouble later, just as you would when you hear a strange noise from your automobile or when you see that tiny bomb on your computer screen!

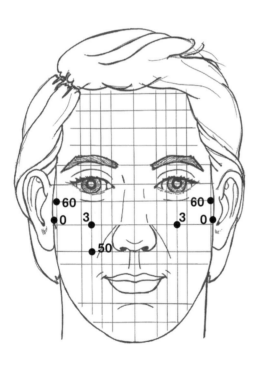

## Pain, Shooting

**3, 50, 60, 0**

These points correspond more particularly to kinds of pain that are difficult to bear such as toothache, sciatica, herpes zoster, or any other similar cause. Naturally you will also stimulate the points corresponding to the root of the pain.

# Paralysis

**37, 51, 60, 63, 64, 73, 74, 97, 98, 0**

**Lower limbs   63, 64, 37, 51**

**Upper limbs   97, 98, 51, 37**

### (see also Paralysis, Facial, and Paralysis, Hemiplegia)

Of course it is impossible to treat a long-standing case of paralysis or one with a traumatic origin. However in certain cases some improvement can be noted by stimulating these points. Paralysis following a cerebrovascular accident or stroke is one of the cases where this technique is effective. In such cases, the earlier the stimulation is performed after the accident, the better the results are likely to be. Of course this must be done in parallel with the requisite medical treatment and reeducation, which should also be undertaken without delay.

Remember to add the massage of the reflex zones affected.

# Paralysis, Facial

**3, 15, 37, 50, 61, 100, 127, 156, 51, 0**

This term is applied to motor problems affecting certain muscles in the face, whether it is a case of total paralysis or a simple loss of feeling in the zones. It is advisable to stimulate these points at length every day. Please note that point **100** located on the right corresponds to the right half of the face. It is the same for the left side.

Please remember that there are reflex zones corresponding to the face itself and massage them at the same time.

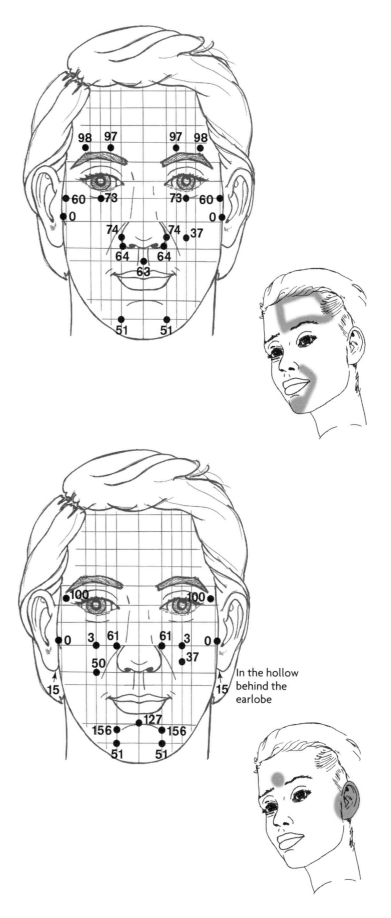

In the hollow behind the earlobe

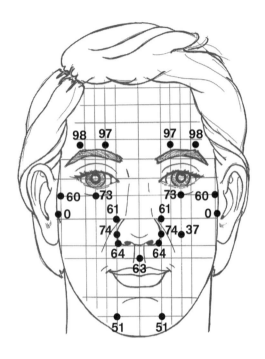

# Paralysis, Hemiplegia
**37, 51, 60, 63, 64, 73, 74, 97, 98, 0**

**Lower limbs  63, 64, 37, 51**

**Upper limbs  97, 98, 51, 37**

Here it is necessary to boost energy. To do this, stimulate all of the points given but concentrate on point 37.

### Special Treatment for Hemiplegia

Apart from stimulating all of the Dien' Cham' points, there is another method for this problem which is also Vietnamese and has been improved upon by Nhuan Le Quang. Highly rewarding results can be obtained with it where the necessary time is taken to practice it correctly. We would advise its use as a complementary measure when the paralysis seems well-entrenched.

This treatment must be applied for eight straight hours. Most often recuperation is complete after these eight hours, but sometimes a second session is necessary. In any case this technique has no risks attached and can only improve the situation of a patient suffering from this serious problem. You should enlist the assistance of one or two other people. The bedroom must be heated as the patient has to stay naked during the whole treatment.

### *Necessary Equipment*

- Several large-sized towels
- Bags of ice
- Six or more hot water bottles
- Blankets
- Scalding hot water
- Chilled cold water
- Plastic sheeting to protect the bed from water

## Preparation of the Patient

It is advisable to restrict food intake during the day preceding this treatment. Only give a minimum to drink, too, because it will be impossible to get up during the eight hours of the treatment.

## Procedure

- Cover the bed with wide plastic sheeting. The patient should be naked and lay on the bed.
- Drench the bath towels with ice cold water and cover his or her head, neck, and shoulders, including the face, just leaving a space for breathing comfortably. Install the bags of ice to slow down the warming of the towels.
- Wrap the legs, feet, and the pelvic area with towels drenched with really warm water. Be careful not to scald the patient and remain within his or her limits of endurance. Install the six or more hot water bottles in order to slow down cooling.
- Maintain this for eight hours, regularly renewing the towels, the bags of ice, and hot water bottles. Sometimes it will only be necessary to dampen the towels from time to time with hot or cold water, according to where they are situated. Always do this with gentleness and after having checked the temperature of the water. This avoids having to move the patient.
- Of course it is advisable to stimulate the patient at regular intervals using Dien' Cham' points during this long session.

Always exercise a lot of patience and understanding with your patient. Even if the seriousness of the problem really merits the effort of performing this long session, it must be recognized that it is hardly very pleasant to be cared for in this way. Speak to him or her beforehand and make the decision together after having explained the procedure in detail. During the session use encouragement all the time because the patient must feel accompanied throughout the long hours and everything will turn out for the best.

Remember to listen to the patient when he or she complains. The water may well seem quite bearable to your hands but feel much too hot applied to the stomach or abdomen. Try to adapt and help him or her to stand the maximum of heat in the lower part of the body, and cold on the upper part. Ice is also sometimes felt as something disagreeable, but it is really worth trying!

Modulate the stimulation of the reflex zones concerned, that is to say by treating the side corresponding to the paralyzed limbs of the body. (The right side of the face treats the right side of the body and the left treats the left side of the body—nothing could be simpler!)

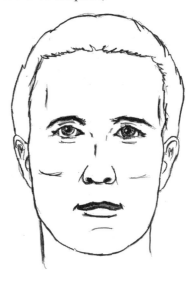

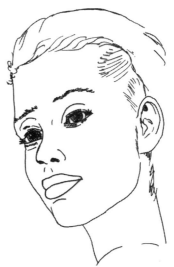

For you to fill in.

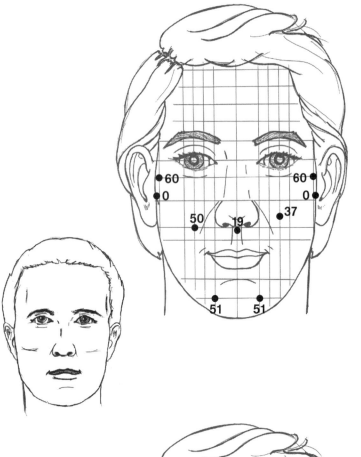

## Paresthesia (loss of feeling)
### 19, 37, 51, 60, 50, 0

Pins and needles, tingling, numbness, hot and cold sensations, the impression of having legs made of jelly, and so on: whatever the origin of such symptoms of paresthesia, it is possible to improve them by stimulation of these points, which also act on the pins and needles sometimes felt on waking. Of course this does not replace a visit to a physician in order to find out the causes and receive treatment.

In addition, stimulate the reflex zones corresponding to the area where there is loss of feeling; fingers, hands, arms, feet, legs, face, and so on. No zones have been indicated here because they will change according to the body part affected.

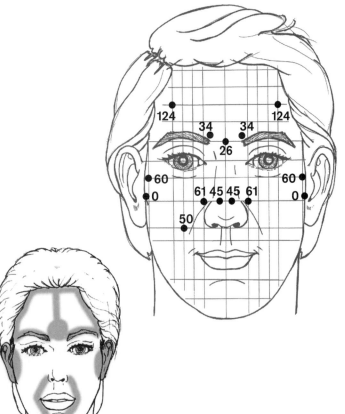

## Parkinson's Disease
### 50, 60, 45, 26, 61, 124, 34, 0

This sickness is a very big handicap for sufferers and is above all characterized by a specific kind of trembling and muscle rigidity. It is often linked to age, but there are other forms that follow slow-acting viral infections, such as typhus. Long and frequent stimulation of these pressure points attenuates the generalized trembling and muscular rigidity.

Also massage the zones corresponding to the head, face, upper and lower limbs, in order to provoke the circulation of energy. Also practice the Basic Session several times per day if necessary, in order to relax the nervous system and generate the vital energy needed to fight this sickness.

# Pectoral Angina
## 1, 3, 100, 106, 73, 61, 19, 60, 0

**(see also Heart Insufficiency)**

These points allow treatment of the disagreeable symptoms of pectoral angina—chest pain and a feeling of oppression and suffocation usually located on the left side of the thorax—which can sometimes spread to the neck, the jaw, and the left arm. The points should be stimulated every day and in certain cases more often. You can quickly soothe a bout of pain by pressing strongly on point **19**, and then rubbing the indicated zone with your finger until the pain disappears.

However do not neglect the warning sign that your body has given you. Make an appointment with your physician to find out exactly what is going on.

Vitamin E from a natural source is an excellent preventive remedy for cardiovascular diseases. In cases where there is a suspicion of risk, or if you are over fifty years old, you should take some daily. The advised daily dose is 400 mg per day or more if necessary.

Monitor your food intake and avoid stress!

Reconsider your dietary habits and do a little more exercise!

In addition to the points indicated, treat these zones. Generally speaking the points are located within the zones.

# Periods, Irregular
## 124, 37, 26, 63, 50, 7, 0

This problem, which is common in adolescence, usually stems from poor energy distribution leading to an erratic hormone function. The sequence given allows good results to be obtained. Also remember to check for a correct digestive system. Sometimes it is necessary to add the Relaxation points (**124, 34, 8, 0**), as the influence of the nervous system

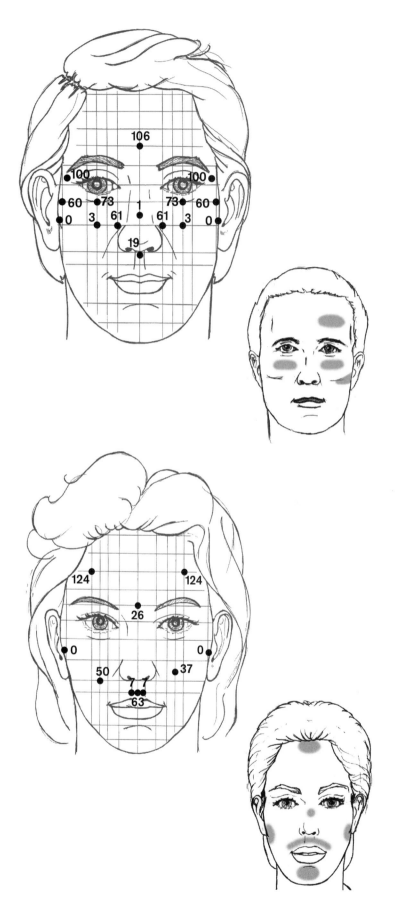

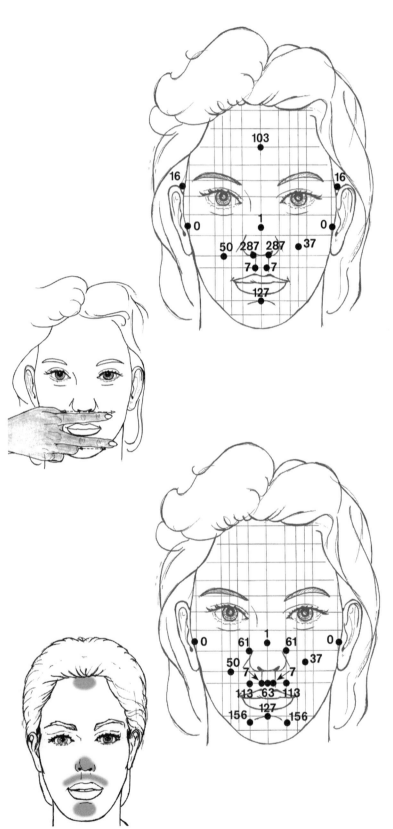

is great on this sort of problem. It is also advised to supplement the diet with vitamin E, either in wheat germ oil or taken as a food supplement.

Stimulate the reflex zones of the whole of the endocrine system every day.

## Periods, Over-Abundant
### 16, 103, 50, 37, 287, 7, 127, 1, 0

More and more women suffer from over-abundant bleeding during their periods which leads to tiredness, iron deficiency, and many other complaints. The problem is often linked to the presence of an IUD or coil, but can also be linked to a hormonal imbalance which should be treated. These points can be stimulated several times per day during the period as necessary. Generally speaking menstrual bleeding returns to normal quickly.

**Please note:** point **16** quickly reduces secretions and limits hemorrhage.

You may add the stimulation of the region around the lips by following the procedure described in Contraception.

## Periods, Painful (dysmenorrhea)
### 127, 156, 63, 7, 61, 1, 50, 37, 0

### Simplified procedure
### 37, 7, 113, 0

These two sequences can be practiced at the same time or one after the other. The second has the advantage of being easily memorized and usable anywhere, discretely. You will be surprised at the relief that this simple massage will bring!

There is also another easy procedure that is practical to use in case of need. Tap the curve of the chin with the index, middle, and ring fingers.

Also these other reflex points and zones to may stimulated several times per day if necessary.

# Perspiration, Excess

## 124, 34, 60, 19, 61, 50, 127, 87, 51, 16, 0

This sequence of points treats the causes of the most common cases of excess perspiration. Regular stimulation of them will enable you to avoid discomfort and inconvenience when the summer comes.

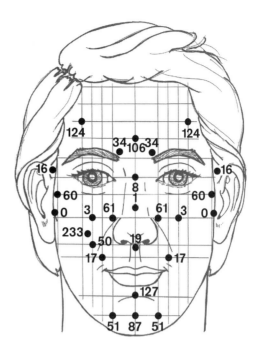

- To treat this problem generally: points 0, 8, 17, 50, 60, 61, 106, 124, 233
- For excess perspiration from the feet: points 1, 50
- For excess perspiration from the hands: points 1, 3, 50

# Pneumonia

## 26, 3, 61, 7, 8, 73, 60, 14, 0

Pneumonia is an infectious sickness that is due to the pneumococcus bacterium. It is characterized by an acute inflammation of the lung, affecting one lobe in particular. Symptoms include high temperatures, coughing, breathing difficulties, and pain in the chest. The points indicated can afford effective relief but a physician must be consulted all the same. Perform this stimulation for a few minutes several times per day.

Also stimulate reflex zones corresponding to the lungs on the cheeks and the forehead.

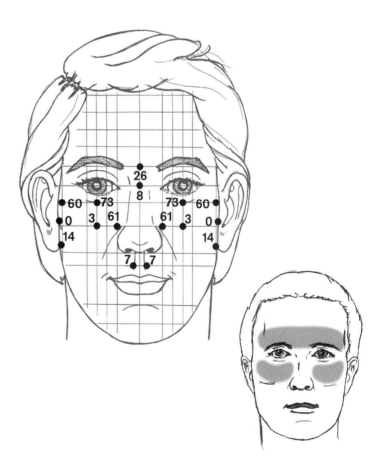

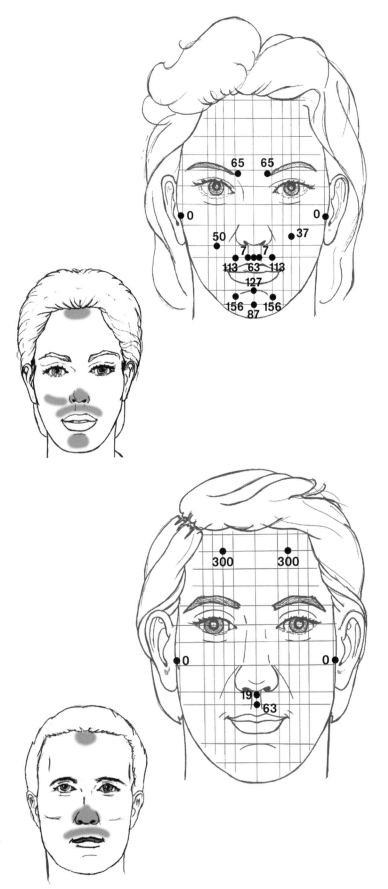

## Pregnancy
### (especially to promote pregnancy in case of difficulties)
**7, 113, 63, 127, 0**

### As well as
**127, 156, 87, 50, 37, 65, 0**

These pressure points have already served to obtain a much wanted pregnancy for many women! Stimulate them daily until the desired result is forthcoming. You should also advise your partner to stimulate points enabling enhanced fertility (see Sexuality).

You may practice Dien' Cham' throughout your pregnancy, with caution. It will allow you to overcome minor pain and problems that occur on a day-by-day basis without having to resort to drugs or medicine, which always have some consequences. Just remember that certain pressure points assist the process of giving birth and avoid them until the appropriate moment! You will find the necessary information in chapter 5, devoted to the correspondences for each point.

> **Warning**
> From the seventh month, avoid stimulating points located under the nose!

## Premature Ejaculation
**19, 63, 300, 0**

These points increase sexual energy, which will allow you to fight effectively against this particular symptom and all other forms of sexual weakness. Pressure points related to sexual toning up can be usefully added (see Impotence and Sexuality).

# Prostatitis

**7, 113, 65, 73, 156, 87, 0**

### As well as
**22, 37, 63, 0**

Prostatitis covers all of the problems caused by hypertrophia or abnormal enlargement of the prostate gland, which affects many men after the age of fifty. Inflammation of the prostate gland is hard to bear, with painful and frequent urination and high temperatures accompanied by violent shivering. Whatever the precise nature of the problem, try stimulating these points regularly. The second shorter sequence can be practiced briefly during the day and every time it seems necessary.

To fight against frequent and painful urination, add points **126, 43,** and **300**.

Also massage the reflex zones located on the upper lip, the chin, and the hairline.

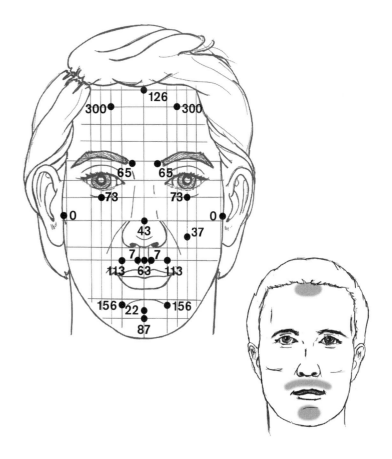

# Pruritis

**17, 50, 3, 60, 0**

### As well as
**26, 3, 61, 60, 50, 87, 0**

### (see also Itching and Scratching)

This irritation is the reason why we scratch the skin. It is generally caused by a skin lesion such as eczema or psoriasis. However there are cases of pruritis that are independent of such lesions. Pruritis of the anus and vagina can be caused by excessive heat or dampness or wearing of synthetic underwear, or linked to an allergy (soap or toilet paper for example). In all of these cases you are advised to regularly stimulate these few points, and this will bring appreciable relief.

In addition to the reflex zones shown here, also stimulate the zones that relate to the site of the trouble.

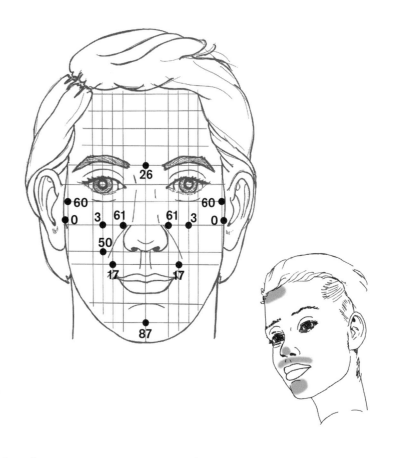

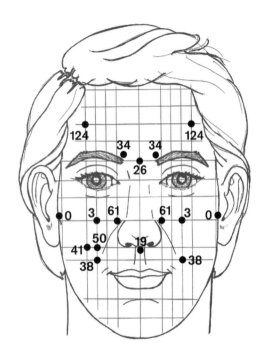

## Psoriasis
### 34, 124, 19, 50, 26, 61, 3, 41, 38, 0

This skin condition, which is difficult to get rid of and sometimes hereditary, is usually situated in specific zones such as the elbow, knee, and scalp, but sometimes covers the whole body. It consists of shiny, dry scales over red skin, which tends to bleed easily. It is very often linked to stress and can be improved thanks to the points indicated, which should be stimulated twice per day for several minutes. It is also necessary to check on diet and exclude any food type that may worsen the chronic state of toxicity, which is the origin of all skin conditions.

Also stimulate the reflex zones that are in relation with the site of the trouble: scalp, elbow, knee, and so on.

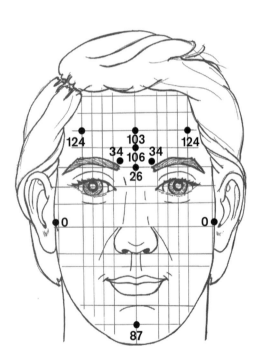

## Psychological Troubles
### 87, 103, 106, 124, 34, 26, 0

Psychological troubles of all kinds can be helped by stimulating these points. This will assist in cases of nervous depression, memory loss, difficulty in concentrating, aggression, oversensitivity, a temper tantrum in a child, withdrawal, and so on. It is necessary to perform this massage for a few minutes daily over a long period, without satisfying oneself with just a slight improvement.

## Ptosis of the Bladder

### 22, 87, 126, 0

The descent of the bladder has similar causes to that of the uterus and is treated in the same way (see below). It is also advised to interrupt urination at regular intervals in order to reinforce the muscles and fight against the tendency to incontinence, which is developing.

Add these reflex zones corresponding to the bladder, and widen your scope a little to include adjacent zones.

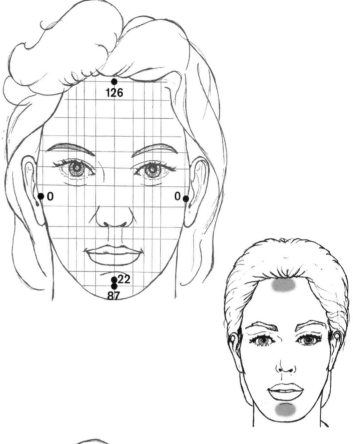

## Ptosis or Prolapse of the Uterus

### 22, 87, 103, 19, 63, 156, 127, 0

The weakening of the muscles of the pelvic floor (caused by a difficult birth or a surgical procedure, for example) provokes this "descent of organ" called ptosis: the neck of the uterus can descend into the vagina, causing incontinence, risk of infection, and various problems with periods and during sexual intercourse. It is necessary to tone up the pelvic floor by doing certain exercises (like the contraction of the pelvic region and perineum), completing this by frequently stimulating the given points.

As often as possible massage the uterine reflex zones found on the upper lip, forehead, and the chin. In addition to the recommended complete session, you can also perform brief massages using the knuckle of a finger several times per day.

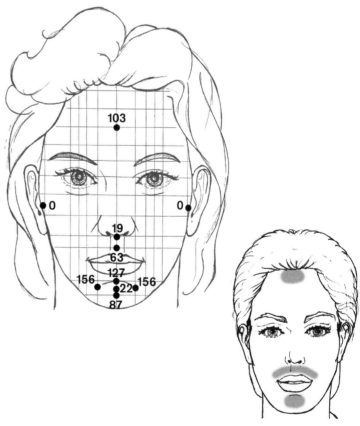

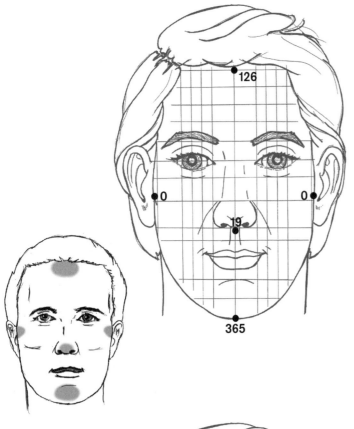

## Rectum
### 19, 126, 365, 0

Any and all of the problems linked to the rectum, like piles, anal fissure or fistula, pruritis, and so on, can be improved by stimulation of these points. It is advised to practice this massage several times per day until the troubles disappear (see also Hemorrhoids).

Also stimulate these reflex zones.

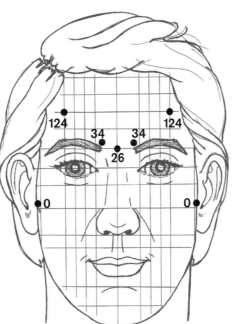

## Relaxation
### 124, 34, 26, 0

Most sicknesses result from blocked energy, which in turn is caused by stress, nervous tension, tiredness, and a lack of health-restoring sleep. You should remember that high-level nervous tension, especially if it lasts, weakens the immune system. This is why it is important to know how to relax, and learning this is the best way of preserving your health capital and regenerating the body. These few pressure points, linked to the points used for toning up, are part of the basic session you should do every day.

# Resuscitation (reanimation)
## 19, 127, 26, 124, 34, 0

Pressure point **19** is well known to proponents of martial arts. It is one of the main so-called Kuatsu (or resuscitation points) that are greatly effective in cases of loss of consciousness, drowning, and respiratory standstill. While you are waiting for help from the emergency services, press this point hard using your thumbnail if you have nothing else, until consciousness returns.

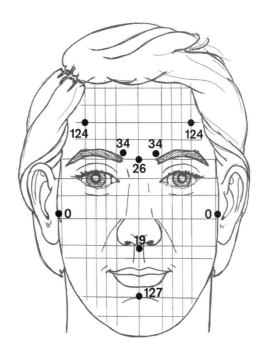

# Salivation, Insufficient
## 14, 0

This can usually be solved by gently tapping point **14** to start salivation. In any case, have your physician check the state of your pancreas; an imbalance there can be a cause of this anomaly.

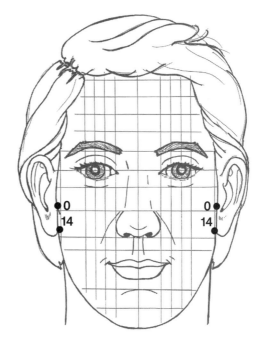

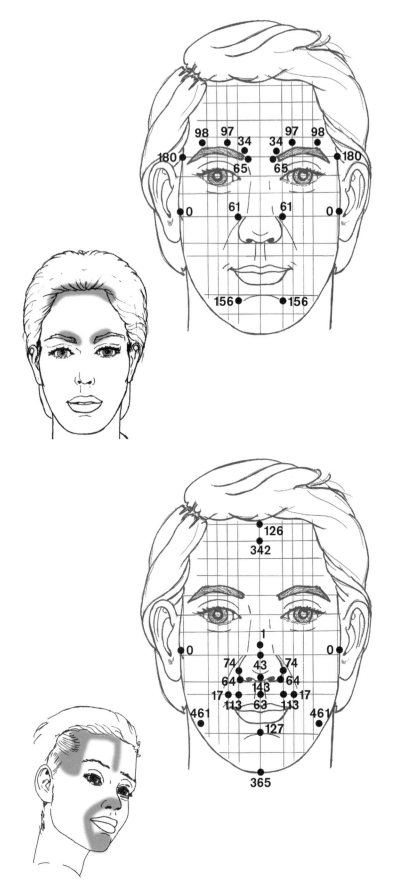

## Scapulohumeral Periarthritis
### (or "Frozen Shoulder")
### 98, 180, 61, 34, 65, 97, 156, 0

This type of rheumatism outside the joints can affect the totality of the fibrous tissues of the tendons enveloping the shoulder joint. It is a version of what is called periarthritis. This can happen following a case of tendonitis or be linked to cervical arthrosis or cervico-brachial neuralgia. This disease is painful and is a serious handicap. It can be helped considerably by stimulation of these points, which should be performed for a few minutes running, two or three times per day.

At the end of my conferences I always ask if someone in the audience is suffering from scapulohumeral periarthritis. There is always one person who has had the sickness for several years. I take the opportunity to make a quick demonstration, and take pleasure in my modest success. The person is always amazed to find that the condition is improved in less than a minute, when he or she has been taking anti-inflammatory drugs for years!

Remember to search for the most sensitive spot within the zones given. Sometimes it is necessary to go a little above or below the point indicated, often under the edge of the orbit. Make sure to gain good purchase so that your instrument cannot slip toward the eye!

## Sciatica
### 17, 1, 126, 342, 0

### As well as
### 461, 43, 63, 365, 64, 74, 113, 127, 143, 0

All of the above points correspond to sciatica. You can start with the first set of points and continue with the second to treat this problem. Try to find out precisely which points have the most rapid effect. You should also check which ones are the most sensitive and work mainly on these.

You can establish your own personalized schedule in this way. However this should not stop you from consulting an osteopath or a chiropractor!

In addition to stimulation of these points (including point **17** which has an anti-inflammatory effect), also: massage the nostrils, corresponding to the buttocks; around the nostrils, corresponding to the groin; and the nasogenian creases, which are the small creases that link the corners of the nostrils with the corners of the mouth. Repeat this stimulation as often as necessary until an improvement is felt.

In a case of an acute attack, three or four short sessions performed at intervals of a few minutes will procure real relief, and will last on average four hours, which is not such a bad result! Renew this as soon as the pain returns. Two or three days of massage are generally needed to treat sciatica.

## Secretions (decreasing)
### 106, 126, 63, 7, 17, 1, 50, 61, 15, 16, 51, 22, 0

All of these points contribute to decreasing body secretions produced in excess. They can be used to diminish superfluous perspiration (hot flashes), to calm fits of crying, reduce symptoms of a head cold or overabundant expectoration during bronchitis. (It should be noted however, that in some cases, it is better to allow the body to eliminate without interfering!)

These points (above all point **16**) decrease or stop bleeding wherever it is located: nose bleeds, piles, hemorrhage from the uterus following child birth or caused by fibroids, and so on. Of course it is not necessary to stimulate all these points. Just choose those that seem the most effective in your case or alternate them.

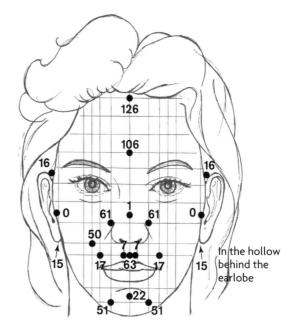

In the hollow behind the earlobe

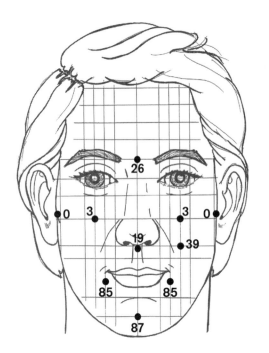

## Secretions (increasing)
### 26, 3, 39, 85, 19, 87, 0

Do you never perspire? Does your stomach not secrete enough acid? Are your periods insufficient? Do you produce too little urine? You may need to increase your body's secretions. Please note that point 0 always acts as a regulator as for other cases. It increases secretions when necessary and decreases them when they are excessive. If you are not sure about your own judgment, have confidence in point 0. This way you will allow the body to regulate itself, which is often better than a possibly incorrect stimulation.

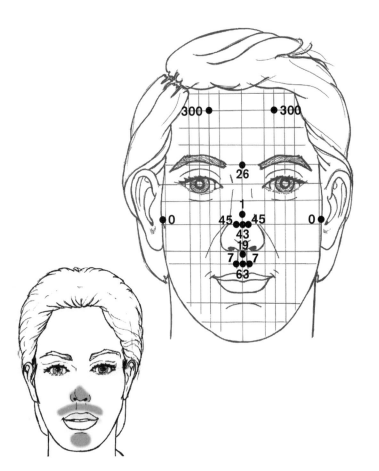

## Sexuality
### 1, 7, 19, 43, 45, 63, 300, 0

These points stimulate the life energy and increase sexual energy in both men and women. The gain in energy is considerable especially if your problem is linked to tiredness or overwork. If on the other hand, you think that stress or excess nervous tension is the problem, start by stimulating the Relaxation pressure points and then add one of these sequences:

- In case of difficulties with an erection, points 63 and 300.
- To boost sexual desire, points 63 and 300.
- To pacify and cool down desire, stimulate point 26.

Both men and women should stimulate these reflex zones situated around the mouth.

## Shaking
### 45, 1, 50, 60, 124, 34, 0

These points can calm all cases of shaking. Its origin is of little importance. Use these points whether the shaking is caused by tiredness, susceptibility to cold, or the tremor in aging persons, which is sometimes associated with Parkinson's Disease (see above) or even linked to an infectious sickness.

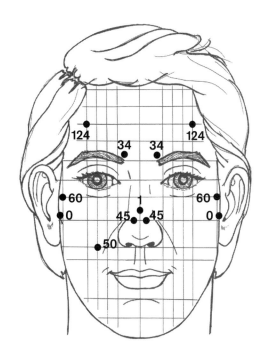

## Shingles, Herpes zoster
### 17, 300, 124, 64, 61, 60, 3, 38, 50, 0

This problem is caused by the chickenpox virus, which has been lying dormant in the body since childhood. In adults it provokes a sharply burning sensation, which is always situated on one side of the body, on the level of the ribs, the chest, or sometimes in the back. Shingles are usually accompanied by a high temperature, headache, and general tiredness. Although the problem is usually benign, the eyes are sometimes affected, in which case it is advisable to quickly consult an ophthalmologist. The stimulation of these points brings very real relief. Repeat it several times per day until the lesion disappears. A little vitamin E or aloe vera can also be applied.

Also remember to stimulate the zones on the face corresponding to the part of the body affected.

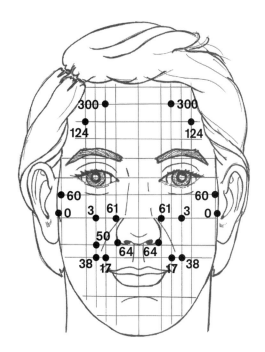

## Shock

**19, 26, 124, 34, 43, 0**

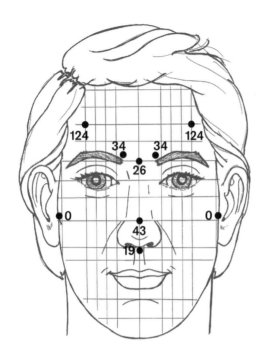

These points should be memorized for cases of accidents, and physical or psychological shocks, leading to the medically-defined state of shock, which can even result in death. First signs are paleness, a weak and rapid pulse, superficial, irregular breathing, visible anxiety, and agitation. Sometimes the patient is thirsty and liable to vomit. If nothing is done quickly, unconsciousness follows, and arterial blood pressure drops dramatically.

## Shoulder, Frozen, Pain in
### (see Scapulohumeral Periarthritis)

## Shyness, Fright

**124, 34, 8, 0**

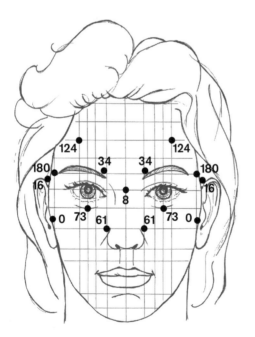

These points—which are relaxation points—are often enough to restore confidence in the affected person. However, if they are found to be insufficient and if the shyness is accompanied by a feeling of oppression with a knotted stomach or solar plexus, difficulties in breathing easily, and an emotional, irregular heartbeat, you can add points 180, 73, 61, 16, 0.

# Sinusitis

## 26, 50, 61, 65, 8, 124, 126, 106, 0

Sinusitis is most often linked to an allergy and is an infection that can be either acute or chronic. It can be the source of intense discomfort or pain in the forehead and even provoke high temperatures. In acute cases of sinusitis, stimulate these points several times per day and then continue the treatment with just one daily massage.

You may also practice the massage indicated under Cold.

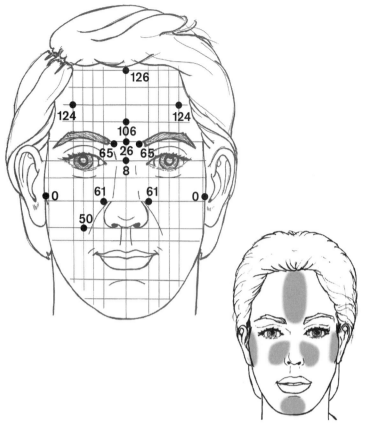

# Skin Problems

## 26, 61, 3, 19, 0

These points allow attenuation of all kinds of skin problems, from acne to eczema, psoriasis, mycosis, and so on. Stimulation of them increases natural defenses, soothes inflammations, and promotes elimination or evacuation. Also refer to each of these sicknesses individually, for each of which a specific series of points have been given.

Remember that it is necessary to drain the emunctories correctly. Overloaded liver, kidneys, and colon all contribute a great deal to skin problems.

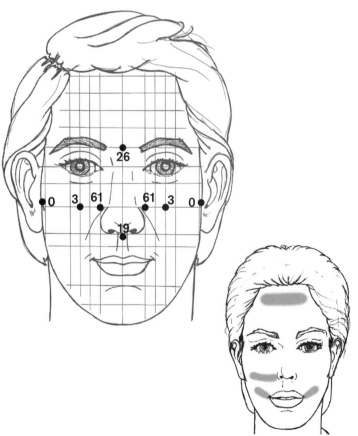

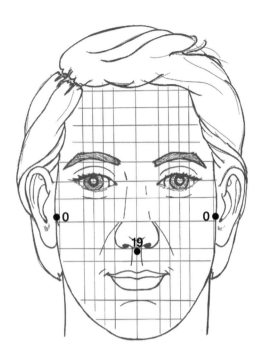

## Sleepiness
### 19, 0

The stimulation of these two points, which are always readily accessible, will be of great service in cases where you need to boost your vigilance. It can be useful when you are driving (though it may still be advisable to take a break) or in other life situations.

**Please note** that to tone up, you should stimulate point **19** upward (downward the effect is relaxing and calming).

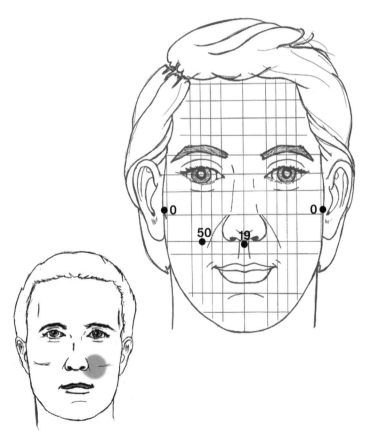

### Following a meal
### 19, 50, 0

This sequence is useful if you feel an uncontrollable desire to sleep following a heavy meal, or if you need to recover dynamism in the afternoon. Stimulate these points, which will put you back on top form quickly and restore your vigilance.

**Please note** that to tone up, you should stimulate point **19** upward (downward the effect is relaxing and calming).

## Smoking (stopping)
### 50, 19, 3, 60, 85, 127, 300, 61, 14, 124, 34, 26, 0

These days everyone knows the ravages of tobacco smoking. However, not so many people manage to give up this horrible habit! Many youngsters start smoking before puberty and this makes stopping a lot more difficult when the individual reaches adulthood. In the case where you are trying to give up smoking and feeling tempted, or suffering withdrawal symptoms, points **14** and **61** will help. It is advisable to stimulate these points several times per day, every time that the need is felt.

During the day, if you have not remembered the pressure points carefully, use this simplified method and massage the following vigorously: the nostrils, in front of the ears, the area between the lower lip and the chin, and the chin itself. Also frequently stimulate the Relaxation points described in the Basic Session given in chapter 3.

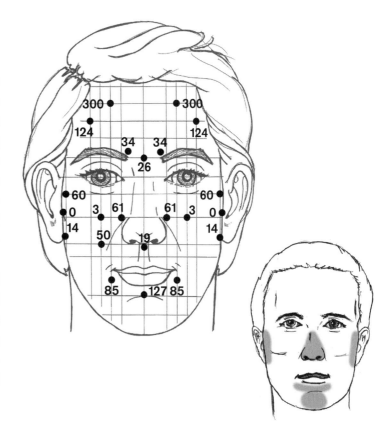

## Solar Plexus
### 180, 73, 61, 3, 0

How many times have you heard one of your friends or family complain that his or her solar plexus feels knotted, or felt this way yourself? This signifies stress, worry, anxiety, and nervous tension, with all of the attendant consequences on health and equilibrium, should the situation last! These pressure points unblock the solar plexus. They help a person to relax and breathe more easily. It is important to free up the solar plexus in order to allow improved circulation of energy to the surrounding organs: liver, gallbladder, stomach, pancreas, spleen, small intestine, and the heart, which are generally the first affected by blockages.

**Please note:** These points can often provoke perspiration.

Do not forget that wherever there is a projection of the spinal column on the face, you will always find the solar plexus about halfway along.

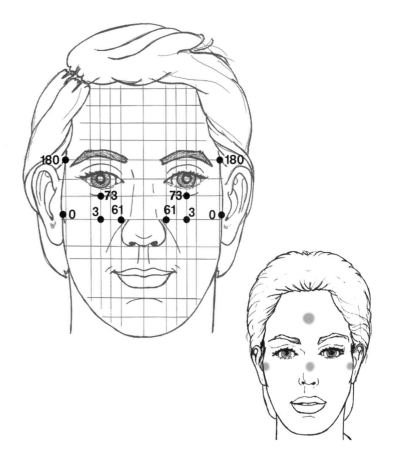

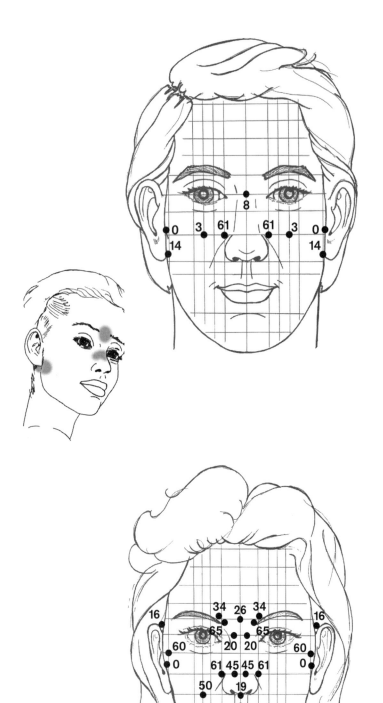

## Sore Throat, Pharyngitis
**14, 3, 61, 8, 0**

A sore throat is a simple inflammation of the throat, which can easily spread to the upper respiratory tract if not treated urgently. Quite often after a seemingly unimportant common cold, you find yourself with a faltering and changed voice and sometimes the voice disappears altogether! It can also happen that you overstrain your voice in one way or another, leading to an inflammation of the throat and making swallowing difficult. A full-blown bout of pharyngitis with a high temperature and a general feeling of sickness is on the way, with the danger of supplementary complications. It is best to do something about it at the first signs. The irritation in the throat will diminish as soon as you stimulate these pressure points.

Remember to take some magnesium chloride as well.[9]

At the first sign of a sore throat, massage the zone behind and below the earlobes. It is simple, quick, and often sufficient to prevent the situation worsening.

## Spasmophilia, Spasms, Fibromyalgia
**61, 16, 19, 20, 63, 87, 0**

**Or**

**65, 60, 50, 45, 34, 26, 0**

**(see also Tetany)**

Nowadays many people suffer from spasmophilia and fibromyalgia in varying degrees. This sickness is related to the metabolism of calcium and the nerve centers of the adrenal complex, and is characterized by various acute symptoms like lipothymia (where the sufferer has a dread of fainting), paresthesia, psychological troubles, intestinal spasms, and cramps. This can even lead to a true case of tetany. Besides the stimulation of these points, a calcium and magnesium supplement is recommended.

# Speech Difficulties
## 8, 14, 60, 65, 0

Difficulties with speaking can have several causes such as blood circulation problems around the brain, tumor, and so on. They are often linked to aging. Point 8 in particular stimulates the area of the brain involved with speech.

Also try these reflex zones, which stimulate the brain function. It is also advisable to check on the state of the liver and the gallbladder, because when there are blockages there, the situation will be worse.

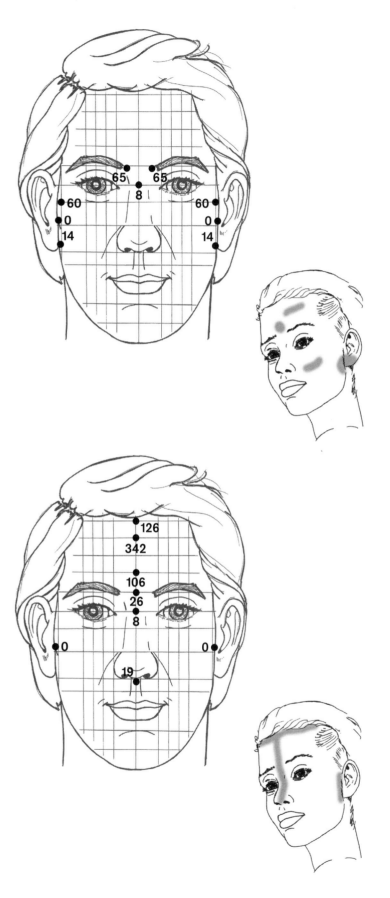

# Spinal Column
## from 19 to 126, 0

Points corresponding to each vertebra can be localized on the face. A spinal column in perfect order is a gauge or proof of good health. Therefore use these points regularly without waiting for backache to occur. If you are suffering at present, stimulate the points given below that are appropriate:

- cervical vertebrae: **8, 26, 106**
- dorsal vertebrae: **19 to 8** (on the bridge of the nose)
- lumbar vertebrae for lumbago: **342**
- stimulation of this series of points unblocks the spinal vertebrae: **126 to 19**

To restore your spinal column to full health or to make it more supple, start by stimulating points **126** and **342,** using small sweeping movements from top to bottom. Then, tapping lightly, move down the forehead and nose. Finally, repeat this moving back up again and finish with point 0 as usual.

Refer back to **Diagram 8** in chapter 2, which shows the main projections of the spinal column on the face.

In addition to the pressure points, you may stimulate all of these reflex zones.

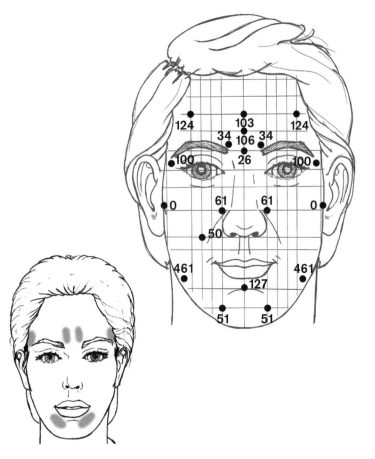

## Sprains
**61, 127, 51, 34, 26, 103, 106, 0**

### Or
**127, 124, 106, 26, 0**

Point **100** corresponds to the wrist, **461** to the ankle, and **50** to sprains of the feet or the hands. In the case of a twist or sprain, always remember to stimulate the pertinent zone, which you will find toward the central part of the chin. Then stimulate all of these points, allowing you to recover mobility of the joint much more quickly.

Add the reflex zones corresponding to the affected joint: ankle, wrist, or knee.

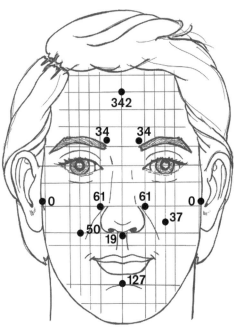

## Stiffness, Aching, and Muscle Cramps
**34, 127, 19, 61, 342, 50, 37, 0**

These points will procure quick relief whether your stiffness is muscular, caused by strenuous physical exercise, or accompanies a fever. Furthermore if you are subject to cramps and various kinds of pain caused by spasms, follow this short program regularly until the troubles disappear. You can also take a magnesium supplement (see also Spasmophilia).

To this program, you may add the zones corresponding to your troubles: the ankles, ribs, back, and so on.

## Stomach
**(see Appetite; Gastritis; Flatulence; Ulcer, Gastric)**

## Stomach Acidity

### 124, 34, 26, 39, 19, 0

This highly disagreeable symptom can be effectively treated using simple facial massage. Repeat this as much and as often as necessary using the rounded end of a ballpoint pen.

In addition to the necessary change in diet, it is naturally important to stimulate the zones corresponding to the stomach. It is advisable to include those tending to eliminate stress, which is often the main culprit for this ailment.

It is good to promote relaxation by stimulating points **124, 34, 26,** and **0**. Then go on to points **39** and **19**, finishing on point **0**. You can repeat this sequence several times a day, preferably before meals, until relief is obtained. If necessary, stimulate the points again after the meal to improve digestion.

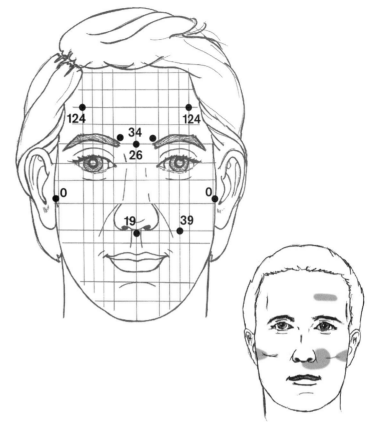

## Stress

### 17, 6, 19, 180, 124, 34, 26, 0

It is important to learn how to manage the stress that affects all of us almost daily. The causes are various: overwork, conflict, difficult or important meetings, examinations, and various worries. It is easy to learn this short sequence of points in order to be able to use it without delay in cases of need. The more you practice this the less you will really need it. Try to remember to perform some controlled breathing exercises at the same time. One exercise is to bring your attention to your breathing in, and then your breathing out, for a few seconds.

With the ends of your fingers bent as if you are about to play piano, tap all of the zones of your forehead for several seconds. You will feel revitalized and relaxed.

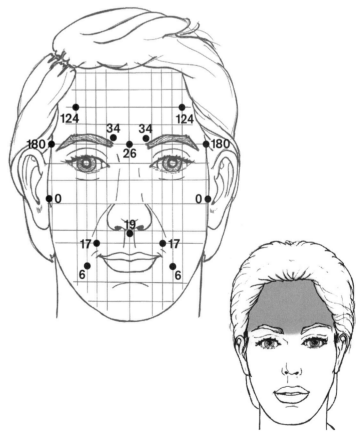

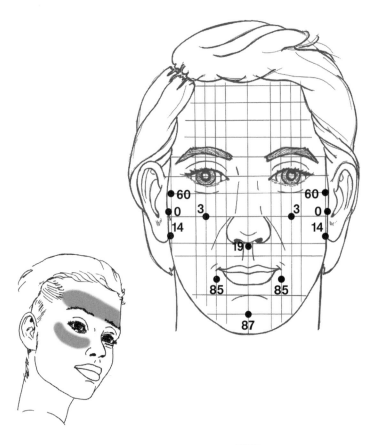

## Suffocation, Feelings of
### 19, 60, 14, 3, 85, 87, 0

This kind of disagreeable feeling can stem from various sources, which should of course be identified and treated: asthma, bronchitis, pulmonary emphysema, pectoral angina, or common spasmophilia. The stimulation of these points and zones will bring a measure of relief quickly.

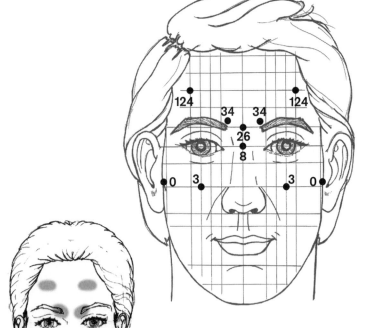

## Tachycardia (fast heartbeat)
### 34, 124, 3, 8, 26, 0

Points 8 and 26 slow the heart down. Point 8 is handily located on the nose, between the eyes, and 34 at the beginning of the eyebrows. You can easily stimulate them with your finger every time it is necessary.

These zones can be used for a quick session in case of necessity.

# Teeth

## 39, 3, 16, 43, 51, 61, 8, 34, 106, 124, 180, 0

All of these points soothe toothache. Choose the ones that seem to correspond the best. In particular:

- point **51** soothes pain
- point **15** corresponds to the jaws
- points **22** and **127** soothe the lower jaw

## Simplified procedure
### 124, 180, 61, 127, 22, 0

Stimulation of these points will not correctly treat a dental cavity or abscess, but will allow you to wait for a dentist's appointment without suffering. The result is obtained after five or ten minutes. You can also obtain relief by rubbing the zones shown on the diagram with the fingers.

You may repeat this short routine during the day as often as you like until the pain has totally disappeared. Another simple way is to lightly massage the root of the nose by pinching lightly.

# Tennis Elbow

## 97, 98, 17, 0

The syndrome of tennis elbow is a form of tendonitis which got its name from a form of overexertion affecting above all tennis players, who performed repetitive, violent actions with the playing arm. However this trouble can also plague people who spend many hours on computers, pianos, or other instruments. The result is pain in the wrist, hands, and forearms.

This is an opportunity to stimulate the reflex zones corresponding to the painful spots: wrists, hands, and forearms.

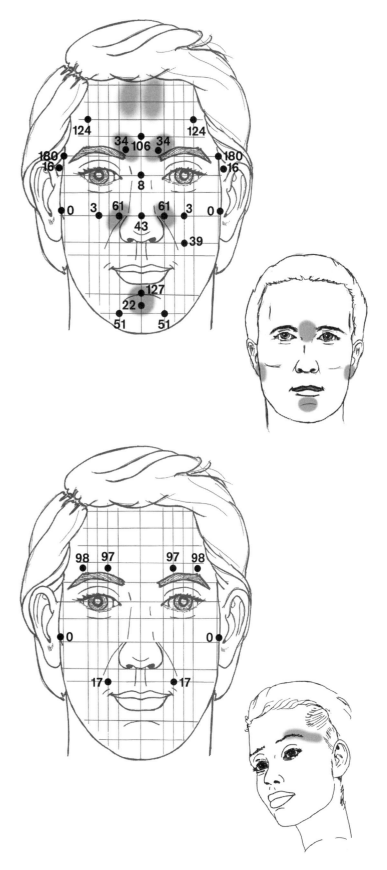

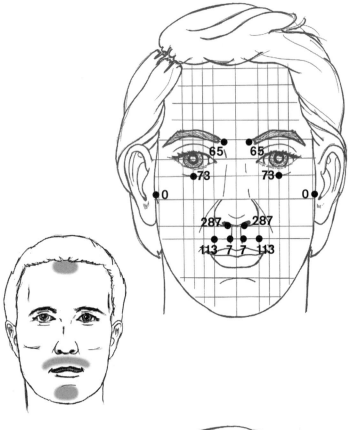

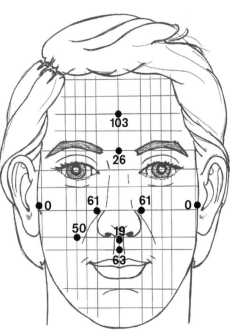

## Testicles
### 7, 113, 65, 73, 287, 0

The points given can be stimulated in all cases affecting the testicles: inflammation, hormonal insufficiency, developmental insufficiency, sterility, and impotence. (Also see corresponding headings.)

Also stimulate the reflex zones located on the chin and center of the forehead, toward the hairline.

## Tetany
### 50, 19, 63, 26, 61, 103, 0

### (see also Spasmophilia)

This is a case of contractions or cramps affecting the extremities (hands and feet). It can spread to the limbs and sometimes even to the abdomen. This trouble is essentially the same as a state of chronic spasmophilia. It usually occurs in cases of abnormally low levels of calcium in the blood due to deficiency in the diet, or in the related parathyroid function. However cases of tetany have also been recorded during certain infectious sicknesses.

Quite naturally you should add the reflex zones related to the parts of the body affected.

# Throat Inflammation

## (see also Sore Throat and Cold, as well as Cough, Laryngitis, and other ENT problems)

Using the index fingers, vigorously rub under the ears as well as vertically and horizontally in front of the lobes, as shown in the figure.

In order to stop the problem right at the start, just use the "gimmick" that everyone knows in Korea:

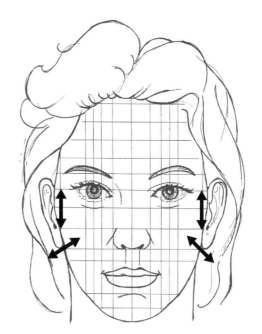

- Apply tiger balm to the neck, shoulders, and spinal column.
- Then scratch these zones thoroughly using the edge of a coin or spoon.

In case of a cough, perform the same procedure on the chest, preferably using white tiger balm.

Pressure points can also be stimulated using the end of a ballpoint pen dipped in tiger balm.

# Thyroid Regulation

## 7, 8, 14, 39, 100, 0

### As well as
### 14, 15, 26, 8, 20, 0

Here it is a question of treating an erratic thyroid function that oscillates from insufficient to over-active. These points can be used without danger, whichever of the two problems affects you most: hyperthyroidism or hypothyroidism. Whatever the case, the problem should be corrected because it can provoke other disorders. Before taking hormone therapy, which is generally for life, try stimulating these points.

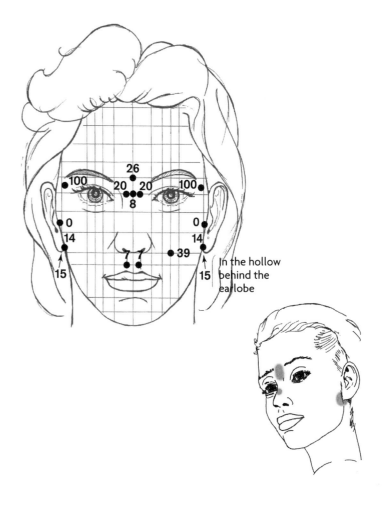

### Hypothyroidism: Add 15 as well as Toning Up points.

If you suffer from hypothyroidism, vigorously massage the angle of the jaw and the nose root. Repeat this several times per day until a result is obtained.

# Tinnitus
## (see Ears, Buzzing in)

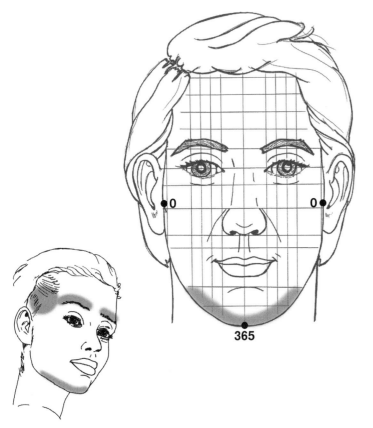

# Toes
## 365, 0, and edge of lower jaw

In the case of an injury, sprain, or fracture of a toe, the stimulation of point 365 should help immediately. From this point, move along the bony edge of the lower jaw, with the big toe in the middle and the toes represented on either side, in order.

There are other points corresponding to the toes. Try to find which are the most responsive.

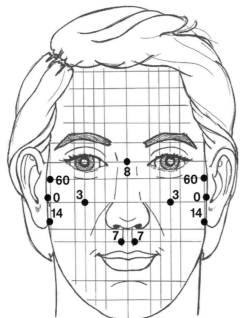

# Tongue Cramp
## 7, 60, 3, 8, 14, 0

Who has never suffered from the disagreeable experience of a tongue cramp that strikes right in the middle of a meal? If you massage points 7 and 60 you will obtain rapid relief.

## Toning Up (general)
### 127, 19, 26, 103, 126, 1, 0

These points form part of the Basic Session of Dien' Cham' that has been dealt with previously. They will boost life energy, tissue formation, maintenance, and replacement. They also warm up the body and prepare the body's natural defenses. It is therefore extremely useful to stimulate these points, which are easy to remember due to their alignment on the face centerline. This can be done as soon as you awake, during the day in case of tiredness, or whenever you just lack a bit of punch. These points are recommended for people suffering from obesity as well as from hypothyroidism.

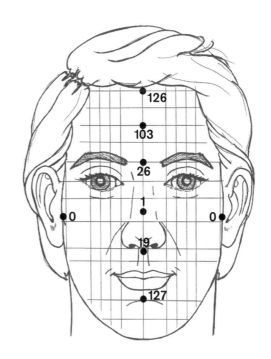

## Tonsillitis
### (see Sore Throat)

## Ulcer, Gastric
### 61, 64, 74, 39, 34, 17, 0

### (see also Gastritis)

An ulcer manifests by a sharp pain in the few minutes following a meal. This pain is accompanied by nausea, vomiting, and even bleeding. The consumption of tobacco and alcohol, certain medicines, excess coffee or tea, overwork, stress, and worry are all conducive to gastric ulcers. The points given here favor healing of the ulcerated stomach lining. Their anti-inflammatory and anti-infectious qualities are very useful with this kind of problem, especially if it is linked with the presence of bacteria.

In case of hemorrhage from the stomach: points 37, 16, 61, 50, 0.

Also stimulate reflex zones corresponding to the stomach, on the left of the nose and on the forehead.

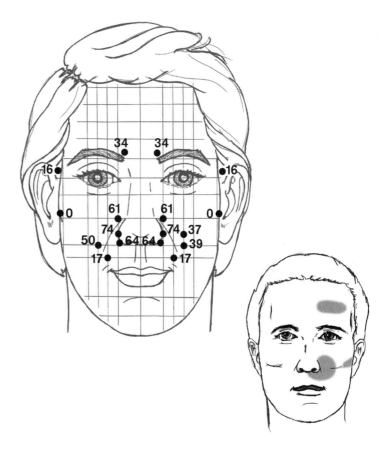

## Ulcer of the Mouth, Thrush, Aphtha

**8, 14, 15, 0**

Stimulate these few points as soon as the ulcers start appearing or for any trouble affecting the mouth. Also advisable is a mouthwash using magnesium chloride (about 0.70 ounce for a quart of water) and eating lighter foods!

To these points you can also profitably add the digestive zones which are obviously linked to this disorder; stomach, gallbladder, and intestines.

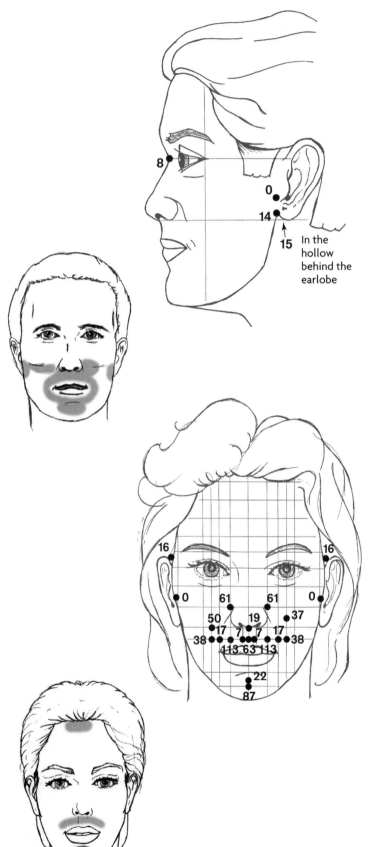

## Uterine Fibroids

**7, 19, 63, 16, 17, 22, 87, 0**

**As well as**

**7, 113, 63, 38, 50, 37, 61, 0**

This common complaint is linked to hormonal imbalance. Instead of resigning yourself to this as well as the allied problems such as over-abundant periods, untimely bleeding, period pain, and tiredness associated with anemia, just try these points, which are often very effective and can help you to avoid surgery. Vertically sweep all of the area above the upper lip and add the points on the chin. Point **16** will control hemorrhage due to the presence of a fibroid. Often points **7** and **113** will also help them disappear.

# Uterine Problems

**63, 19, 22, 87, 287, 0**

**Or**
**7, 37, 65, 113, 156, 0**

**(see also Uterine Fibroids, Periods, and Ptosis or Prolapse of the Uterus)**

These points can be stimulated whatever the problem with the uterus. Cases of fibroids, ptosis, endometriosis, menorrhagia or excess bleeding during periods, amenorrhea or abnormal absence of periods, dysmenorrhea or pain during periods, can all be improved in this way. Please refer to the various entries for these. These two series of points can be used alternately with those found on the relevant pages.

Of course you should also stimulate the reflex zones located on the upper lip, nostrils, chin, and top of the forehead.

# Vaginal Discharge, Leucorrhea

**1, 3, 7, 43, 61, 37, 63, 87, 127, 22, 287, 16, 0**

This unpleasant problem of a white discharge can be improved by regular stimulation of these points. This results in an astringent effect, which is linked to the hormone regulating system. Point 0 stimulates life energy in fact. To this we can add a general stimulation of the genital organs described in Contraception in order to treat the problem as a whole.

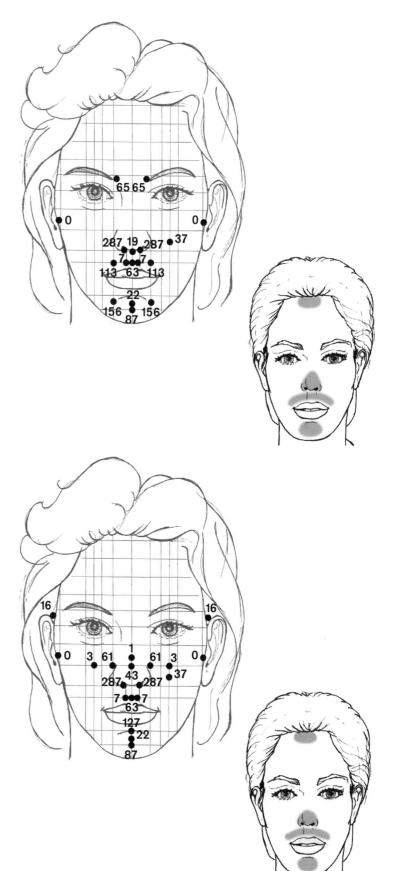

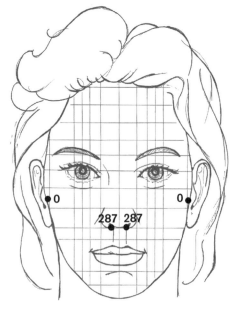

## Vaginal Dryness
### 287, 0

This disagreeable phenomenon, which is often linked to menopause or one of the after effects of surgery, can easily be corrected by stimulation of this point.

Also practice massage of the zones around the lips and nostrils as indicated under Contraception. Results should be excellent!

Before sexual relations:

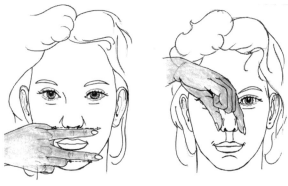

- Using the index and middle finger of the right hand, rub the area surrounding the mouth about 200 times, back and forth.
- Pinch the nostrils at the base and move toward the tip of the nose about 200 times.

You should feel an agreeable warmth in the pelvic zone.

## Vaginal Inflammation
### 61, 60, 37, 50, 17, 38, 63, 7, 87, 0

There are few problems that are as disagreeable as this burning sensation in a sensitive place! Most of the time this kind of inflammation is linked to mycosis or sometimes an allergy. A tendency to vaginal dryness can also be the cause.

Stimulate these points for a few minutes. You should also remember to wear white cotton underwear, take a vitamin E supplement and stop using soap for intimate hygiene.

Local application of a little St John's Wort oil generally soothes this kind of problem.

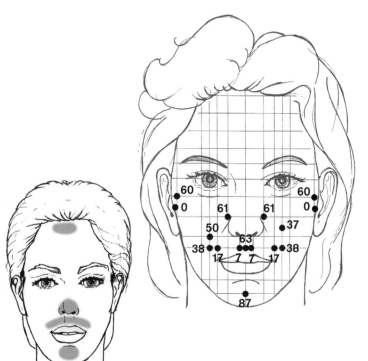

# Vaginitis, Vaginismus
## 19, 63, 50, 156, 127, 0

Vaginitis is an inflammation of the vagina. Vaginismus consists of a painful muscular spasm in the vagina, which makes sexual relations so painful they are often impossible. The most frequent causes are psychological, such as bad or frightening past experiences related to surgery, childbirth, or sexual aggression. The symptoms include vaginal dryness and showing lack of sexual desire for a partner. In addition, physiological problems, like a cyst or metritis, can provoke a deep-seated pain. The stimulation of these points can help attenuate the pain, but where necessary you should also treat the causes by reference to the relevant entry.

Also perform the massage indicated under Contraception a few minutes preceding sexual intercourse. Results are usually excellent after a few sessions.

Also stimulate reflex zones located on the chin, high on the forehead, nostrils, and upper lip.

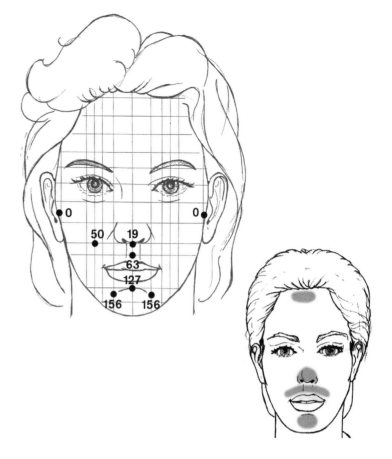

# Varicose Veins
## (see Legs, Blood Circulation)

# Vertigo, Dizziness
## 63, 34, 106, 65, 60, 8, 0

Most of the time dizziness or vertigo is benign but it can also be an advance sign of a more serious sickness. Consult a physician if symptoms persist or if the vertigo is accompanied by nausea and vomiting. Common benign causes include rapid changes of position, anemia, low blood pressure, poor blood circulation around the brain, excessively hot weather, and high altitude. In all of these cases stimulation of these points will be useful.

# Voice, Loss of
## (see Laryngitis)

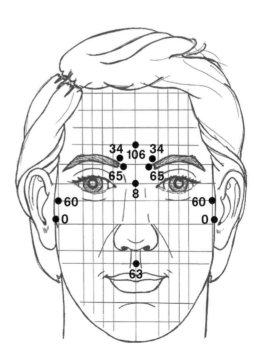

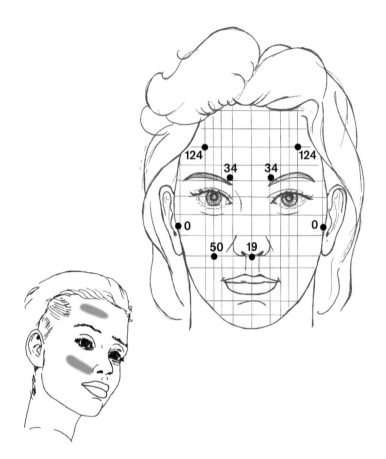

# Vomiting
## 50, 19, 34, 124, 0

There are many causes of vomiting, including overeating or drinking, if the stomach is sensitive, tainted food that the body is naturally trying to reject, a blocked appendix, kidney stones, gastro-enteritis, and various other infectious conditions. The body is just attempting to eliminate toxins and mucus that is bothering it. There is also the case of the well-known morning sickness of pregnant women during the first few weeks.

Stimulation of the points indicated effectively stops vomiting but it is not always the best course of action. Sometimes it is better to do nothing, even encouraging the vomiting by stimulating the end of the nose. (If you are treating someone else, remember to stand to the side and not opposite!) We must try to use our natural intuition and wisdom.

### Provoking Vomiting: Point 19

This point can provoke the vomiting or stop it, depending on the case. This property renders the point very useful, such as in the case of a child that has got something stuck in his or her windpipe, and who seems to be suffocating. In this case it is recommended to strongly stimulate this point, which will provoke rejection of the object.

### Warning
If you are pregnant avoid stimulating point 19!

## Warts

### 26, 20, 50, 3, 51, 0

These small but ugly-looking growths can often be made to disappear by using these points often. Stress often plays a role in warts, especially the flatter kind (verruca plana). Remember to regularly massage the Relaxation points given in the Basic Session in chapter 3.

It is also advisable to supplement your diet with a calcium and magnesium complement. It is often effective to apply fresh sap from the Greater Celandine or fig.

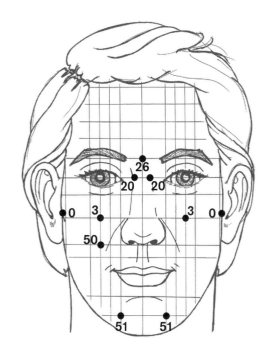

## Water Retention

### (see Cellulitis)

## Worms, Intestinal; Tapeworms

### 19, 41, 43, 45, 3, 38, 39, 126, 127, 130, 365, 0

All of these points favor the elimination of intestinal parasites, which often appear in children, but also sometimes adults. With this goal in mind it is also important to stimulate the liver function as well as the gallbladder, as these are often a contributory cause when these parasites have developed. Stimulation is more effective if performed in the evening. Point **127** is particularly advised in cases of tapeworm because it favors expulsion. Massage should last at least ten minutes.

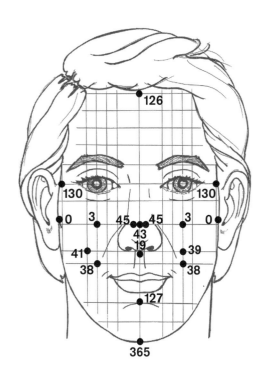

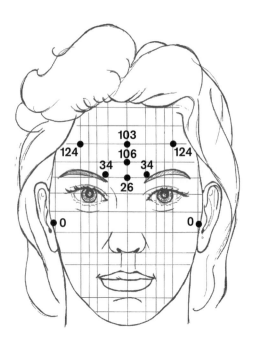

## Wrinkles
### 124, 34, 26, 103, 106, 0

A simple facial massage will have the important benefit of erasing newly appearing wrinkles and attenuating those that are already deep. This is in addition to the general toning up of the body it procures. This stimulation can be performed with the end of the fingers, a ballpoint pen, or a roller, and will make you look healthier as it improves local blood circulation. Do not worry about making blotchiness worse. On the contrary, it will be improved by massage of the points advised for blood circulation difficulties. Do not hesitate to use them as often as possible!

# 5

# Correspondences, Effects, and Indications for Dien' Cham' Points

This chapter is devoted to the correspondences, main effects, and main therapeutic indications for the points in this book, taken one by one. As mentioned earlier, contrary to other kinds of reflexology, each Dien' Cham' point has several correspondences with multiple effects.

Often it will be handier for you to consult this chapter during your sessions, rather than search **Diagram 1** for a point you have forgotten. On the other hand, it would be premature for you to read this during your first steps. You would also be ill advised to try to memorize all of the information set down here.

Remember that while facytherapy includes 500 reflex points just on the face, Dien' Cham' only has 57! I have retained the numbers traditionally reserved for these points in order to forestall confusion. So do not be surprised to find some missing when, for example, we jump from 3 to 6, 26 to 34, or even from point 365 to 461!

For each point you will find the following:

- The various correspondences, in bold type
- The main effects
- The main indications, which are usually several
- Details regarding point location and advice on how to massage with respect to direction, kind of stimulation, and so on in italics

Each point is also illustrated with a diagram showing precisely where it is located. This will enable you to locate each point easily and without error.

# 0

**Solar plexus, kidneys, ears, eyes, mouth, nose, spinal column, adrenal glands, arms, legs, genitals, stomach**

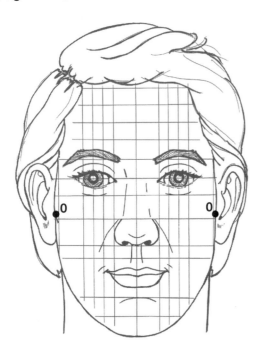

This is the point with which a session should begin—above all in cases where the person is tired or weak—and always ends it. It regulates all body functions. If you have stimulated a point excessively which did not need it, or if you make a mistake, by for example increasing blood pressure in someone with high blood pressure, this point will enable you to correct yourself. Therefore please get into the habit of terminating on this point, located in front of the ear, systematically. Remember to stimulate it if you obtain a reaction that appears too strong.

*This point is located in the hollow in front of the ear. However most of the time it is better to massage the whole zone vertically.*

- *From top to bottom, if you want to relax everything, make everything peaceful*
- *From bottom to top, if you primarily want to tone up*

## Main Effects

- Regulates blood pressure, whether low or high
- Relaxes the nervous system
- Regulates the heartbeat
- Relieves pain
- Helps digestion
- Tones up the veins by contracting them
- Slows down perspiration when it is excessive
- Stops hemorrhage
- Stops the nose from running and other excess secretions
- Warms up the body
- Tones up the body
- Helps uterus contraction during childbirth and in cases of hemorrhage from the uterus
- Increases natural defenses
- Increases sexual energy
- Tones up the kidney function
- Stimulates the life force

## Main Indications

- Tiredness
- Asthenia
- Sexual weakness
- Premature ejaculation
- Colds
- Chills
- High blood pressure
- Low blood pressure
- Lumbar pain
- Spots or pimples
- Perspiration of the hands
- Perspiration of the feet
- Tachycardia
- Ears (deafness, buzzing, and earache)
- Eyes (problems with sight)
- Sinusitis
- Allergies
- Nicotine poisoning
- Drug side effects
- Drug rehabilitation
- Paralysis

- Stomach
- Vaginal discharge
- Burns or scalding from hot water

# 1

## Lumbar vertebrae, adrenal glands, sexuality

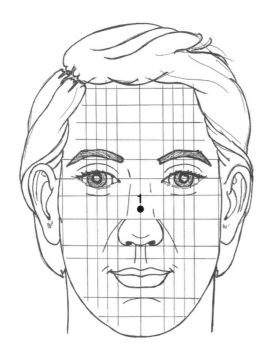

**Main Effects**
- Relaxes
- Regulates the heartbeat
- Increases sexual energy
- Decreases loss of secretions
- Relieves lumbar pain
- Increases blood pressure–hypertensive effect
- Increases energy
- Tones up the body
- Warms up the body

**Main Indications**
- Physical tiredness
- Nervous exhaustion
- Irregular heartbeat: arrhythmia, tachycardia
- Heart fatigue
- Lumbar pain
- Difficulties in straightening body
- Weak sex drive
- Vaginal discharge (leucorrhoea)
- Over-abundant periods (hypermenorrhoea)
- Abdominal pain
- Diarrhea
- Piles

This point can be of great use if you are always tired and suffer from chronic low blood pressure. Stimulating this point raises the blood pressure by two or three points in just a few seconds! (This is why we warn against its use in subjects with high blood pressure. In this case it would be dangerous to stimulate this point.)

*This delicate point (located on the end of the nose in the center of a small depression) must be stimulated alone with a small amplitude rubbing movement on the spot, preferably with the rounded end of a ballpoint pen.*

> **Warning**
>
> Do not stimulate this point in cases of high blood pressure.

*always tired and suffer from chronic low blood pressure.*

*To raises the blood pressure*

*not for High Pressure*

## 3
### Lungs, heart (only on left side), temples, chest

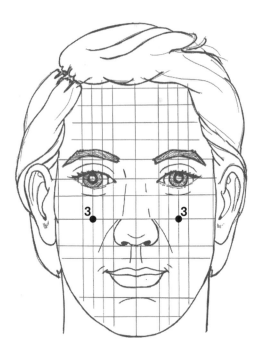

This point will be very useful if you often have bronchitis or lung ailments, heart trouble, or if you want to give up smoking.

Stimulation will enable you to rapidly lower your blood pressure by several points if you are suffering from high blood pressure.

*Massage this point using sweeping movements toward the ears or stimulate it individually.*

### Warning
Do not stimulate this point in cases of low blood pressure.

## Main Effects
- All cardiac troubles
- Relaxation
- Drops blood pressure (hypotensive effect)
- Drops temperature, useful in cases of high fever
- Dissipates energy
- Reduces secretion from the mucous membranes
- Eases pain
- Diuretic
- Helps breathing

## Main Indications
- Insomnia
- Muscular cramps or spasms
- High blood pressure
- Colds with fever
- Headaches
- Chest pain
- Facial paralysis
- Pain in temples
- Asthma
- Coughing
- Hot breath
- Toothache
- Sinusitis
- Blocked nose
- Hot, dark-colored urine
- Constipation with urinary deficiency
- Excessive perspiration from the hands
- Skin problems
- Swollen face
- Eyesight problems
- Red eyes
- Stinging eyes

## 6

### Calves, heart

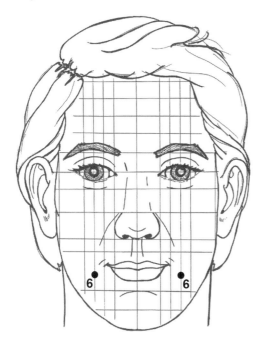

This is another useful point to know in cases of chronic tiredness and low blood pressure.

*The point can be stimulated alone, especially in cases of low blood pressure, or associated with point 85 in a small sweeping movement toward the center of the chin.*

> **Warning**
>
> Do not stimulate this point in cases of high blood pressure!

### Main Effects

- Rapidly increases blood pressure in the arteries
- Relieves pain in the calves
- Improves eyesight
- Tones up the body
- Stops hemorrhage
- Tones up the heart

### Main Indications

- Low blood pressure
- Calf muscle cramp
- Diminished eyesight
- Tiredness

## 7

### Pancreas, ovaries, prostate gland, genitals and their functions, uterus

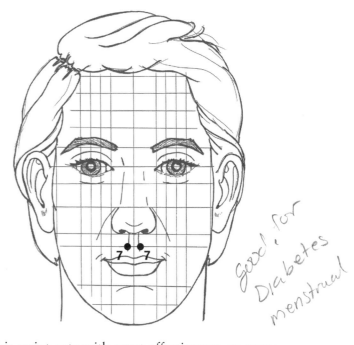

Good for
Diabetes
menstrual

This point acts with great effectiveness on menstrual or period problems, calms cystitis, and helps with digestion, useful when too much food has been consumed or cases of sugar abuse. People with diabetes will find it beneficial to use this point regularly.

*This point is located on the axis passing through the center of the nostrils. Using a sharp instrument or the rounded end of a ballpoint pen, you can either massage the point by itself, or perform a sweeping movement vertically or horizontally over the whole area situated between the upper lip and the bottom of the nose.*

## Main Effects

- Bolsters natural defenses
- Improves blood circulation
- Frees up energy circulation
- Warms up the body
- Procures natural anti-inflammatory effect
- Regulates secretions
- Eliminates toxins
- Relieves abdominal pain (periods, ovaries, prostate glands, with tendencies to spread to the thighs)
- Increases sexual energy

## Main Indications

- Diabetes
- Allergies
- Over-abundant and irregular periods
- Painful periods
- Inflammations
- Vaginal discharge (leucorrhea)
- Ovaries
- Prostate gland
- Thigh pain
- Cystitis
- Low sexual energy
- Sinusitis
- Digestive problems
- Flatulence
- Colitis
- Blockages of the tongue
- Goiter

# 8

## Heart, cervical vertebrae, throat, thyroid glands, neck, jaws, teeth, tongue

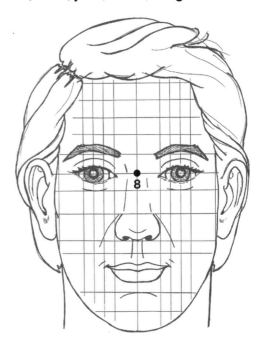

This point—which is located on the Heart Meridian—slows the heartbeat, which is useful for tachycardia, lowers blood pressure, unblocks cervical vertebrae, and treats sore throats. It also helps to regulate the thyroid function.

*Steady your fingers on the nose and stimulate using small circular movements. Be careful not to slip toward the eyes!*

> **Warning**
> Do not stimulate this point in cases of low blood pressure!

## Main Effects

- Relaxes
- Reduces blood pressure
- Drops body temperature
- Regulates perspiration
- Promotes free circulation of energy
- Relieves cervical and back pain caused by inflammation
- Regulates cardiac function

**Main Indications**

- Insomnia caused by nightmares
- High blood pressure
- Cervical vertebrae pain
- Blockages at level of neck, stiff neck
- Inflammation of the tongue
- Speech difficulties
- Inflammation around jaws
- Gingivitis
- Sore throat
- Sinusitis
- Goiter, thyroid problems
- Troubled eyesight
- Irritability
- Irregularity of heartbeat
- Heart problems

## 14

### Ears, throat, parotid glands, hypothyroidism (or thyroid insufficiency)

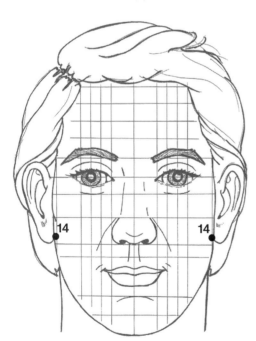

This point treats deafness and earache, and unblocks the jaw (MTA).

*This point is located at the junction of the earlobe and the face and must be massaged horizontally just under the lobe.*

> **Warning**
>
> Do not stimulate this point in cases of low blood pressure!

**Main Effects**

- Analgesic
- Lowers body temperature
- Reduces blood pressure
- Anti-inflammatory
- Helps digestion
- Promotes salivation
- Relaxes

**Main Indications**

- Stomachache
- Toothache
- Pain in jaw
- Headache
- Head cold with fever
- Malaria
- High blood pressure
- Goiter
- Coughing
- Laryngitis
- Earache
- Inflammations of face
- Indigestion
- Difficulty with swallowing
- Loss of appetite
- Insomnia

## 15
### Ears, jaws, spinal column, gums

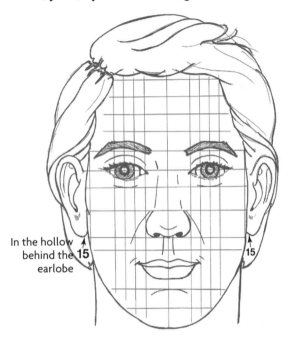

In the hollow behind the earlobe **15**     **15**

When this point is stimulated it reduces blood pressure by three or four points and so it is important to avoid this point in cases of low blood pressure! It is also effective in cases of thyroid gland insufficiency.

*This point is located in the hollow just behind the earlobe between the jaw and the base of the skull. It can be stimulated alone, or in association with point 14. If you wish to do the latter, massage the two points by rubbing horizontally, then vertically. Finish up with point 0.*

### Main Effects
- Strongly reduces blood pressure
- Lowers body temperature
- Relaxes
- Relieves pain
- Anti-inflammatory
- Irrigates the brain

### Main Indications
- High blood pressure
- Perspiration caused by high blood pressure
- Bouts of flu
- Malaria
- Insomnia
- Headaches
- Gingivitis
- Ear problems, earache
- Deafness
- Buzzing in the ears
- Blocked jaws, MTA
- Feeling cold
- Spinal column
- Hypothyroidism

## 16
### Ears, hemorrhage, heart, eyes

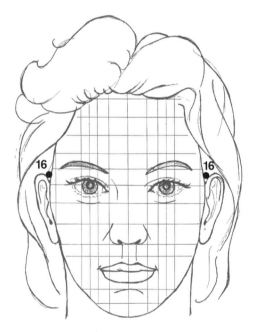

**16**     **16**

The stimulation of this very important point rapidly decreases or stops excess loss of body fluids such as internal or external hemorrhage, over-abundant menstrual loss, possibly provoked by fibroids, excessive perspiration, runny nose, outbursts of crying, and so on.

*Stimulate this point by massaging in small circles, with a finger or end of a ballpoint pen.*

## Main Effects

- Regulates secretions
- Regulates muscular contraction
- Relaxes muscles
- Lowers body temperature
- Reduces blood pressure
- Relieves eye pain
- Relieves headaches
- Stops hemorrhage of all kinds
- Anti-inflammatory

## Main Indications

- Excess crying
- Excess perspiration
- Internal and external hemorrhage
- Insomnia
- Fever
- Head cold
- High blood pressure in the eye causing pain
- High blood pressure
- Headache
- Toothache
- Pain around eyes
- Cervical vertebrae pain
- Insect bites
- Blocked arm

# 17

## Adrenal glands, colon, kidneys, thighs, hips (action similar to corticoids)

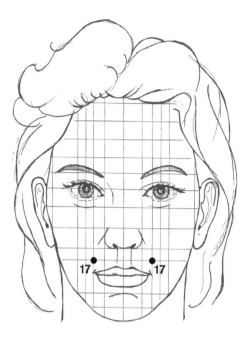

Stimulation of this point liberates what can be called natural corticoids, with well-known anti-inflammatory qualities. The relationship with the pelvic area means that it has many uses.

*You can stimulate this point by vertical sweeping movements, either independently of any others, or in association with all of the points located in the area.*

### Warning

Do not stimulate this point in cases of cancer (above all of the stomach)!

## Main Effects

- Warms up body
- Tones up kidneys
- Regulates blood pressure
- Reduces secretions
- Dissolves mucus
- Stops hemorrhage

- Anti-allergic
- Antibiotic
- Anti-infectious
- Relieves pain from inflammations
- Boosts body energy
- Calms pain from colitis
- Calms acute pain
- Calms itching
- Relaxes thighs and hips
- Regulates muscular contraction
- Relaxes muscles

**Main Indications**
- Allergies
- Infections
- Sensitivity to cold
- Colitis
- Colitis with spasms
- Diarrhea and dysentery
- Running nose
- Productive cough
- Excess perspiration
- Excess menstrual flow
- Hemorrhage from uterus
- Gynecological problems
- Neuralgia
- Rheumatism, arthritis
- Asthma
- Weak kidney function caused by fatty deposits
- Tiredness, asthenia
- Low blood pressure
- Overwork
- Stress
- Apathy and laziness
- Pruritis
- Eczema
- Burns
- Herpes zona

# 19

## Heart, lungs, nose, liver, stomach, colon, lower abdomen, corresponds to Yang Governing Vessel

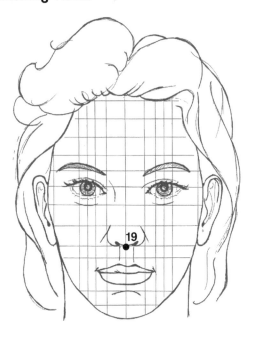

This point can be of great utility. It increases blood pressure and energy, calms stomach pain and constipation, stops hiccups and vomiting, and provokes contraction of the uterus. It also has the effect of rejecting foreign items swallowed in error, which can be useful for many parents! It is well known by those that practice judo, as it is a resuscitation point, which boosts and tones up the heart. Do not hesitate to use it in cases of fainting.

*Points located under the nose must be stimulated vertically.*

### Warning

Do not stimulate this point in cases of high blood pressure!

Stimulation of this point is prohibited in the case of pregnant women, unless they are about to give birth (in which case it favors contractions).

## Main Effects

- Regulates cardiac function
- Produces and increases secretion of adrenalin
- Resuscitates
- Tones up
- Facilitates breathing
- Brightens the mind
- Warms up body
- Increases energy
- Arouses Chi
- Increases sexual energy
- Develops virility
- Stimulates gastric secretions
- Promotes peristaltic movements of intestines
- Regulates muscular contractions
- Facilitates or stops vomiting
- Increases contraction of the uterus

## Main Indications

- Cardiac problems
- Drug-induced shock
- Fainting
- Resuscitation after drowning
- Suffocation following choking on an object
- Epilepsy
- Difficulty with breathing or asthma
- Sleepiness
- Lack of energy
- Nervous depression
- Sexual weakness
- Stomach pain
- Colitis
- Constipation
- Piles
- Giving birth
- Nausea, vomiting
- Lumbar pain
- Drugs (helps elimination of poisons)

# 20

## Cervical vertebrae, throat, eyes, neck, parathyroid glands

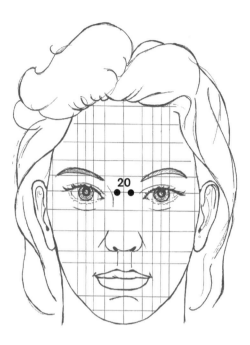

This point acts mainly on problems of decalcification.

*It is located on both sides of point 8 (at the center of the nose root), a short distance away. Stimulate this point with the rounded end of a ballpoint pen, or the steel tip of a roller.*

*You can also simply squeeze these points between thumb and index finger for a few seconds.*

## Main Effects

- Remineralizes
- Stimulates parathyroid glands
- Soothes the eyes
- Stimulates circulation around brain
- Soothes the throat
- Relieves tension in the neck
- Relaxes

**Main Indications**

- Osteoporosis
- Demineralization
- Headaches
- Circulation around brain
- Rickets
- Fractures of various sorts
- Tired eyes
- Sore throats

**Main Effects**

- Arouses the Chi
- Stops excessive secretions
- Relieves bladder pain
- Tones up bladder
- Soothes prostate trouble
- Strengthens natural defenses
- Boosts energy
- Soothes pain in pelvic region
- Calms colic pain

## 22

### Bladder, teeth, pelvic region, prostate gland, small intestine, uterus

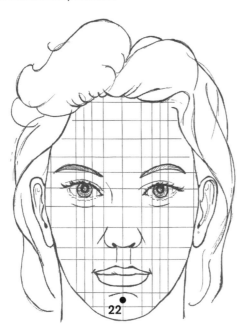

**Main Indications**

- Painful diarrhea
- Dysentery
- Dental pain, above all in lower jaw
- Flatulence
- Indigestion
- Cystitis (associated with point **17**)
- Ptosis or descent of the bladder
- Ptosis of the uterus
- Excess menstrual flow
- Irregular periods
- Prostate trouble
- Vaginal discharge or leucorrhoea
- Difficulties with urination
- Tiredness, asthenia
- Apathy

This point has an action on all problems relative to the bladder: inflammation, cystitis, ptosis or descent of the bladder, urinary incontinence and bedwetting, and so on.

*You can stimulate this point alone, or perform vertical sweeping movements over the zone linking point 22 with point 87.*

## 26

**Cervical vertebrae, throat, sinus, pituitary gland, parasympathetic nerve, pineal gland**

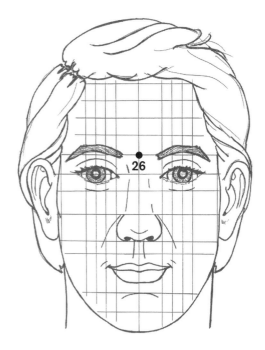

This is the point corresponding to the third eye. It calms an agitated mind, but can also refresh it and acts on psychological balance in general. However, I advise you not to stimulate it too much! This special point has so many indications and is so reactive that overstimulation can easily produce an effect opposite of the one desired. Try with a short stimulation, then adapt. This point acts like aspirin on pains and fevers.

*Stimulate using repeated small movements, from the top down.*

> **Warning**
>
> Do not stimulate this point in cases of low blood pressure!

### Main Effects
- Relaxes
- Soothes pain
- Antiseptic
- Soothes itching
- Regulates heartbeat
- Strongly reduces blood pressure
- Rapidly reduces body temperature
- Moderates spasmophilia
- Increases diuresis
- Increases secretions
- Detoxifies
- Promotes elimination of alcohol
- Calms sexual craving

### Main Indications
- Insomnia
- Neurasthenia
- Memory lapse
- Epilepsy
- Trembling
- Parkinson's disease
- Hiccups
- Spasms, tetany
- Headaches
- Burns
- Grazes
- Tachycardia
- High blood pressure
- Fever
- Head colds
- Giddiness or dizziness
- Malaria
- Anuresis (difficulties with urination)
- Blocked nose
- Eczema
- Itching
- Alcohol poisoning
- Nausea
- Asthma
- Snake bites
- Bee or scorpion stings
- Anesthesia point (cauterization of the nose, tonsils)

## 34
**Shoulders, arms (along the eyebrows from point 34), feet, sinuses, eyes, heart, optical nerve**

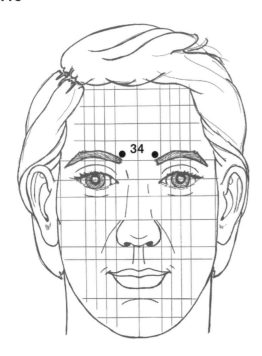

This point relaxes the nervous system and promotes sleep (for use in cases of insomnia).

*The region between points 34 and 180 should be stimulated by repeatedly lightly pressing along the eyebrow, moving from the center and along the orbit.*

### Main Effects
- Calms the nervous system
- Soothes pain
- Improves eyesight
- Relaxes muscles
- Regulates cardiac function

### Main Indications
- Insomnia (in association with point **124**)
- Nervous depression
- Headaches

- Pain in feet and toes
- Shoulder pain
- Stomachache and gastritis
- Toothache
- Poor eyesight
- Cramps and spasms
- Vomiting and nausea
- Arrhythmia
- Tachycardia

## 37
**Spleen, blood circulation, digestion, prostate gland, trigeminal nerve**

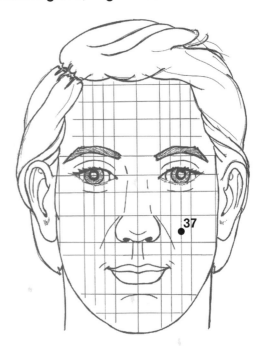

This point is located on the Spleen Meridian and is useful in cases of a depressed immune system, heavy legs, and lack of energy.

*Massage the point alone, or vertically, associating it with point 39. To stimulate these points together, press the ballpoint pen upward and obliquely inward.*

## Main Effects

- Increases natural defenses
- Stops hemorrhage
- Promotes circulation of blood
- Promotes circulation of energy
- Improves digestion
- Soothes pain in the region of the spleen
- Dissolves mucus
- Corrects urinary problems

## Main Indications

- Heavy periods
- Hemorrhage stomach (associated with points **16, 61,** and **50**)
- Heavy legs and arms
- Insensitivity of legs and arms
- Pins and needles
- Nervous tiredness
- Physical tiredness
- Difficult digestion
- Mucus
- Bedwetting
- Incontinence
- Water retention, edema
- Coughing
- Asthma
- Heavy head
- Facial paralysis
- Facial neuralgia
- Anemia

# 38

## Knees, thighs, ribs, middle fingers, kidneys, colon, and antibiotic effect

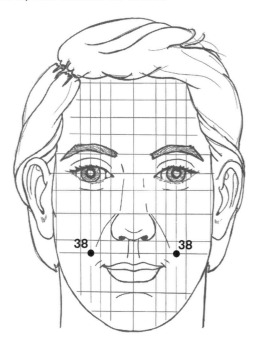

Apart from the beneficial effects in dealing with typical knee problems like arthrosis and accidents, stimulation of this point liberates natural antibiotic substances. This is of great use in cases of infection of many kinds, wherever they happen to be located.

*This point should be stimulated obliquely, toward the corners of the mouth. The "knee" zones stretch over an inch or so from the corners of the mouth when you smile, toward the ears.*

*You can also vigorously massage the two sides of the mouth vertically, and then incorporate point 38.*

## Main Effects

- Stops inflammation
- Detoxifies
- Helps intestinal transit
- Soothes thigh pain
- Soothes rib pain
- Soothes knee pain

- Connects to the middle finger
- Alleviates flatulence (intestinal wind)
- Fights against infection

**Main Indications**
- Inflammatory skin ailments
- Boils and abscesses
- Earache
- Sinusitis
- Gingivitis
- Constipation
- Thigh, rib, knee, or middle finger pain
- Difficulties voiding intestinal wind following an operation (together with point **19**)
- Fever
- Lumbar pain

# 39
## Stomach, colon, thyroid gland, trigeminal nerve, breast, index finger

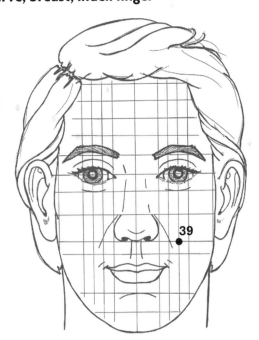

This point is located on the Stomach Meridian and improves all problems related to digestion

such as gastritis and heartburn, or excess stomach acidity.

*This point is often associated with point 37, located just below. Perform small downward massage movements from top to bottom.*

**Main Effects**
- Soothes stomach
- Soothes pain linked to stomach tumors
- Helps digestion
- Index finger pain
- Anti-inflammatory
- Reduces blood pressure
- Reduces fever

**Main Indications**
- Stomachache
- Slow digestion
- Index finger pain
- Acne
- Gingivitis
- Inflammation of the lips
- High blood pressure
- Toothache
- Facial neuralgia
- Facial paralysis
- Foot pain caused by sciatica
- Nose sicknesses
- Sinusitis
- Runny or blocked nose
- Mastitis
- Mastitis following pregnancy (together with point 73)
- Stimulates production of milk
- Thyroid trouble
- Lack of appetite

## 41

### Gall bladder (even after surgical removal), cholesterol

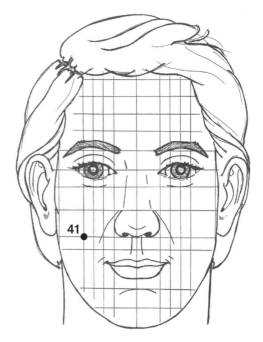

This point is a good regulator of digestion and cholesterol level.

*A small horizontal rubbing movement at the level of the base of the nose will associate it with point 50, corresponding to the liver. If you want to stimulate this point alone, push in the end of your instrument or ballpoint pen obliquely upward.*

### Main Effects

- Relieves pain
- Regulates stomach acid production
- Alleviates stomach pain
- Alleviates liver pain
- Alleviates gall bladder pain
- Regulates secretion of bile
- Regulates cholesterol level
- Reduces blood pressure
- Soothes cervical vertebrae pain
- Soothes pain around shoulders
- Brightens eyes
- Decreases allergic reaction

### Main Indications

- Migraine
- Constipation
- Rib pain
- Stomach pain
- Liver problems
- Gall bladder trouble
- Jaundice
- Bitter taste in mouth
- Cholesterol (together with point 50)
- High blood pressure
- Cervical vertebrae pain
- Pain around shoulders
- Bilateral headaches
- Troubled eyesight
- Rheumatism
- Allergies
- Eczema
- Insomnia

## 43

### Teeth, lumbar vertebrae, coccyx, kidneys

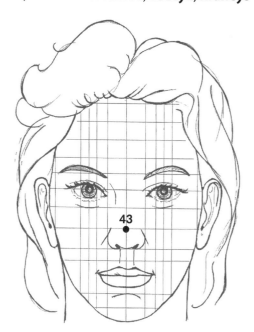

This is a useful point in all cases presenting kidney or lumbar problems. It improves recovery and convalescence following infectious sickness or a surgical procedure. It is the same as the acupuncture point called "Door of Life" (Ming Men or 4 GV).

*This point can be stimulated with a ballpoint pen or the end of a roller. It is generally associated with point 45.*

## Main Effects
- Warms the body
- Tones up life force energy
- Provides strength to a weakened body
- Strengthens gums and teeth
- Tones up kidneys
- Soothes lumbar region
- Soothes lumbar pain
- Increases sexual energy

## Main Indications
- Lumbago
- Lumbar pain
- Dental pain related to kidneys
- Gingivitis
- Chronic tiredness
- Cold feet and hands
- Painful periods
- Piles with hemorrhage
- Colitis with diarrhea (cold kidneys)
- Sciatica
- Incontinence at night
- Bedwetting
- Excess urine
- Nephritis
- Renal colic
- Sexual weakness
- Sperm leak
- Vaginal discharge (leucorrhea)

# 45

## Ears, lumbar vertebrae, coccyx, stomach, kidneys

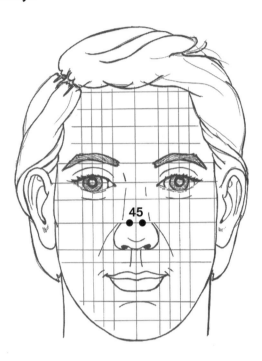

This point acts powerfully in cases of renal problems, in the same way as the previous point, with which it is often associated. It is also a good ally for the relief of persons affected by Parkinson's disease.

*As previously, this point should be stimulated with the rounded end of a ballpoint pen or with the rounded point at the end of a roller. It is generally associated with point 43.*

## Main Effects
- Tones up the body
- Regulates muscular contraction
- Relaxes and calms
- Soothes lumbar pain
- Soothes earaches
- Assists digestion
- Tones up kidneys
- Increases sexual energy

**Main Indications**

- Neuralgia
- Spasmophilia, fibromyalgia
- Constipation
- Trembling
- Parkinson's disease
- Tiredness
- Sexual problems
- Impotence
- Apathy
- Gastritis
- Slow digestion
- Earache
- Deafness
- Nephritis
- Renal colic
- Incontinence
- Bedwetting

## 50

**(Only on the right side!) Liver, lymph system problems, legs**

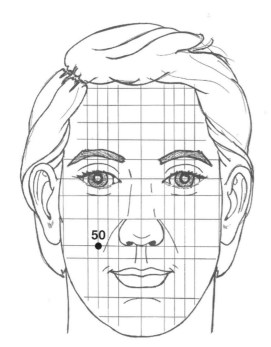

This point is located on the Liver Meridian. Stimulate it for any liver problems including hepatitis. It tones up the liver function and facilitates drainage of stasis in the lymph system: edema, water retention, and ganglions. It also stops hemorrhage and lowers blood cholesterol.

*This point can be associated with point 41, as described above.*

> **Warning**
>
> Do not stimulate this point in cases of high blood pressure.

**Main Effects**

- Regulates muscular contraction
- Stimulates natural defenses
- Relaxes the nervous system
- Lowers cholesterol level
- Soothes pain
- Increases blood pressure
- Increases energy
- Calms allergies
- Stops hemorrhage
- Dissipates poisons and toxins
- Anti-inflammatory
- Regulates perspiration
- Helps digestion
- Regulates blood circulation
- Soothes liver and gall bladder pain

**Main Indications**

- Facial paralysis
- Sprains
- Twisted foot or hand
- Insomnia
- Epilepsy
- Rib pain
- Cervical vertebrae pain
- Twisted neck
- Pain at crown of head
- Low blood pressure

- Allergy
- Hemorrhage
- Heavy periods
- Rheumatism
- Eczema
- Perspiration from feet and hands
- Slow digestion
- Indigestion
- Flatulence
- Piles
- Liver problems
- Weak gall bladder
- Gallstones
- Swollen stomach
- Blocked nose
- Eyesight problems
- Poor eyesight
- Cholesterol

## 51
**Feet (above all the soles), toes (along the chin), big toe (along edge of chin, in center)**

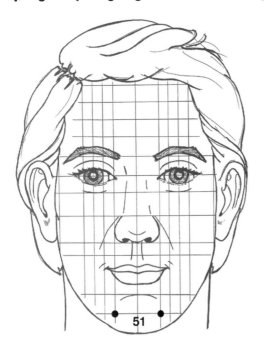

In addition to the problems directly linked to this zone, this point is also useful for relaxing

and soothing excess of yang in the head. Keep in mind that the cause of headaches is usually excess yang energy moving upward and accumulating. Stimulation of these points allows this energy to descend.

*To precisely locate these two points, place your closed first three fingers (index, middle, and ring) in the center of the chin, on the protuberance.*

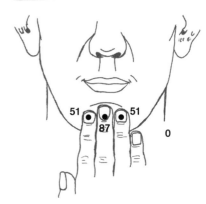

- *point 87 is in the middle, under the middle finger*
- *point 51 is on each side, under the index and ring fingers*

*To stimulate this point press your instrument upward. You can also sweep this zone to cover all of the points.*

### Warning
Do not stimulate this point in cases of low blood pressure!

### Main Effects
- Relaxes
- Reduces fever
- Reduces blood pressure
- Soothes pain in the arms
- Soothes pain in the legs
- Soothes headaches
- Disperses energy
- Regulates blood and energy

## Main Indications

- Insomnia
- High blood pressure
- High blood pressure in the eye
- Headaches caused by high blood pressure
- Pain in arms, legs, or head
- Cold feet
- Feeling loss, or pins and needles in feet
- Pain in soles of feet
- Pain in toes
- Asthma
- Coughing
- Dental pain

# 60

**Eyes, heart, lungs, chest, breasts, forehead, tongue, face, arms, forearms, hands, middle fingers, bladder**

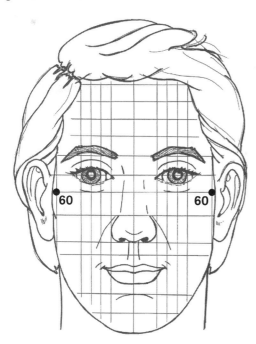

In the case of problems with the eyes, this point is often associated with point **130**, located just above it. The "lung zone" is not limited to this point alone, but starts at the base of the nostril

and crosses the cheek. Concerning this point, the heart is only found on the left.

*According to the case, you can stimulate this point alone, associate it with point 130, or stimulate the whole region between it and the nostril.*

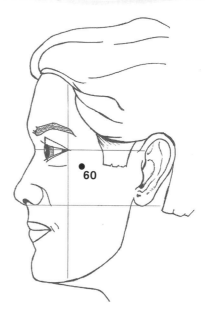

## Main Effects

- Soothes problems in arms and forearms
- Soothes pain in hands
- Soothes problems located in the face
- Soothes pain in breasts
- Reduces temperature
- Warms up body
- Regulates perspiration
- Helps give up smoking
- Clears lungs
- Frees up breathing
- Improves eyesight
- Regulates heartbeat
- Tones up heart
- Relaxes
- Soothes bladder problems
- Anti-inflammatory
- Strengthens body
- Regulates Chi
- Relaxes

**Main Indications**

- Worry
- Facial neuralgia
- Shooting pain
- Paresthesia or loss of sensation
- Loss of sensation in limbs or fingers
- Leukoplasia
- Headache behind forehead
- Arm and forearm pain
- Arm and forearm pain following fracture
- Spasms of tongue
- Arthrosis of hand
- Arthrosis of fingers
- Mastitis
- Cysts on breasts
- Bronchitis
- Tobacco smoking
- Respiratory trouble
- Dyspnea
- Asthma
- Trembling
- Parkinson's disease
- Tiredness
- Apathy
- Cardiac problems
- Inflammation
- Arthritis of arms and hands
- Cystitis
- Urinary problems
- Convalescence
- Sensitivity to cold
- Blood circulation
- Restores blood composition
- Vertigo
- Defective memory

# 61

## Lungs, liver, heart, stomach, spleen, thumbs, trigeminal nerve

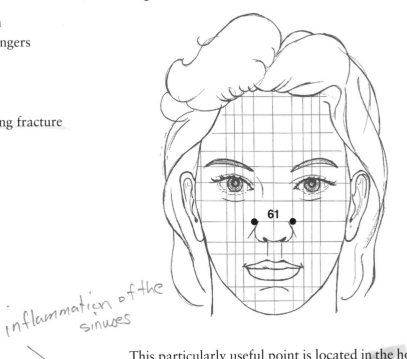

*inflammation of the sinuses*

*bleed heavily*

This particularly useful point is located in the hollow above the nostrils. It warms up the body and promotes secretion of natural endorphins. It is used in cases of sinusitis and blocked nose. It stops hemorrhage, soothes pain, and decreases or stops a runny nose in case of rhinitis.

*Massage this point using small rubbing movements the length of the nostrils.*

**Main Effects**

- Produces endorphins
- Regulates perspiration
- Soothes pain
- Warms up body
- Regulates heartbeat
- Reduces blood pressure
- Regulates muscular contraction (relaxes)
- Anti-inflammatory
- Detoxifies
- Promotes free circulation of energy
- Dissolves mucus
- Stops hemorrhage generally

**Main Indications**

- Excessive or insufficient perspiration
- Abdominal pain
- Drug withdrawal symptoms
- Headaches
- Stomachache
- Gooseflesh
- Heart rhythm abnormalities
- High blood pressure
- Facial paralysis
- Skin problems
- Eczema
- Vaginal inflammation
- Inflammation of the cervix
- Leucorrhea
- Inflammation of the throat
- Tonsillitis
- Asthma
- Thumb pain
- Nose bleeds
- Gastric ulcer
- Oppression
- Sciatica
- Nausea and vomiting
- Goiter
- Fever
- Coughing
- Blocked nose
- Head cold
- Congestive states

# 63
## Colon, pancreas, uterus, stomach

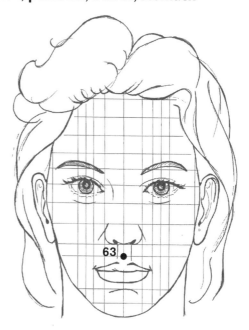

Useful in cases of constipation, indigestion, and various types of pain. Massage this point in cases of vertigo. It stimulates contractions of the uterus and is therefore very useful during childbirth, when it also prevents and stops hemorrhage from the uterus.

*Stimulate this point with your ballpoint pen.*

**Contraindication**

Pregnant women (except during childbirth).

**Main Effects**

- Regulates vaginal secretions
- Regulates production of saliva
- Increases sexual tone
- Provokes erection, sexual desire
- Stimulates natural defenses
- Soothes spinal column pain
- Soothes pain in uterus
- Soothes stomach pain
- Regulates muscular contraction (particularly of uterus, hands, and feet)

- Promotes circulation of energy
- Warms up the pancreas, stomach, colon, and uterus

**Main Indications**
- Frigidity
- Impotence or difficulty with erection
- Dizziness and giddiness
- Epilepsy
- Nervous trembling
- Stomach pain
- Dry or bitter mouth
- Low blood pressure
- Sciatica
- Childbirth
- Hemorrhage from uterus after childbirth
- Period pain
- Irregular periods
- Uterus and vagina pathologies
- Spinal column pain
- Diabetes
- Seasickness

# 64

## (Located at the lower outer edge of each nostril) Groin, hip, stomach, tongue, throat

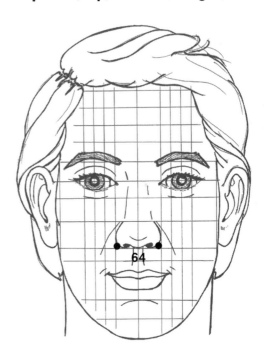

This point is really useful in cases of sciatica, complementing points given in the Practical Dictionary.

*Preferably stimulate this point with a ball-point pen or the rounded tip of a roller handle.*

**Main Effects**
- Calms groin pain
- Calms stomach pain
- Regulates muscular contraction

**Main Indications**
- Sciatica
- Groin pain
- Decalcification of the hip
- Gastritis
- Paralysis of lower limbs
- Tongue or throat pain

## 65

**Cervical vertebrae, neck, ears, eyes, sinuses, nose, brain, ovaries, shoulders**

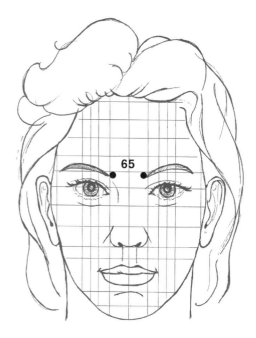

This point is in relation with the Bladder Meridian and is precious in case of vertigo, headaches, and problems related to blood circulation around the brain.

*Stimulate the point either alone, or associated with point 34, on the line of eyebrows.*

### Main Effects

- Relaxes
- Soothes cervical vertebrae and shoulder pain
- Soothes headaches above all at eyebrows
- Unblocks nose
- Soothes earache
- Promotes good circulation of blood around brain
- Improves eyesight
- Soothes bladder problems

### Main Indications

- Headaches linked to periods
- Irregular and painful periods
- Cystitis
- Dizziness and giddiness
- Heavy eyelids
- Eye problems
- Incontinence
- Prostate trouble
- Cervical vertebrae and shoulder pain
- Arthrosis in shoulder
- Scapulohumeral periarthritis
- Sinusitis
- Deafness
- Earache and ear problems
- Stiffness and torticollis in neck
- Head cold and blocked nose
- Jaw pain
- Difficulty concentrating
- Defective memory
- Pain on Bladder Meridian

## 73

**Eyes, lungs, breasts, ovaries, kidneys, heart, head, chest, shoulders, back, arms, legs, bladder**

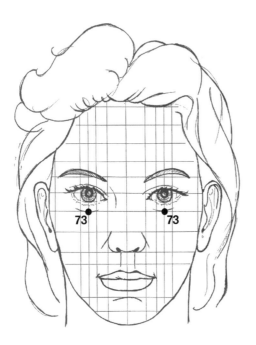

This point is useful in cases of coughs, mastitis, cysts on the breast or ovaries, problems with eyesight and conjunctivitis, and so on. It promotes lactation when breast-feeding.

*It is located on the lower edge of the orbit, on the bony mass. It is delicate, so stimulate it using a tiny twisting movement.*

### Main Effects

- Relaxes
- Soothes breast inflammation
- Soothes chest inflammation
- Calms eye irritation
- Promotes lactation
- Tones up
- Promotes blood circulation
- Frees up energy
- Warms body

### Main Indications

- Cardiac fatigue
- Breast problems, mastitis, cysts
- Pectoral angina
- Insomnia
- Dry coughing
- Kidney pain
- Prostate trouble
- Ovary pain
- Urinary problems
- Pain in shoulders and arms
- Pain in orbits
- Eye weakness
- Kidney stones
- Heavy head (cold)
- Irregular periods

## 74

**Groin, liver, stomach, ears**

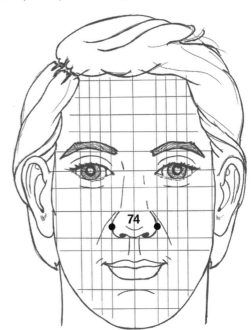

This point is linked to point **64**, next to it, in cases of sciatica and stomachache.

*It is located on the curve of the nostril, and should be stimulated with the steel tip on a roller handle, a round instrument, or the fingernail.*

## Main Effects

- Calms groin pain
- Calms stomach pain
- Soothes the liver
- Increases contraction of the leg muscles
- Tones up veins

## Main Indications

- Headaches due to indigestion
- Lower limb paralysis
- Gastritis
- Poor digestion
- Groin pain
- Sciatica
- Hiccups
- Buzzing or tinnitus in ears
- Deafness

## 85

### Ureters, little fingers, bladder

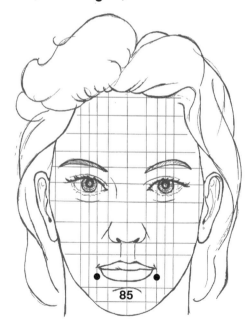

This point controls excretion and therefore urinary problems and water retention. (Remember that the kidneys are projected on either side of the mouth along the nasogenian crease.)

*The massage should usually be performed by associating this point with the kidney zones using a vertical movement, up and down, on either side of the mouth.*

## Main Effects

- Reduces fever
- Freshens the body
- Reduces blood pressure
- Diuretic
- Promotes secretions
- Drains the body
- Eliminates poisons and toxins
- Reduces cholesterol level
- Frees up breathing
- Soothes little finger
- Soothes pain from cystitis

## Main Indications

- Hot flashes
- High blood pressure
- Water retention
- Edema
- Cellulitis
- Kidney stones
- Urinary problems, lack of urine
- Cystitis
- Dry coughing
- Dry nose
- Excess cholesterol
- Tobacco smoking
- Alcoholism
- Drug taking
- Intoxications
- Asthma
- Problems with little finger
- Calf muscle pain

## 87

**Bladder, neck of uterus, ovaries, testicles, prostate gland, crown of the head, neck, occiput**

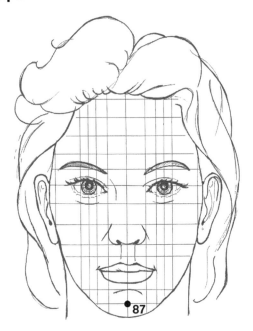

This point is useful for all bladder problems (ptosis, incontinence, bedwetting), ovary problems (cysts, inflammation, malfunction) and also prostate problems. (It is equivalent to acupuncture point 3CV.)

*This point is found exactly in the center of the fleshy part of the chin. It is a point that can be stimulated alone using a rubbing movement, or in conjunction with point 22, using vertical sweeping movements from top to bottom.*

### Main Effects

- Frees up the neck
- Reduces body temperature
- Initiates descent of Chi
- Disperses and circulates energy
- Soothes pain at crown of head
- Soothes occipital pain
- Diuretic
- Regulates production of urine
- Soothes prostate pain
- Frees up breathing
- Antispasmodic
- Provokes contraction of uterus and bladder
- Detoxifies

### Main Indications

- Head injury
- Torticollis
- Stiff neck
- Headaches
- Psychological trouble
- Sunstroke
- Heatstroke
- Water retention
- Cystitis
- Asthma
- Respiratory problems
- Spasmophilia
- Cramps
- Painful periods
- Prostate trouble
- Impotence
- Frigidity
- Bladder ptosis
- Ptosis of the uterus
- Ovarian cyst
- Fibroid
- Incontinence
- Bedwetting
- Poisoning
- Feelings of suffocation
- Fever
- Hot flashes
- Menopause
- Cold extremities

## 97

### Eyes, sinuses, arms, elbows, shoulder blades, shoulders, feet, big toe

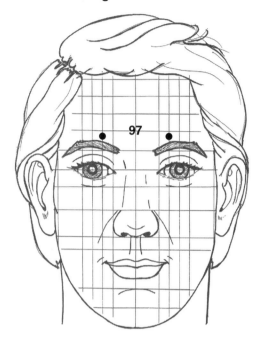

This point is for eyesight trouble, sinusitis, pain in the arms or in the shoulders, tennis elbow, epicondylitis of the elbow, or any other pain in this area.

*These points are often stimulated at the same time as points 65, 34, and 98, using sweeping movements along the eyebrows.*

### Main Effects
- Soothes shoulder, arm, elbow, and foot pains
- Soothes problems in joints
- Soothes pain in shoulder blades
- Useful in case of problems with a big toe
- Improves eyesight
- Facilitates intestinal transit

### Main Indications
- Tennis elbow
- Poor eyesight
- Pain in the arms, shoulders, or shoulder blades

- Pain in lower limbs
- Paralysis of upper limbs
- Sinusitis
- Blocked nose
- Constipation
- Fracture or sprain of big toe

## 98

### Eyes, elbows, shoulder blades and arms

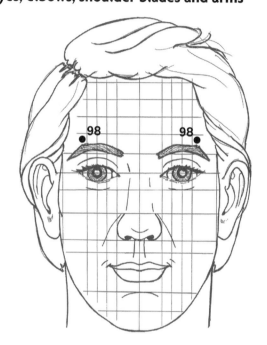

The indications are almost the same as for the previous point.

*Stimulate it horizontally with a sweeping movement outward.*

### Main Effects
- Improves eyesight
- Soothes arm and elbow pain
- Facilitates intestinal transit

### Main Indications
- Tennis elbow
- Insomnia

- Constipation
- Poor eyesight
- Pain in the arms
- Dorsal vertebrae pain

## 100
**Eyes, neck, occiput, wrists, thyroid glands, corresponding sides of the face: point 100 on the right = right side**

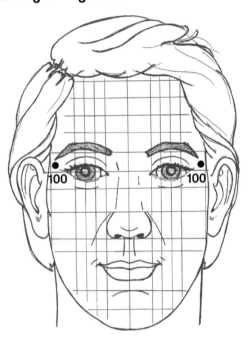

This point specifically concerns eye pain and optical migraines, but it also deals with thyroid gland problems.

*Massage this point located on the bony edge at the end of the eyebrow, with gentle rubbing movements, while steadying yourself on the eyebrows. You can also vertically sweep the zones toward point 130, or simultaneously stimulate points 180, 100, and 130.*

**Main Effects**
- Soothes eye pain
- Relaxes nervous system
- Soothes temples and cervical vertebrae
- Soothes wrists
- Regulates blood pressure
- Strengthens heart
- Regulates heartbeat
- Reduces fever
- Circulates energy in corresponding side of face

**Main Indications**
- Heart fatigue
- Optical migraines
- Dizziness
- Eye pain or problems
- Facial paralysis
- Facial hemiplegia
- Fever
- Insomnia
- Torticollis
- Cervical vertebrae pain
- Occipital pain
- Accidents or pain in the wrist: fracture, sprain, or arthrosis
- Pain in knees
- Basedow's disease or goiter
- Thyroid problems

## 103

**Crown of the head (22GV in Chinese system), forehead, eyes, spinal column, brain, liver, pituitary gland**

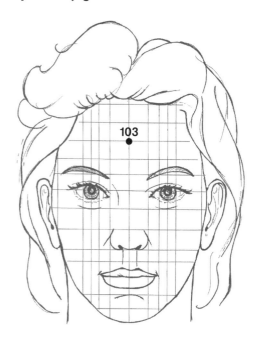

This important point tones up the memory, regulates functioning of the hormonal system, and stimulates the chakras.

*To stimulate points located on the forehead, tap them with the ends of your fingers or perform downward sweeping movements from the top downward.*

### Main Effects

- Improves memory
- Relaxes
- Tones up
- Regulates the Chi
- Regulates blood composition
- Soothes pain at crown of head
- Soothes backache
- Clears mind
- Stops superfluous secretions

### Main Indications

- Nervous depression
- Physical tiredness
- Epilepsy
- Pain at crown of head
- Memory loss
- Pain in spinal column
- Piles
- Prolapsed uterus
- Poor eyesight
- Head injury

## 106

**Spinal column, cervical vertebrae, throat, eyes, sinuses, crown of head, neck, occipital region, forehead, shoulder blades**

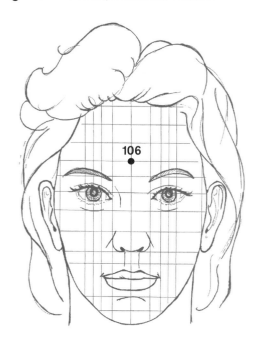

This point frees up circulation around the brain and promotes concentration. It is used to soothe many problems relative to the head.

*Perform same stimulation as for previous point.*

## Main Effects

- Relaxes
- Tones up
- Soothes jaw pain
- Soothes dental pain
- Soothes cervical vertebrae pain
- Regulates heartbeat
- Regulates perspiration
- Unblocks the nose

## Main Indications

- Heart problems
- Insomnia
- Cervical vertebrae and forehead pain
- Toothache
- Excess perspiration
- Blocked nose
- Goiter
- Worry

## From point 8 to point 106 (passing through point 26): cervical vertebrae

It is very often useful to link these points to treat cervical arthrosis, headaches, eye problems, memory loss, circulation around brain, thyroid dysfunction, and so on.

*Perform sweeping movements in zone 8–106, and then along the eyebrows, zones corresponding to shoulders and arms.*

# 113

## Pancreas, prostate gland, ovaries, uterus, and pneumogastric nerve

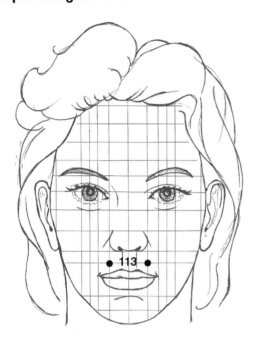

This point acts positively on diabetes, cystitis, digestion, and period pain. It can also help with most sexual problems.

*It can either be stimulated alone with a ballpoint pen, or be included in a massage stimulating the whole zone between the base of the nose and the upper lip. In the latter case perform sweeping movements over the zones linking points 17, 113, and 7, toward the center of these zones.*

## Main Effects

- Stimulates natural defenses
- Soothes pain in ovaries
- Soothes prostate trouble
- Soothes pain in thighs
- Equilibrates function of pancreas
- Promotes digestion

**Main Indications**

- Ovarian troubles
- Prostate troubles
- Thigh pain
- Indigestion
- Diabetes
- Pancreatic disorder
- Sciatica
- Asthma
- Colitis
- Goiter

# 124
## Gall bladder and bile duct (on right), spleen (on left), brain

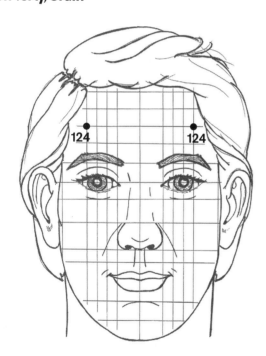

This point is a basic point for relaxation and toning up.

*Perform horizontal sweeping movements of half an inch to an inch over this point.*

**Main Effects**

- Calms nervous system
- Soothes pain
- Decreases perspiration
- Decreases allergies
- Strengthens body
- Regulates Chi

**Main Indications**

- Pain in dorsal vertebrae, lumbago
- Drug withdrawal symptoms
- Asthenia, nervous fatigue
- Insomnia
- Deficient memory
- Headaches
- Dental pain
- Cold perspiration
- Epistaxis (nose bleeds)
- Sinusitis
- Psoriasis
- Skin problems
- Convalescence

## 126
### Crown of the head, spinal column, coccyx, anus, rectum, bladder, nose, and brain

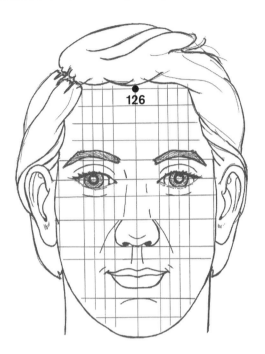

The stimulation of this point and the zone along the hairline also soothes lumbar pain including lumbago.

*In cases of lumbar pain, lightly tap the forehead along the hairline, or perform small vertical sweeping movements over the area.*

*Together the points from 126 to 19 unblock the spinal column. Therefore you can stimulate them by covering this whole zone from top to bottom, or bottom to top, according to your intuition. In one direction energy rises and in the other it descends.*

> **Warning**
> Do not stimulate this point in cases of high blood pressure.

### Main Effects
- Increases blood pressure
- Causes Chi energy to rise
- Soothes pain in head and coccyx
- Slows down secretions
- Helps burping (for example in babies)

### Main Indications
- Low blood pressure
- Pain at crown of head
- Piles
- Frequent urination (prostate trouble)
- Head colds
- Sinusitis
- Pain in coccyx
- Lumbago

## 127
### Small intestine, heel, ankle, upper part of uterus, pelvic region, relations with Yin Conception Vessel

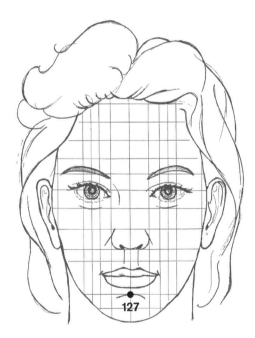

This point is located in the center of the hollow between the mouth and the chin. It should be stimulated in case of period pain, menopause, and problems with sexuality in general. It also acts on colitis with spasms and diarrhea, if treated at the onset.

*Points stimulated on the chin must be stimulated vertically downward.*

## Main Effects
- Powerfully relaxes nervous system
- Warms the abdomen
- Regulates peristaltic movements
- Tones up
- Causes Chi energy to rise

## Main Indications
- Insomnia
- Perspiration from hands and feet
- Asthenia
- Nervous fatigue
- Asthma
- Shock caused by medicines
- Indigestion
- Gastritis
- Stomachache, cold stomach
- Leucorrhea (vaginal discharge)
- Period pain
- Drug withdrawal symptoms
- Tobacco smoking
- Bout of chattering teeth
- Dental pain (lower jaw)
- Facial paralysis
- Sciatica
- Heel pain
- Cervical vertebrae pain
- Heavy feeling in head (especially the forehead)
- Dysentery, diarrhea
- Tapeworm
- Pain preventing head from leaning backward

# 130
## Eyes, hands, and wrists

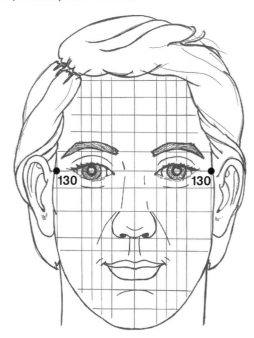

This point is the correct one for treating migraines.

*Vertically massage this point, which is found in a hollow just behind the orbits. It can be associated with point 60.*

## Main Effects
- Soothes inflammation of the eyes, ears, arms, hands
- Contracts the iris
- Brightens eyesight

## Main Indications
- Eye problems
- Earache and pain in ear
- Pain in arms, hands, fingers
- Problems in metacarpals
- Headaches and migraines
- Pain in temples
- Pain in feet (on the Gall Bladder Meridian)

## 143
**Colon, rectum, coccyx**

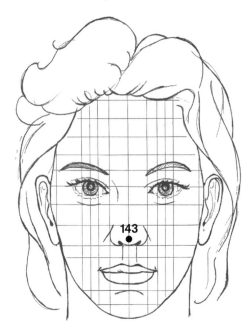

This point acts mainly with respect to intestinal problems and the coccyx.

*Stimulate this point, located just under the tip of the nose, with the ballpoint pen. (Not to be mixed up with point 19, which is at the base of the nose.)*

### Main Effects
- Facilitates intestinal transit
- Reduces fever, refreshes generally
- Soothes pain in coccyx
- Provokes descent of Chi
- Provokes perspiration
- Lowers blood pressure

### Main Indications
- High blood pressure
- Pain in coccyx
- Dorsal pain
- Sciatica
- Piles

- Constipation
- Fever without perspiration
- Hot flashes

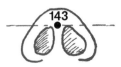

View from below nose

## 156
**Calves, heart, ovaries, testicles, prostate gland, colon**

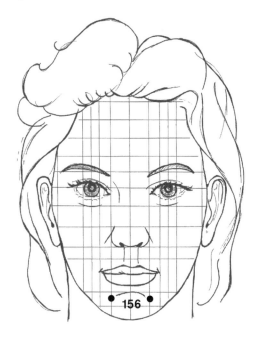

This point allows treatment of problems related to the ovaries and prostate gland, besides many other applications.

*This point is located on either side of point 127 and can be associated with it by performing a horizontal sweeping movement, following the upper limit of the chin.*

## Main Effects

- Regulates hormone functions
- Regulates menstrual cycle
- Regulates circulation of the blood
- Regulates circulation of energy
- Regulates blood pressure
- Regulates digestion
- Soothes period pain
- Soothes ovaries, prostate gland
- Regulates heartbeat
- Tones up natural defenses
- Increases resistance of body
- Soothes legs, feet, knees, eyebrows, neck, cervical vertebrae, shoulders

## Main Indications

- Cramp in calf
- Leg and knee pain
- Pain in eyebrow
- Facial paralysis
- Blocked cervical vertebrae
- Constipation
- Pain in pelvic region
- Ovarian pathologies
- Prostate trouble
- Impotence
- Frigidity
- Period pains
- Irregular heartbeat
- Tachycardia
- Blocked nose
- Perspiration (feet and hands)
- High or low blood pressure

# 180

## Solar plexus, temples, thumbs

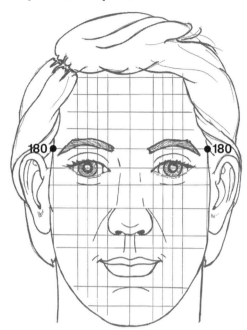

This point relaxes and acts on the region around the solar plexus, as well as certain migraines.

*Please note: Stimulation of this point can sometimes provoke perspiration or leave the hands damp.*

*Massage point moving toward the ears.*

## Main Effects

- Anti-inflammatory
- Reduces fever
- Provokes perspiration
- Lowers blood pressure
- Soothes temples
- Soothes thumb
- Relaxes solar plexus

## Main Indications

- Bronchitis
- Influenza without perspiration
- Pain in temples
- Pain in thumbs

- Tonsillitis
- Sore throats, throat infections
- Pain in solar plexus
- High blood pressure
- Inflammation of the eye, conjunctivitis
- Dental pain
- Migraines

*Each point can be stimulated separately, if it is necessary to treat for a problem with a finger. On the other hand if you want to soothe the eyes or improve eyesight, it is best to stimulate all of these points using vertical sweeping movements. Point 100 can be incorporated in this sequence.*

## 177
**Ring finger, eyes**

## 185
**Index finger, eyes**

## 191
**Little finger, eyes, elbow, heart**

## 195
**Middle finger, eyes**

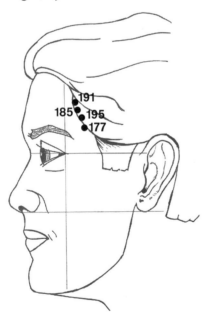

These points can be dealt with together as they are all found on the temples, close to each other, and have common characteristics. As they concern the fingers and eyes, their indications do not require stating.

## 197
**Knees, kneecaps, liver, eyes**

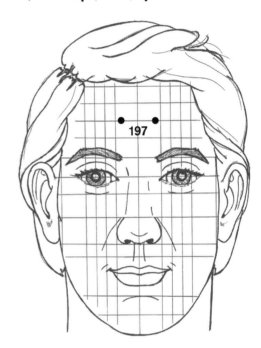

This point is next to point **103**. It can be stimulated vertically. It should be noted here that there are also knee reflex zones at the corners of the mouth.

### Main Indications
- Any knee problem
- Arthrosis of knee
- Ligament trouble
- Hepatitis
- Poisoning
- Optical migraine
- Poor eyesight

## 233
### Liver

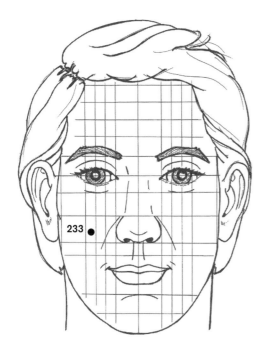

This point is complementary to points **50** and **41**.

*This point can be stimulated at the same time as its neighbors, points **41** and **50**, located just below.*

### Main Effects
- Detoxifies
- Lowers cholesterol level
- Warms up body
- Drains
- Stimulates natural defenses
- Soothes liver and gall bladder pain
- Regulates perspiration
- Regulates blood circulation

### Main Indications
- Hepatitis
- Liver congestion
- Sluggish gall bladder
- Gall stones

- Alcoholism
- Drug dependency
- Piles
- Distension
- Cholesterol
- Excess perspiration
- Poor circulation
- Rib pain

## 287
### Ovaries, testicles, vagina

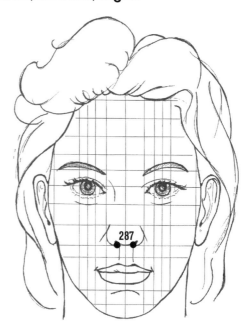

The effects and indications of this point are similar to those for points **19**, **7**, and **113**.

*It is found above the upper lip at the entrance to each nostril, on the same line as point **19** and close to points **7** and **113**. This point can be stimulated alone or linked to neighboring points. In the latter case, vertically massage the upper lip as far as points **7** and **113**.*

### Main Effects
- Stops hemorrhage from uterus
- Regulates genital functions

- Regulates vaginal secretions
- Reduces vaginal discharge
- Frees up energy
- Warms up body
- Eliminates toxins
- Soothes menstrual problems
- Increases sexual energy

**Main Indications**
- Heavy and irregular periods
- Pain in ovulation
- Mastitis
- Vaginal discharge
- Hemorrhage from uterus
- Piles
- Prostate trouble
- Impotence
- Bursitis
- Sexual weakness
- Gynecological inflammations
- Vaginal dryness

# 300

## Kidneys, lumbar region, index finger, sexual drive

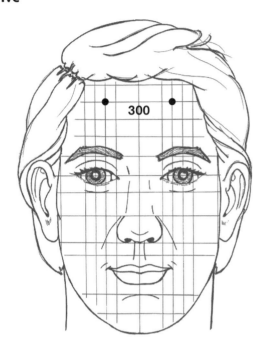

This point is mainly related to kidney problems, lumbar pain, and sexual problems.

*It should be swept using horizontal movements with a ballpoint pen or the knuckle of the index finger.*

**Main Effects**
- Tones up kidneys
- Tones up sexual drive
- Facilitates erection
- Soothes kidney pain
- Soothes lumbar pain
- Soothes index finger pain

**Main Indications**
- Tobacco smoking
- Lumbar pain
- Neuralgia
- Nocturnal urges to urinate
- General physical tiredness
- Low sexual energy

## 342
### Spinal column, colon, lumbar vertebrae, cold feet

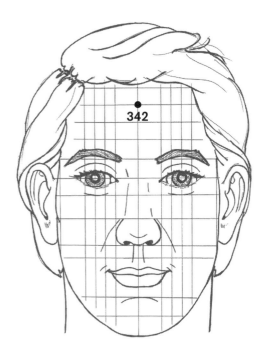

This point is one of choice for lumbago, and should be stimulated as soon as the first symptoms appear. (Please remember that the cervical vertebrae are located at point **26**, and the dorsal vertebrae on the bridge of the nose).

*Points 126 and 342, both corresponding to the lower back, are usually stimulated in the same movement. To stimulate points 126 and 342 together, stimulate them from top to bottom using small movements, then descend lightly tapping along the forehead and nose, then move upward again, finally finishing on point 0.*

### Main Effects
- Soothes spinal column
- Equilibrates intestinal function
- Warms up soles of feet

### Main Indications
- Lumbar pain
- Lumbago
- Flatulence
- Colitis
- Cold feet

## 365
### Toes, anus, crown of the head, neck, occipital region

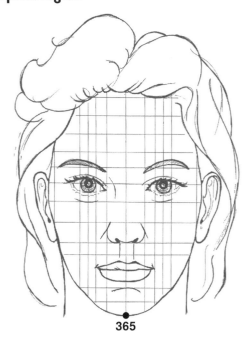

This point, which has the special capacity of healing you from head to toe, soothes anything from a headache to a painful toe!

*In the same way as the area related to point 126 extends along the hairline, this point's area of influence stretches along the lower jawbone on both sides. Sensitivity at any point will guide you to the precise zone concerned; remember that the big toe is closer to the center with the smallest furthest away.*

### Warning
Do not stimulate this point in cases of high blood pressure.

## Main Effects

- Regulates muscular contraction
- Regulates intestinal peristaltic movement
- Tones up
- Increases blood pressure
- Regulates secretions

## Main Indications

- Diarrhea
- Piles
- Pain in feet
- Lumbago
- Sciatica
- Pain in buttocks
- Cystitis
- Pain in rectum

# 461
## Heel, ankle

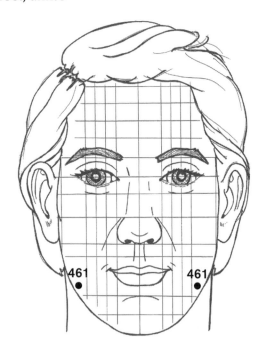

If you twist your ankle stimulate this point straightaway, or as soon as possible, to avoid the unnecessary consequences of a real sprain (pain and swelling, and so on).

*This point is located on the lower cheeks, on the edge of the lower jawbone. It can be stimulated with the steel tip, a knuckle, or using a sweeping movement of the end of a ballpoint pen.*

> **Warning**
>
> Do not stimulate this point in cases of low blood pressure!

## Main Effects

- Soothes the heel
- Lowers blood pressure

## Main Indications

- High blood pressure
- Pain in heel
- Painful ankle
- Twist or sprain
- Sciatica

# 560
## Lumbar vertebrae, kidneys

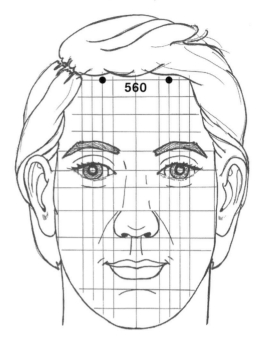

**Main Effects**
- Soothes lumbar pain
- Soothes kidneys
- Regulates evacuation

**Main Indications**
- Lumbago
- Pain at crown of head
- Urinary problems
- Incontinence
- Enuresis
- Prostate trouble
- Piles
- Pain in coccyx

This point is complementary to point **126** which is close by.

*This point can be stimulated at the same time as point **126**, by small vertical sweeping movements following the hairline.*

# 6

# Advanced Dien' Cham':
# Personalized Sessions

This chapter is devoted to advanced Dien' Cham', which is the most interesting form of practice. It has been written primarily for therapists, as well as people possessing knowledge in the field of physiology. Even if you do not have that kind of training, I encourage you to try to do what you can all the same. There is no risk that you will make a serious blunder, as each point will be tested beforehand! The only risk is not being able to go very far with it. It is always worth trying to see what you are capable of.

Chapter 4 showed you the effectiveness of the method and proposed certain model sequences for rapid sessions. Although there are other choices of points and zones for the given conditions, the components given were based on the reflex points and zones most often used for the cases described and those which have given the best results on a majority of people in my own experience. Even when you have learned how to choose the best components for a session for yourself, you will still have recourse to chapter 4 for a long time, as, with it, the application of Dien' Cham' requires no preliminary work or head scratching. I expect that you may also on occasion give a photocopy of a useful page to a family member or friend that you would like to help.

Now let us consider the process of tailoring a session to the needs of a specific person, by determining the reflex points and zones that will give the best results, out of the hundreds of possible combinations. You will find all of the references that you need in this book. However, it is very important that you follow my path step-by-step for this training. My experience during training courses has shown that you only have to disregard one piece of vital information for comprehension to be lost and the rest of the job spoiled.

## WORKING IN PAIRS

Initially it is advisable to do the training process described in this chapter with another person. Later of course it will be possible to practice on yourself, but for this step it would complicate matters and you may well make a lot of unnecessary errors. During my courses trainees always work in pairs and they usually prefer this. It allows them to test things for themselves by taking turns, and to confirm that everything has been correctly assimilated and understood.

You should allow two hours for this session the first time. If, however, you are just determining a treatment for one of the partners, it will take less time. After you have gained a measure of experience, a maximum of about twenty minutes will be sufficient.

## MATERIALS

In addition to this book for reference, you will need sheets of paper, a pen, a pencil, and an eraser. You will also require several photocopies of empty grids, the models for which you will find at the end of this chapter. You will also need to refer back to the diagrams in chapter 2, so you may want to copy them as well, particularly **Diagrams 1 (both views), 2 (both views), 3, 4, 6, 7. Diagram 1** will aid you in the determination of reflex points and **Diagrams 2, 3, 4, 6, 7** in the determination of reflex zones. And of course you are going to need your favorite Dien' Cham' instrument, specifically a pointed tip such as the writing tip of a ballpoint that has run out of ink, the sharp end of a wooden chopstick, or the rounded end of a small roller. The rounded cap of a ballpoint—which is often good for the stimulation of points and zones—is not suitable for this process, as you are going to test some points and this can only be done with a lot of precision.

To sum up you will need:

- Photocopies of empty grids (models at the end of this chapter)
- Sheets of paper
- A pen, pencil, and eraser
- An instrument with a pointed tip (pen, chopstick, roller end)
- Photocopies of **Diagrams 1 (both views), 2 (both views), 3, 4, 6, 7.**

## CHAPTERS TO CONSULT

For this task, you will find it necessary to refer to certain sections in this book that could be usefully bookmarked beforehand.

Chapter 2: "Reflex Zones and Points: Main Diagrams"
Chapter 5: "Correspondences, Effects, and Indications for Dien' Cham' Points"
Chapter 6 Reference Lists: "The Main Correspondence Points for Parts of the Body, Functions, and Symptoms"

Chapter 5 has the primary advantage of allowing you to easily locate each point. If you attempt to look for them on **Diagram 1**, you risk losing your patience! On the other hand, do not worry about the main effects and therapeutic indications given for each point in chapter 5 for the moment. These will serve you later, when, for example, you want to know why one specific point is often used for various symptoms. Often you will find the correct answer in those lists. For the moment, however, referring to them would complicate matters unnecessarily.

I would advise you to read the Reference Lists at the end of this chapter (see pages 243–245) carefully to have a good idea of what they contain. It is not necessary to memorize anything, though. That is not the aim! But you should realize that in addition to the points corresponding to different parts of the body, there are also some that correspond to various functions, as well as numerous symptoms. It is from these lists that in a short while you will choose points to test.

Now it is time to follow my path step-by-step into the practice of advanced Dien' Cham'.

# 1. IDENTIFYING PROBLEMS TO BE SOLVED

*Here we are not just concerned with relieving symptoms. You are going to learn how to search deeper into the roots of various sicknesses in order to heal them more effectively.*

After a first quick reading of this book, you will no doubt have followed my advice to get your feet wet by applying the various "recipes" in the Practical Dictionary of Therapeutic Sessions in chapter 4. This has probably allowed you to discover for yourself the surprising efficiency of this method, which allies simplicity and rapidity.

Now you are going to decide for yourself the reflex points and zones that best suit the person you are trying to help—including yourself!

## Establish a List of Troubles to Treat

Take a fresh sheet of paper. On this sheet, note down a column listing the various troubles and symptoms affecting your partner, according to her instructions.

For example:

- Frequent headaches
- Poor digestion
- Hot flashes
- Varicose veins
- Insomnia

Try to limit yourself to four or five problems maximum, for the purposes of your first session. If you have fewer, that is even better. Or you can decide to concentrate your efforts on just one symptom to start with, leaving the others until later when the first problems are solved. See what is best for you here!

Write the colon sign (:) after each symptom, like this:

- Frequent headaches:
- Poor digestion:
- Hot flashes:
- Varicose veins:
- Insomnia:

This is done in order to clearly show that you are going to work on what *follows* the colon, and not just the symptoms initially listed! It might seem to be a detail but you will see that it counts!

Now you should note down a location in the body that seems to be the seat of each problem. Keep asking yourself the same question: "Where is this happening?" Some sample possible answers follow (in italics):

- Frequent headaches: *right temple*
- Poor digestion: *stomach, liver*
- Hot flashes: *ovaries, liver*
- Varicose veins: *left and right legs*
- Insomnia: *nervous system, head, and so on*

To this list you can add the possible causes of the symptom indicated. Think laterally. For each, you will be choosing from an array of possibilities. To give you an example, headaches can be caused by accidents or head injuries, but they are also likely to be symptoms of the following: liver or liver plus gall bladder problems, repeated or habitual stress, problems of blood circulation, high blood pressure, or ovarian problems. You should inquire into these kinds of connections in order to understand the messages sent by the body as a request for help! Now go back to the list you have started and add the new information as shown (given here in bold type):

- Frequent headaches: *right temple,* **liver, gall bladder, poor blood circulation**
- Poor digestion: *stomach, liver,* **weak digestive function, stress, constipation**
- Hot flashes: *ovaries, liver,* **menopause**
- Varicose veins: *left and right legs,* **poor blood circulation**

- Insomnia: *nervous system, head,* **nervous tension, digestive problems**

The last phase of this preliminary exercise is to look at the "Main Functions of Points" list and the "Symptoms" list at the end of this chapter to see which entries are most likely to correspond to your problem; then add them to your list. In this way "headaches" will certainly suggest the addition of *pain relief* (from the list of Functions) and *dull pain* (from the list of Symptoms). As for the hot flashes, all you have to note is that there are pressure points that *dissipate heat* (from the list of Functions) and others that relate to *excess perspiration* (from the list of Symptoms). And so the procedure seems clear in this case! Don't you think so?

Sample entries for our example have been added below (in bold italics):

- Frequent headaches: *right temple,* **liver, gall bladder, poor blood circulation,** *assists blood circulation, lowers blood pressure, pain relief, dull pain*
- Poor digestion: *stomach, liver,* **weak digestive function, stress, constipation,** *increases secretions (gastric for example), assists digestion, laxative, digestive troubles*
- Hot flashes: *ovaries, liver,* **menopause,** *disperses heat, assists blood circulation, fever, feeling hot, excess perspiration*
- Varicose veins: *left and right legs,* **poor blood circulation,** *assists blood circulation*
- Insomnia: *nervous system, head,* **nervous tension, digestive problems,** *relaxation*

You now have a list of various possibilities, which it will be interesting to test in order to find the best pressure points, the ones that have the most effect.

## Noting Down the Corresponding Points

Now make a new vertical list of the indications given after the colon for each item on your original list. Example given for headache:

- Right temple:
- Liver:
- Gall bladder:
- Assists blood circulation:
- Lowers blood pressure:
- Pain relief:
- Dull pain:

Here you only need to note down the indications that appear in one of the Reference Lists of points at the end of this chapter (Parts of the Body, Functions, or Symptoms). If, as in my example, you have noted down "menopause" following "hot flashes"—which is logical, as it is a diagnostic term—you do not write this down, because you will not find it in any of the Reference Lists.

When you have finished making your list of indications, go to the Therapeutic Index of Dien' Cham' Point Correspondences at the end of the book and jot down all the points (all!) that correspond.

Example for headache:

- Right temple: 3, 180, but also (for side of face): 41, 180, 100, 61, 3
- Liver: 50, 103, 19, 61, 74, 197, 233
- Gall bladder: 41, 124
- Assists blood circulation: 0, 7, 37, 43, 50, 74, 87
- Lowers blood pressure: 26, 3, 85, 39, 51, 14, 16, 15, 180, 8, 41
- Pain relief: 26, 124, 34, 61, 60, 39, 41, 50, 3, 0, 14, 16
- Dull pain: 41, 60, 34, 61, 14, 16, 0

Do the same with respect to each item on your first list. Do you now see why I advised against doing the work for more than four or five symptoms each time? I know this is a long and tedious process to begin with, but afterward things become easier and much quicker.

## 2. TEST AND SELECT POINTS

As you have seen, some lists contain a great number of points, but your final treatment process will not consist of stimulating all of them! Remember that, for example, there are about twenty points for the eyes, which are usable whatever the ocular problem you have to solve! The idea is to choose from the enormous number of points the ones that are going to be the most effective for the person you are testing.

The procedure is quite simple now. You are going to test all of the points on your partner. This will also be an opportunity to learn a certain number of them in a natural way.

### Working Position

It is preferable to perform this work with the two persons sitting opposite each other, either across a narrow desk or next to a table. Keep **Diagram 1** representing the facial reflex points handy. You will need to refer to it constantly. Place a bookmark at chapter 4: "Using Dien' Cham' for the Prevention and Treatment of Health Problems." Also remember that you are going to need to take notes and work on your lists.

Ask your partner to look straight at you in order to locate the points with respect to the dummy grid. Remember that the vertical lines are based solely on the iris!

> **Warning**
>
> Just because you find a point noted down several times does not mean that it particularly suits the person!
>
> Do not select it before testing it out!
>
> On the other hand, you only need to test it once.

### Testing and Selecting Points

Now you are going to test all the points in your lists, one by one! Of course when you find certain points repeated, there is no necessity to test them more than once.

Using the rounded off point of your little roller, the writing tip of an empty ballpoint pen, or the tip of a chopstick carefully shaped for the purpose, press down strongly, but not brutally, on the point to be tested. Turn the instrument in your fingers as you press. Make sure that the instrument remains at a right angle to the face.

Test all of the points in the list, and note down the most painful ones by drawing a circle round them. Out of a list of, say, ten points, try to retain only between two and four, no more.

Do the same for all of your lists.

If a point is painful on one side of the face and not the other retain it all the same.

Of all those tested it is best to keep just a simple sequence of twenty or so points, chosen from among the most sensitive.

## 3. NOTING DOWN YOUR SELECTION ON THE DUMMY GRID

Take a photocopy of a dummy grid and mark all of your points on it. This will be the session to perform daily until a result is obtained.

Keep a careful record of the previous lists with which you have worked because they will be useful later. As soon as certain points become inactive or painless, that is a sign that a problem has been solved or that you need to change points. At that point, it will be sufficient to repeat the testing of step 2 and change the session as a function of the new results.

# 4. ADDING CORRESPONDING REFLEX ZONES

All that needs to be done now is to add the reflex zones chosen as a function of their correspondences with the part of the body or organ in question. If you take the example of a headache again, to the sequence of selected points you would, by referring to **Diagrams 2** and **3**, add the zones of the head and those corresponding to the liver, and so on.

To give another example, in the case of varicose veins, you can add the zones corresponding to the leg in question and even the precise spot on the leg affected!

# 5. PRACTICING THE COMPLETE SESSION WITH REFLEX ZONES AND POINTS

All that is left is to do a practice session, and then teach your partner to practice it on herself in front of a mirror. Remember that Dien' Cham' sessions always start with a Basic Session!

To perform this kind of session correctly, you should follow the general instructions given in chapter 3, which serve as a good basis for all of the personalized sessions that you will one day practice.

## Example:

- Always start with a Basic Session
- Then work on the points located on the cheeks and cheekbones
- Move along the nose upward
- All the way to the forehead
- Then the eyebrows where necessary
- Down over the temples
- Around the mouth
- Then the chin
- Ending up in the region around the ears
- Not forgetting point 0 to finish

Your personalized advanced Dien' Cham' session is finished!

# REFERENCE LISTS: THE MAIN CORRESPONDENCE POINTS FOR PARTS OF THE BODY, FUNCTIONS, AND SYMPTOMS

## Points for Parts of the Body

The points indicated below are classified as a function of their correspondences with various parts of the body. They are also classified according to their frequency of use.

### 1) Head

brain, 65, 103, 124, 126
crown of head, 103, 106, 126, 50, 51, 87, 365
ear, 65, 45, 41, 0, 14, 15, 16, 74
eye, 103, 16, 34, 50, 3, 6, 0, 60, 65, 73, 97, 98, 100, 106, 130, 177, 185, 191, 195, 197
face, 60, 37
forehead, 106, 103, 26, 60, 39, 61, 51
gums, 15
jaw, 8, 15
lip, mouth, 8, 37, 39, 3, 61, 0
neck, 8, 106, 65
neck, occiput, 106, 26, 65, 87, 365, 127, 8, 100
nose, 126, 65, 26, 61, 39, 50, 3, 19, 7, 0
parotid glands, 14
pituitary gland, 26, 103
side of face, 41, 180, 100, 61, 3
sinus, 26, 34, 65, 97, 106
teeth, 8, 43, 34, 63, 22, 127
temple, 3, 180
throat, 8, 61, 14, 26, 64, 106
thyroid gland, 14, 39
tongue, 8, 60, 64

### 2) Shoulder, Arm

arm, 97, 98, 60, 0, 51, 34, 73
elbow, 98, 19, 97
finger, index, 39, 185, 300
finger, little, 85, 191, 0
finger, middle, 38, 60, 195
finger, ring, 60, 177
finger, thumb, 61, 180, 3

forearm, 98, 60, 0, 51

hand, 130, 60

shoulder blade, 106, 34, 97, 98

shoulder, 34, 98, 65, 73

wrist, 100, 130, 41, 0

The fingers are also projected along the hairline and along the nasogenian crease (from point 61 to the corner of the mouth).

### 3) Pelvis, Legs

ankle, 127, 461

calf, 6, 156

foot, 34, 51, 97

groin, 64, 74

heel, 127, 461

hip, 64, 74 + between ear and cheekbone

knee, 38, 197 + corners of the mouth towards the ear for about an inch or so

kneecap, 39, 156, 197

leg, 6, 50, 156, 0, 73

pelvis, 17

thigh, 7, 17, 113, 37, 38, 50, 3

toe, big, 97, 51, 365

toe, fourth, 51

toe, second, 51

toe, small, 51

toe, third, 51

### 4) Rib Cage

breast, 73, 39, 60

chest, 73, 3, 60

ribs, 38, + nostrils

solar plexus, 180

### 5) Abdomen

above navel, 19, 63, 61, 39, 37, 50

around navel, 127

below navel, 127, 87, 22, 19

### 6) Back

cervical vertebrae, 8, 26, 65, 106

coccyx, 43, 45, 126, 143

dorsal vertebrae, 73, 98, 106

lumbar vertebrae, 1, 43, 45, 342, 300, 560, 0

spinal column, 126, 342, 103, 1, 143, 19, 63, 0

### 7) Organs

adrenal glands, 0, 1, 17 + corners of the mouth

bladder, 85, 87, 22, 26, 126, 3, 60, 73

brain, 124, 103, 126, 34, 26, 65

colon, 342, 98, 19, 17, 143, 38, 39, 63, 156

gall bladder, 41, 124

heart, 60, 8, 34, 106, 19, 3, 6, 61, 73, 156, 191

kidney, 0, 1, 43, 45, 342, 300, 17, 38, 73
    + corners of the mouth

liver, 50, 103, 19, 61, 74, 197, 233

lungs, 26, 3, 61, 19, 60, 73

ovaries, 7, 113, 65, 73, 156, 0, 87, 287

pancreas, 63, 7, 113

penis, vagina, 19, 63, 1, 50, 287, 0

prostate gland, 7, 37, 87, 156

rectum, 19, 143, 126, 365

skin, mucous membrane, 26, 61, 3, 19

small intestine, 127, 22, 34, 8 + around the mouth

spleen, 37, 124, 61

stomach, 39, 37, 50, 61, 45, 63, 19, 127, 0, 64, 74

testicles, 7, 113, 65, 73, 156, 0, 87, 287

ureters, 85

uterus, 63, 19, 22, 87, 0, 7, 113, 127, 287

## Main Functions of Points

The points indicated below are classified according to their traditional functions.

anti-cholesterol, 41, 50, 37, 38, 85, 113, 7, 233

anti-inflammatory, 26, 3, 50, 17, 38, 14, 16, 61, 60, 7

antispasmodic, 61, 16, 19, 63, 87

assists blood circulation, 0, 7, 37, 43, 50, 74, 87

assists breathing, 26, 19, 3, 38, 87, 143

assists digestion, 0, 14, 41, 39, 37, 45, 113

causes Chi to ascend, 126, 103, 1, 19, 127, 22, 6, 37, 50, 0 causes Chi to descend, 26, 3, 143, 51, 87, 14, 15

disintoxication, 26, 3, 85, 87, 143, 7, 50

dissipates heat, 26, 3, 85, 61, 87, 143, 180, 14, 16, 15, 8

diuretic, 26, 3, 85, 87, 37, 38

expectorant, 37, 3, 461, 26

immuno-stimulant, 0, 61, 37, 50, 113, 127, 156, 7, 22

increases blood pressure, 126, 103, 1, 19, 127, 0, 6, 50, 37

increases secretions, 26, 3, 39, 85, 19, 87

laxative, 19, 143, 3, 41, 38, 50

lowers blood pressure, 26, 3, 85, 39, 51, 14, 16, 15, 180, 8, 41

pain relief, 26, 124, 34, 61, 60, 39, 41, 50, 3, 0, 14, 16

reconstitutes, 124, 103, 34, 1, 45, 127, 22, 50, 41, 37, 39, 60, 61

reduces secretions, 103, 126, 63, 7, 17, 1, 50, 0, 61, 15, 16, 51, 22, 287

regulates blood pressure, 0, 17

regulates Chi, blood formula, 124, 103, 34, 19, 63, 60, 0

regulates heart beat, 0, 1, 3, 8, 16, 19, 34, 61

regulates muscular contraction, 19, 63, 74, 64, 45, 50, 39, 87,14, 365, 61

relaxes, 124, 103, 106, 34, 26, 63, 0, 14, 16, 8, 60

stops hemorrhage, 16, 0, 61, 17, 7, 50, 6, 37, 124, 34, 16, 287

tones up, 0, 6, 7, 19, 45

warms up, 1, 43, 0, 19, 17, 7, 50, 37, 127, 61, 15

## Points for Specific Symptoms

The points given here are classified according to the symptoms they relieve:

allergy, 0, 7, 17, 50

burning sensation, 26, 3, 61

digestive troubles, 0, 7, 14, 41, 37, 39, 45, 113

dull pain, 41, 60, 34, 61, 14, 16, 0

excess perspiration, 124, 34, 60, 0, 19, 61

faulty memory, 103, 124, 34, 60, 50, 3

feeling cold, 1, 19, 17, 0, 51, 127, 60, 50, 37, 6, 61

fever, feeling hot, 26, 3, 85, 143, 60, 87, 14, 16, 15

indolence, apathy, 124, 34, 0, 1, 45, 60, 61, 19, 17, 127, 22, 50, 6

itching, stinging, 26, 3, 61, 17

loss of sensibility, paresthesia, 19, 37, 0, 60

neuralgia, 39, 60, 45, 0, 17, 300

oppression, suffocation, 19, 60, 14, 3, 85, 87, 61

pruritis, acute, 17, 50, 3, 26, 0, 124, 34

sexual weakness, 0, 1, 19, 43, 63, 87

sharp pain, 3, 50, 60, 0, 17

skin eruption, 0, 3, 124

tetany, spasms, 50, 19, 63, 26, 61, 103

tiredness, 0, 6, 7, 19, 45

trembling, 45, 1, 50, 0, 60, 124, 34

vertigo, 63, 106, 65, 60, 8

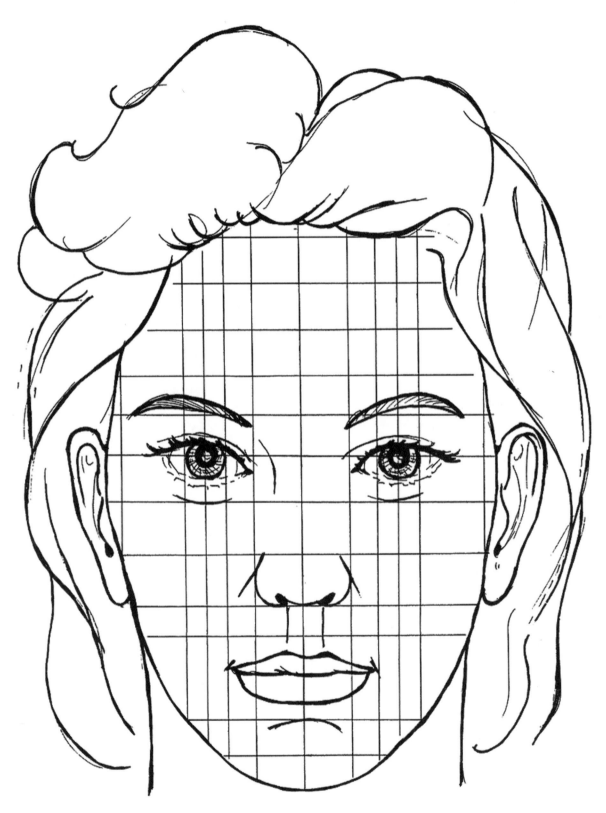

For your individual cases: reflex points

© 2004 Marie-France Muller (may be photocopied for personal use)

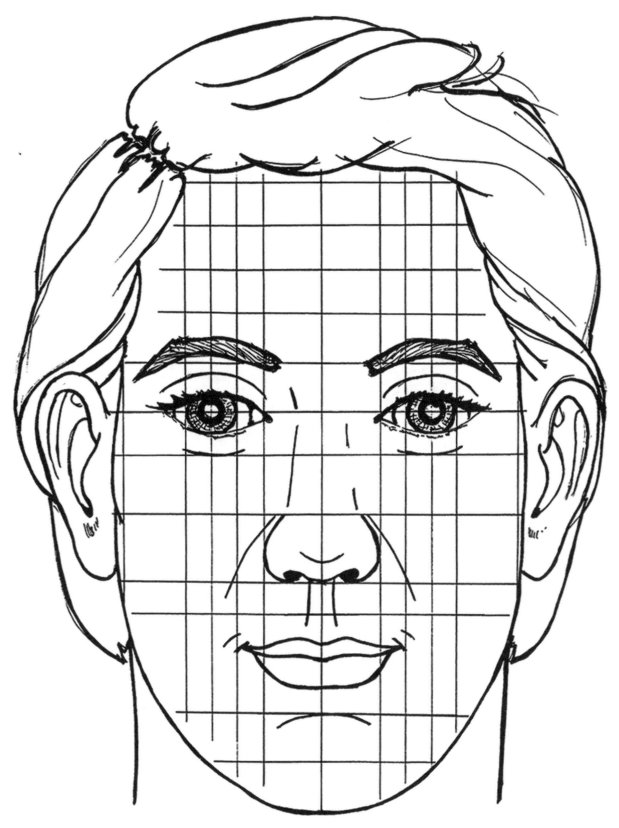

For your individual cases: reflex points

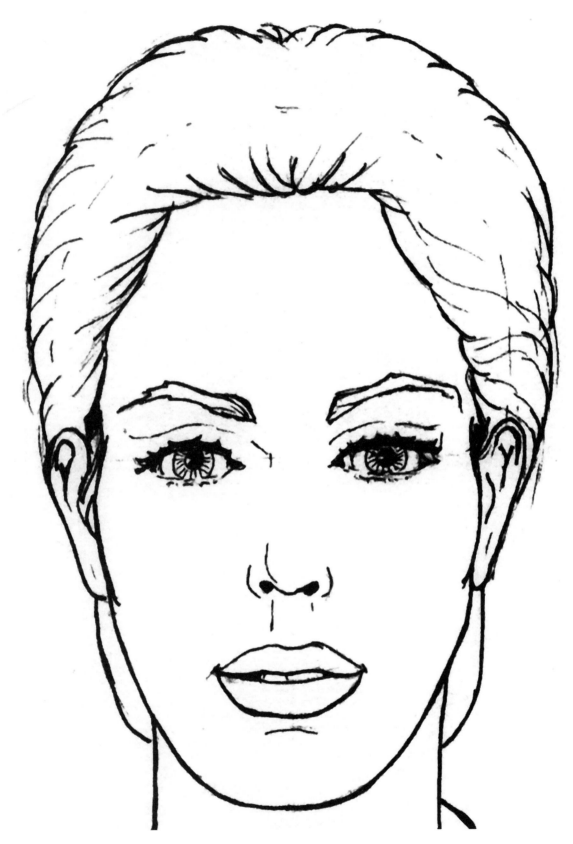

For your individual cases: reflex zones

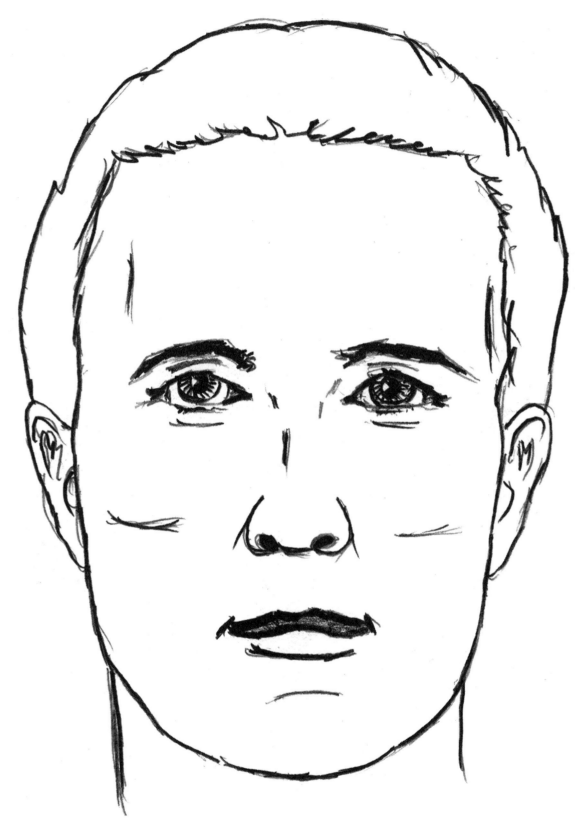

For your individual cases: reflex zones

# 7

# Dien' Cham' for Animals Too!

This method that has come all the way from Vietnam to heal us can give spectacular results on animals, too.

The Dien' Cham' we practice on animals is very similar to that used on humans! We stimulate the same reflex points from equivalent diagrams, just adapting them to the specific morphology of each animal.

Within the scope of this work I will restrict myself to giving you a few useful tips that you will be able to put into practice easily, rather than a full-scale veterinary reflexology handbook! You can refer back to the diagrams in chapter 2, as they are usable on all animals. Also keep in mind the principle of analogy, which works in the same way as for humans. It will quickly allow you to deduce further reflex zones from the ones given.

## A WELL-ACCEPTED METHOD

In Vietnam this technique is widely practiced for treating animals, and in addition they enjoy the attention!

Every evening my husband and I used to have the habit of performing a short session on ourselves to help with tiredness and to prepare for a night's sleep. Our dog watched us doing this and when we finished asked us clearly not to forget him: he wagged his tail, licked the roller that we use a lot, and then presented his muzzle, full of anticipation. You know what it is like: I had no choice but to oblige. I developed a short session for him in which I stimulate the main zones of his muzzle and forehead with the roller and concentrate on areas that correspond best to any problem that he may be having. As for my cats, I prefer using my fingers because the roller scares them somewhat.

You may be practicing Dien' Cham' without knowing it, unintentionally or accidentally. When for example you caress the muzzle of your pet with care and attention, you are treating his or her spinal column, digestive system, lungs, and genital organs. Behind or in front of the ears corresponds to the natural defenses, spinal column, and general physical and psychological balance. The forehead and the eyebrows treat the nervous system, front limbs, and head.

## VARIOUS PROJECTION SYSTEMS

Animals are very similar to us. The same systems of projection have been evidenced, so as you become more familiar with them, it will be gradually easier for you to apply them to your pet. It is true that with animals we generally work on zones rather than points to make things easier. Thus you can avoid having to ask your cat to look straight at you, meet your gaze, and stay in that position without moving, while you fumble with your schematic diagram to better locate pressure points!

### Analogy, Analogy!

On the other hand, analogy works well, and you will be able to find in the face of your pet the same reference points as in your own. The same structure is always found: the forehead, eyes, nose, cheekbones, and mouth. In locating zones, try to establish parallels between features on your own face and your pet's. Dien' Cham' is magic in that it truly adapts to all morphologies and works for all of them.

### Joints

Think of the various reflex zones corresponding to the joints. The head of an animal also contains various angles that generally indicate the relevant locations. Remember that where you find the spinal column you will also be able to locate the thorax and abdomen with all of the internal organs.

### Forehead Reflex Zones

The forehead of most animals is a splendid reflex zone as it is vast and easy to access. To determine the various specific zones, keep in mind a hori-zontal line passing in front of the ears, following the curve of the forehead. It is analogous to the line clearly identifiable in humans, the hairline. The lower line of the forehead passes through the upper eyebrow. Halfway between these two lines you will find the solar plexus and the line separating the thorax and abdomen.

It might be easiest for you to visualize a superimposition of **Diagram 9** onto your pet's forehead, whatever its length. Study again the various diagrams of zones on the forehead and get into the habit of applying them in this case too. The various projections of the legs (**Diagrams 1, 4, and 5**) will often be of great use to you.

### General Projection of Body on Face

In practicing on your pet, you will especially want to use a projection of the body that is equivalent to **Diagram 2** (see Figures 7.1 and 7.2 below), in addition to certain basic zones with main reflex points and indications as per **Diagram 1**.

You will quickly learn to recognize the zones and your pet will show you where to go! Be sure of that! You will be surprised at the results obtained in just a few seconds and your caresses will quickly become therapeutic treatment, which will motivate you to spend some time doing them. What better could a cat or dog dream of?

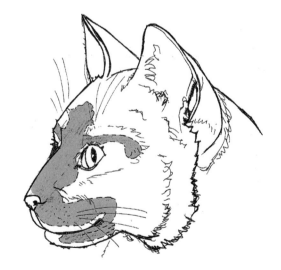

Figure 7.1. Projection of body on the face of a cat

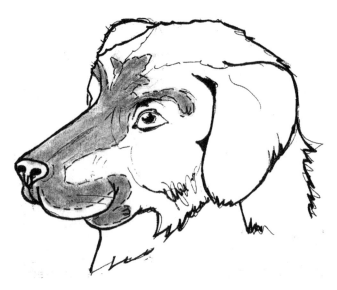

Figure 7.2. Projection of body on the face of a dog

## LOCATING REFLEX POINTS

It should be relatively simple to locate reflex points if you keep the following in mind. Whether your pet is small or big, has a long muzzle or a flattened one, is a cat, dog, or dwarf rabbit, the same reference points apply. Just follow the diagrams and adapt them to its morphology. Here are a few rules that should be observed:

- The nose (which is the central part of the muzzle), represents the spinal column. The coccyx is found toward the nose tip and the neck at the nose root, between the eyes. Between these two points all of the vertebrae are represented.
- Moving up from the nose tip, the lumbar vertebrae, together with the kidneys, intestines, and genital organs are represented.
- Above them are the dorsal vertebrae, together with the bronchial tubes, lungs, and heart.
- At the nose root are the cervical vertebrae, with the throat and the thyroid glands.

Interesting results can be obtained by stimulation of the entire zone along the muzzle in cases of accident, paralysis, arthritis, blocked kidneys, digestive problems, or breathing trouble. Make

sure that you particularly stimulate points directly related to the problem. On either side of the muzzle, you will find reflex zones corresponding to the pelvis (toward the tip of the nose), the ribcage (toward the center), and the neck (on the upper part).

- The bony parts above the orbit of the eye are analogous to the arch of the eyebrows. Toward the nose root, they correspond to the shoulders. The central parts correspond to the back legs, and the area close to the temples corresponds to the paws and digits. Stimulation of this zone has a calming effect and quiets anxious animals or those under stress.
- The forehead is an area that is relatively important and you can stimulate the whole zone together, even if you do not know the correspondences exactly. The center corresponds to the head and cerebral functions.

We can also find the spinal column on the forehead, together with practically all of the body's reflex zones, along a central line starting at the nose and ending between the ears (see **Diagrams 9 and 10** of the forehead). Of course you should not hesitate to stroke this region in particular!

- Around the tip of the nose corresponds to the pelvic area. It is recommended to stimulate this a lot in cases of paralysis, accidental wounds, or hip dysplasia. Be careful not to stimulate the tip of the nose itself; your pet would not be very pleased!
- The philtrum located between the base of the nose tip and the upper lip constitutes a very important point which can even save the life of your pet. It is a reanimation point and tones up the body generally. It should be stimulated in cases of shock, major tiredness, and low natural defenses. If it is stimulated at length it provokes vomiting, useful if your dog has the habit of swallowing anything that comes into range!

During the Basic Session (see below) stimulate it gently so that your pet will get used to it and the resulting boost of vital energy. In this way you will have little problem stimulating it much harder in more serious circumstances.

- The zone from the philtrum (under the nose) to the corners of the mouth corresponds to the thighs but also the intestines. The stomach is represented on the upper part; toward the right the liver; toward the left, the spleen.
- The corners of the mouth correspond to the knee joints and to the tarsus, as well as the kidneys. The zone extends from the corners of the mouth upward a little way in the direction of the ears.
- The zones from the corners of the mouth to the center of the chin correspond to the legs, the metatarsus, the feet, and the digits, located at the center of the chin. This is very useful in cases of fractures. Frequent stimulation of these reflex zones promotes bone growth or ossification and better recovery, even if the limb is plastered.
- It is important to stimulate the zones around the ears. This zone corresponds to point 0 in humans! As these zones have multiple corre-

spondences, they are the necessary termination point for any Dien' Cham' session. It is not by chance that these are the zones preferred by all animals. Which pet owner has never scratched behind the ears of his cat or dog?!

# THE BASIC SESSION: A PERFECT STROKE

These few indications should allow you to easily transform time spent stroking your animal into therapeutic sessions to better care for your pet. A basic session that you can use for your daily stroke is shown on Figure 7.3. It is analogous in every way to the session that you have learned to practice on yourself or on another person.

Please note that here the hairline is replaced by an imaginary line over the top of the head from the bases of the ears. You will want to exercise logic when adapting this advice to the specific morphology of your pet.

## Basic Points

These few reflex zones are generalized from the points given in **Diagram 1** in order to make them easier to massage. You will quickly recognize the main basic points that you already know how to find and use on yourself or another person. Adapting them to your four-legged friend requires no change in technique.

Base yourself on the eyes and the eyebrows, then search for the cheekbones and the jawbone. It is quite like humans in fact.

Do not become discouraged by differences in morphology. The nose of a Shi-Tzu can be massaged in the same way as a German Shepherd. One of the noses is shorter, that is all. In the same way, the shape and the direction of the ears changes nothing with respect to their correspondences. Point 0 is located in the center of the line passing in front of the orifice of the ear, no matter whether the ear is pointing to the front or to the back!

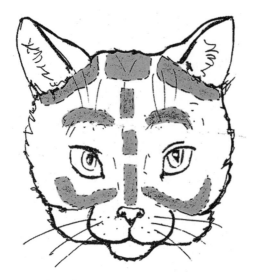

Figure 7.3. Stroking therapy session

Whatever the case, with the help of Figures 7.4 and 7.5 (see below) you should be able to give your first session on an animal quite easily. Why don't you begin with showing them the session you are planning to give them by doing it on yourself? It will reassure them a lot and relax you at the same time, which is doubly beneficial.

Be kind and reassuring and above all remain calm! Remember that your pet is always liable to show to the world what you are feeling in secret. Our cats, dogs, and horses precisely reveal our inner souls and hidden emotions! It is excellent feedback!

With a little practice you will quickly be able to adapt the therapeutic advice given in the Practical Dictionary in chapter 4 to your pet. A coryza in a cat is treated with the same points as those used for influenza in humans, and skin problems react to the points indicated for humans.

Remember that this technique is usable as a complement to any other therapy, which it can assist. Do not hesitate to use it regularly! If you adopt a kitten or a puppy it is best to get into the habit of giving it sessions as young as possible. Your efforts will be amply paid back later on!

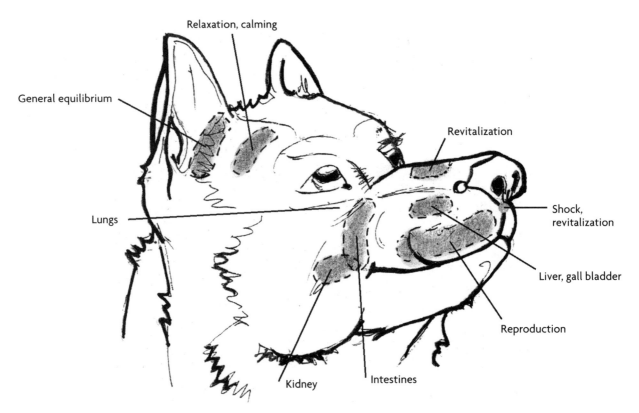

Figure 7.4. Basic pressure points (profile)

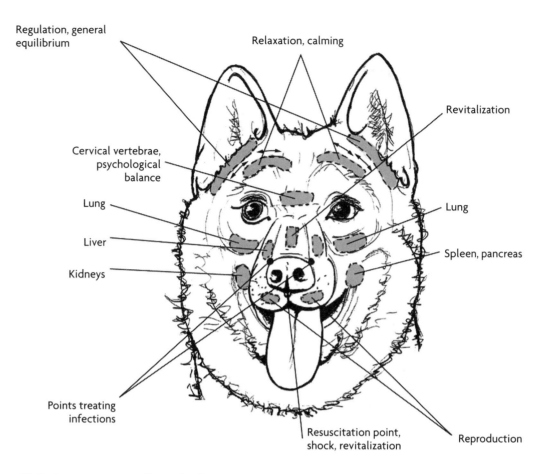

Regulation, general equilibrium

Relaxation, calming

Revitalization

Cervical vertebrae, psychological balance

Lung

Lung

Liver

Spleen, pancreas

Kidneys

Points treating infections

Resuscitation point, shock, revitalization

Reproduction

Figure 7.5. Basic pressure points (front view)

# HORSE REMEDIES

This technique can also be used for treating horses effectively. In fact a bigger roller exists, making the task easier, as long as the sight of this new instrument does not frighten your jumpy steed.

Many problems of legs and feet can be treated in this way. It is the same thing with back problems; good results have been obtained in some cases where all other treatments have failed. Ideally, in case of a fall or an accident, it is best to treat right away, as restoring correct blood and energy circulation around the lesion often diminishes the consequences of the injury. Stimulation should in this case last for several minutes.

If your horse complies, it would be good to practice a rapid general stimulation equivalent to the Basic Session regularly. You could integrate this after a ride or lesson and the usual grooming! The horse's power of recuperation would certainly be improved as well as its natural defenses and nervous system.

## How to Stimulate

The easiest method of stimulation for a horse is to firmly massage or tap the reflex zone with the tip of the finger. If you have a toothed roller it can be passed gently over the zones chosen. The animal will enjoy the light scratching. Obviously you must avoid using any kind of pointed instrument, even well-rounded, because horses can be skittish and a clumsy movement could cause damage!

The session can last from one to ten minutes,

depending on the receptivity of the animal. It can be performed at any time. In case of digestive troubles it is preferable to perform the stimulation after meals.

In the same way as for humans, in case of a pregnant mare, it is advisable to avoid Dien' Cham' except in emergencies.

When you have learned to master these basic techniques for treating animals there will always be time to go further if you want. But with just this much you will have already avoided many health problems with your pet and also helped it get over certain ailments.

# Conclusion

# Some Last Advice

In this book you have all of the necessary fundamentals of Dien' Cham' to soothe and relieve all kinds of pain, to treat health problems as they arise, and even to work on chronic cases. I feel confident that you will be pleasantly surprised by the simplicity and efficiency of this reflexology system. Before I leave you I would like to return to one or two points that seem to me to be of utmost importance.

## GOOD HEALTH DEPENDS ON A GOOD CIRCULATION OF ENERGY

After reading these books I hope that you have understood that your health depends on the correct circulation of energy, that all pain is due to a blockage of energy, that all tiredness slows and reduces the energy flow, and that all physical problems result from disturbances to energy levels in the body. When you have a good level of energy, it is impossible to fall sick or even catch a cold. It is only when you allow tiredness to take over or let worry invade your consciousness that sickness strikes. It can start with a common cold. Then you may feel tired, catch a sore throat, develop a fever, and then a cough. Bronchitis, asthma, backache, stiff neck and shoulders all become possible. Various diseases and sicknesses can start developing and cause trouble at the level of the weakest organ or function. It is desirable to ensure energy circulation, bring it into balance, and give it a boost, so that the body is capable of healing itself.

## ABOVE ALL ENSURE THAT PAIN DOES NOT BECOME ENTRENCHED

One of the main things to understand about Dien' Cham' is that it empowers every-one and anyone to remove sickness right from the outset, soothe pain before it takes hold, or stop a cold, wherever you happen to be at the time, just using your fingers or a simple instrument, without having to wait until you arrive back home.

In France and in Western countries in general everyone seems to be programmed to be sick. We wait to become sick and then we make an appointment with our physician or doctor. Then we swallow our medicines. The result is that we drag our health problems, aches, and pains around with us, sometimes for years. This seems to be the case for backache, often called the sickness of the century, because no one appears to be able to soothe it, with the exception of a few well-trained osteopaths. But all that it is necessary to make it disappear is a few strokes of a pen. Everyone can learn to practice this on him or herself instead of letting the pain become entrenched.

This reasoning is the opposite of that held by many people, including physicians and therapists who advise doing nothing for pain until a proper diagnosis has been made. A cold for them is simply the elimination of toxins. There is a logic to these attitudes because pain certainly is an alarm bell and a common cold is a form of detoxification. If you follow such advice, however, you will no doubt learn that you are the one who pays the price for letting the trouble become entrenched. When a physician eventually comes to diagnose your trouble and gives a name to your sickness—such as a case of arthrosis, rheumatism, polyarthritis, lumbar or cervical pain, or a certain type of inflammation—it may well be too late to heal the problem effectively.

Just because a physician happens to be able to give a name to your pain hardly means that he is able to treat it and make it disappear in just a few days by using allopathic medicines, or a series of massages at the physiotherapist. Sometimes a surgical operation or procedure is proposed, accepted, and performed—but without a satisfactory result! In any case you are very likely to have to swallow all kinds of allopathic drugs (like antibiotics, corticoids, and anti-inflammatory medicines), sometimes for months or years, and your pain will be with you all that time! You have a lot more chance to relieve the pain and its cause if

you have recourse to an energy-based therapy like acupuncture, shiatsu, faith healing, foot or hand reflexology techniques, color therapy, magnetotherapy, osteopathy, homeopathy, herbal medicine, naturopathy, or nutritional therapy, and so on. However it will take you a few sessions or a few months of treatment to obtain good results.

Instead of all that, all you need to do is to use your ballpoint pen to stimulate points on your face as soon as troubles appear and stop the pain from establishing itself. It is up to you to choose!

## WHY IT IS NECESSARY TO TREAT A COLD RIGHT FROM THE START

At first glance there is nothing to worry about. Common colds generally disappear by themselves after one or two weeks without treatment. It is the same for an allergy that only occurs at certain times of the year, or when certain substances are in the immediate environment.

If, however, you do not have a good constitution, a cold can bring other problems. This is often the case with rhinitis, influenza with streaming nose, and the beginnings of a fever. In less than an hour you can be feeling awful with no strength or energy. The runny nose provokes a heavy loss of trace elements (as do diarrhea, bleeding, and excess perspiration). Several complications can develop, such as high fever, exhaustion, breathing difficulties, aches and pains, coughing, bronchitis, and—for the unlucky ones—bouts of asthma for the rest of their lives!

## ABILITY TO CARE FOR ONE'S OWN HEALTH

This method will help you to keep in mind several factors:

- Pain can be relieved in an easy, natural way, without it being necessary to take medicines that poison the body

- The problem can be removed right at the beginning, avoiding all later complications
- Good health depends on the circulation of energy and not on the effects of chemical medicines.
- You can learn to be your very own physician so that you can care for and heal yourself and retain your choice of therapy. This will not stop you from going to a physician if you think it is necessary. However if the allopathic treatment brings no result, you have the option of trying Dien' Cham', which is more natural and traditional. You have nothing to lose and everything to gain!

## START BY MEMORIZING THE REFLEX ZONES

Many people cannot or do not want to look after themselves. They want others to deal with their problems and find it easier to swallow a pill rather than try to determine which points to stimulate. That's their problem!

Other people are really interested in taking care of themselves but they find many methods too complicated. With Dien' Cham' things become easier. It is not necessary to learn all of the points; just thirty of them allow much to be done. Actually, all that is needed to soothe all kinds of sicknesses is to know the reflex zones of the face. You then have to sweep the particular area broadly with a pen and—when you happen on a sensitive point—press a little more deeply to obtain immediate relief.

For example, in the case of pain in the elbow, which is difficult to treat with other methods, it is enough to sweep the arches of the eyebrows to find a painful spot at the top. If you insist a little at that spot you will obtain immediate relief of the elbow pain. It is possible to obtain the same immediate unblocking of the cervical vertebrae by correctly stimulating the root of the nose between the two eyes.

## SIMPLER THAN THE CHINESE ENERGY SYSTEM

Whenever anyone hears about energy they naturally think of the Chinese energy system with yin and yang and the network of meridians. Chinese medicine—acupuncture and herbal medicine in particular—is greatly effective for treating a majority of sicknesses, and is especially effective with pain. Many of the natural methods that have been recently discovered or revived are based on the Chinese tradition, whether it's a case of using the meridian structure or of working with yin and yang energy. (For some additional information, please see Appendix 1 on Chinese Facial Reflexology.)

However, Chinese medicine is highly complex, requiring much knowledge and practice and many years of study before any kind of mastery can be achieved. (Some physicians study acupuncture for three years and consider that it is sufficient, leaving aside the Chinese pulse-taking technique that they believe to be some kind of inscrutable Chinese puzzle that takes up too much time! But they have not really mastered the system.)

With Dien' Cham' it is not necessary to know about yin and yang or pulse-taking to obtain good results. There is an alternative to knowing the meridians which in fact everybody knows already: the nervous system which is present all round the body, each organ having its own energy, the nervous flux.

## THE NERVOUS FLUX, A NEGLECTED ENERGY

Many people try to treat themselves by relaxation, meditation, positive thinking, visualization, concentration, or prayer. All of these techniques rely on the general relaxation of the nervous system, allowing better circulation of the nervous flux, which sometimes guides you by thought to the problem area. In this way certain types of pain, tension, and anxiety can be relieved.

Sometimes even bleeding can be stopped or a tumor made to disappear! But these techniques seem much too simple to be credible. The same is true of Dien' Cham' where all you have to do is to simply stimulate facial reflex zones and points to obtain an immediate improvement. It might seem too easy to be true perhaps, but whether you believe it or not matters little! It really does work! And this book gives you all the guidance you need to experiment with it for yourself.

Years of experience have shown me that to treat something efficiently it is not always useful to search for the sick organ using the pressure points. Sometimes it is enough to use the Basic Session to relax the central nervous system and then boost the nervous flux using the toning up points. It is simple, quick, and effective. It is only then that it is possible to think about the patient's problems and stimulate the specific reflex points and zones concerned.

## EVERYONE CAN PRACTICE DIEN' CHAM'

There is no age limit for practicing Dien' Cham'. From two to one hundred and two years old, anyone can do it, anywhere, in any position, sitting, lying, or standing. You can even teach children to soothe themselves using this simple method instead of programming them to take medicines at the first sign of sickness! They will adopt it quite willingly.

It cannot be stressed enough, however, that other factors for good health should never be neglected: a well-balanced diet, correct and easy breathing, a healthy life, if possible away from sources of atmospheric and electromagnetic pollution and negative waves of all kinds, liable to disturb your home or your workplace. A life that is in harmony with nature and your divine self is also an important factor for your good health and equilibrium.

## BE CAREFUL! NO FANATICISM!

This is an extraordinary technique and you have probably already accomplished the first few steps along this path leading to enhanced health. Perhaps you have already had your first results. Very good! But be careful, no fanaticism! If the results using Dien' Cham' are hardly debatable, do not make this technique the universal panacea. When the situation demands it, do not hesitate to turn to conventional medicine.

> ### In Case of an Emergency Call a Physician!
>
> If for example you are worried that your child is having a bout of appendicitis, first call for a physician. This does not prevent you from stimulating related zones, as well as the points corresponding to infections, while you are waiting for help. In this way you will provide real assistance without putting his or her life in danger.
>
> Do the same in all cases of emergency: first call for help and then practice Dien' Cham' during the interval, in particular the resuscitation points, which can even help you to save a life. In all cases common sense must prevail.

## TO MAKE FURTHER PROGRESS YOU MUST PRACTICE

The best way to make progress is to practice as often as possible. Believe me when I tell you that many opportunities will present themselves. To begin with most practice will be on yourself, using a mirror to better locate points, then on your friends and family. Plenty of practice will enable you to make a surprising amount of progress quickly!

Don't forget that you can even give Dien' Cham sessions to your animals! When I stimulate my face or the face of my one of my close circle, our big dog never misses the occasion to ask for his own session. He picks up his nose and responds to my practice with obvious pleasure, whether I use my fingers, a ballpoint pen, or a roller. I rub his muzzle, forehead, and around his ears, until he gives the signal that he has had enough by moving away contentedly. He always looks really satisfied.

## IMMEDIATE RESULTS

As for results, these should be obtained during the first session when you are working on a specific case, and relief should be almost instantaneous. After more than twenty years of practice using this technique, I am able to affirm that failure can never be ascribed to the technique itself.

If your session is not having any results, there are only three possible reasons:

- Your localization of points is only approximate, incomplete, or incorrect.
- You have not stimulated the points corresponding to the case in question.
- Your stimulation was badly done, either too short (you should count ten to twenty seconds per point) or too light or superficial. The latter is the most common problem.

This method works not for psychological reasons, but because it is based on the natural reflexes of the human body reacting to correct stimulation. Here we are reminded of the control panel analogy again! You should bear in mind that since circulation is the source of life, stagnation is the source of death. Dien' Cham' is an effective way of correcting energy circulation when it is blocked or slowed.

Movement is life and the whole universe is governed by movement; this is one of the most infallible laws of nature. We receive our creative force from the earth, the sun, and water, which are all in constant motion. Thanks to these forces we grow, get old, and die. Nothing is immutable or unchanging, and our vitality increases or decreases as a function of the quality and quantity of our energy. Impermanence is the golden rule!

By stimulating the correct points, Dien' Cham' shows us how to keep our body in motion and conserve the specific rhythm of each of its parts. If circulation slows, pain manifests; this is nature's alarm bell to warn us of disorders and functional trouble in the body.

It is up to each of us to know about our body and its reflexes and learn Dien' Cham' to help the body to react. In this way you will progress and naturally want to gain more knowledge in this science of energy that has been practiced for thousands of years.

My wish in writing this book is for you to take charge of your health at all levels of your being. If you develop the habit of daily practice of this reflexology massage, you will avoid many sicknesses and be able to detect troubles as they arise. Is this not the goal of all therapy?

*I would now like to wish you excellent results, the very best of health and vitality, for you, your family, and friends.*

# Appendix I

# Chinese Facial Reflexology

## ACUPRESSURE

Acupressure is an alternative to classical acupuncture in which the use of needles to stimulate certain points located on meridians—energy pathways in the body—is replaced by manual massage.

In China, this therapeutic method was long practiced on children in preference to acupuncture. This type of massage started to become widespread during the time of the Ming dynasty emperors of the fourteenth to seventeenth centuries. Many traditions have taken account of the idea that the microcosm mirrors the macrocosm, which is the basis of all reflexology. It was the same in ancient China where it was considered that each part of the body—eye, nose, ear, mouth, face, foot, hand, and so on—contains the energy projection of the whole body. The techniques were considered to be emergency medicine, procuring relief for a patient while awaiting the doctor, and also for family health, preventing sickness and treating symptoms as soon as they arose.

- **Acupressure or Do-in** is like acupuncture in that it is practiced on the whole body. However, we will only examine acupressure with respect to the face, in keeping with the focus of this book. In ancient China this kind of auto-massage was known as Tao-yin and was very commonly practiced by peasants and also monks.
- **Ji-jo,** meaning "first aid" in Chinese, is a method of acupressure that concerns pressure points and is capable of helping enormously in most common cases. The points are acupuncture points that are stimulated by the fingers. It is better not to think of the term "first aid" in its Western meaning, because the aim is simply to quickly relieve a minor pain or symptom.

> **Warning**
> Chinese massage or acupressure is not recommended for subjects with serious cardiac conditions or pregnant women.

## Harmonizing Yin and Yang

As with all of the universe, the human body is instable and permanently seeking balance. According to the Chinese tradition, a sickness is always explained by an energy imbalance between yin and yang. A lack or an excess of one of these inevitably ends up with repercussions on one of the body organs if nothing is done to remedy the situation. Chinese massage, like acupuncture, is essentially designed to prevent sickness by harmonizing the circulation of energy in the body to ensure correct functioning. Keep in mind that the basic goal of Chinese medicine is to maintain people in good health and not, as in the West, to wait until sickness strikes to intervene. If these techniques are practiced regularly they stimulate the body's natural defenses and ward sickness off.

# PRACTICING ACUPRESSURE

This appendix does not pretend to be a thorough work on acupressure, which is relatively well known and has been described in many books. Here we are just presenting a few facial massage techniques, capable of complementing the Vietnamese method to which this book is dedicated.

The acupressure techniques use the following methods of stimulating either acupuncture points or reflex zones close to them.

- pushing a fingernail into the point as if it were a needle
- pressing more or less strongly on the zone
- applying pressure using a wooden rod or ballpoint pen
- massaging the point or the zone with the finger ends in a circular motion
- rolling the skin between the fingers
- lightly and slowly touching the skin, which improves blood and energy circulation

You can increase the effect of the stimulation by rotating your fingers or instrument. Depending on the direction of rotation, you can either tone up, concentrating energy at one point, or disperse energy where there is an excess:

- **To tone up,** exert pressure rapidly and energetically around the point, rotating the fingers clockwise. You can also massage the point by exerting sufficient pressure to pull the skin clockwise over the spot.
- **To disperse energy,** press down long and deeply while making counterclockwise rotations. Alternatively practice a deep massage, rotating on the spot in a counterclockwise direction.

## Facial Reflex Zones in Chinese Massage

You will be able to find these zones on Figure A1.1. They are less extensive than those in other systems because they only surround and follow points located on the meridians. The Chinese define twelve main pathways of energy in the body, each connecting a series of specific acupuncture points. The points are places where the energy of the channel rises close to the surface of the skin. Many, but not all, of the meridians involve the face.

The technique is simple enough: all you have to do is to massage for a few seconds the various zones that correspond to your appraisal of the situation. You can cease the stimulation as soon as you sense an improvement.

- The larynx reflex zone is in the middle of the forehead, close to the hairline.
- Just below you will find the windpipe, or trachea.
- In the middle of the forehead are the lung and bronchial tubes.
- Between the eyes is the heart reflex zone.
- In the middle of the bridge of the nose are the liver and gallbladder reflex zones.
- The spleen is projected on the bridge of the nose, just before the nostrils.
- The ears are projected on each side of the bridge

of the nose, in a small depression located half an inch or so away from the inner corner of the eye.

- The digestive system is projected to the left of the nose close to the edge of the nostril.
- The male and female genital organ point is located just below the base of the nose. This is also a point allowing resuscitation (Kuatsu) and corresponds to point 19 in Dien' Cham'. (It is also the 25GV—Governing Vessel—point.)

## Facial Acupressure Points

We are now going to take a look at a few points and zones likely to allow you to quickly relieve your familiar little aches and pains, but only the most common. You will be able to practice these massages on yourself as well as on any other person.

- Massage the central part of the forehead with the index and middle fingers from the hairline to the beginning of the nose between the eyebrows. Make small circular movements upward and downward along this axis.
  *Indications:* any respiratory troubles such as bronchitis or asthma.

- At the Yin-Tang point between the eyebrows, pinch the skin until it reddens, using the index finger and the thumb. This point is one of the "peculiar" pressure points not located on one of the meridians.

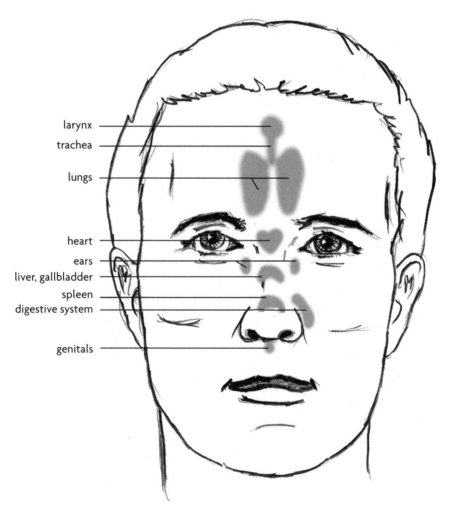

larynx
trachea
lungs
heart
ears
liver, gallbladder
spleen
digestive system
genitals

Figure A1.1. Acupressure zones

*Indications:* headaches, insomnia, sinusitis, dizziness, and hangovers!

- Find the points located on either side and at the base of the nose, where the bone and cartilage meet. Massage them deeply.
  *Indications:* these two points relieve nasal congestion in the case of a cold and serve to fight against the habit of smoking.

- Press down deeply on the points located on either side of the nostrils, where they meet the cheeks (OG1).
  *Indications:* colds, chills, sinusitis, flu, and laryngitis.

- Stimulate point **19** (25GV in Chinese system) at the base of the nose, by briskly digging a fingernail in. This point can be used in an emergency while waiting for help when the victim has lost consciousness, or is having, or liable to have, an epileptic fit. In this case do not forget to place an object between the teeth to prevent the person from biting his or her tongue.
  *Indications:* fainting, seizures, heat stroke, and also effective in cases of continued sneezing!

- Stimulate the point located in the tiny hollow about one inch forward of the tragus, the fleshy protrusion at the front of the ear.
  *Indications:* toothache in the upper jaw.

- Point 24 GV (Governing Vessel) located at the tip of the nose, permits you to attenuate the effects of drunkenness, although it is better to abstain from drinking in the first place!

- Point 2GB (Gall Bladder), located halfway between the ear and the arch of the eyebrows, can be stimulated in the case of eye trouble.
  *Indications:* near-sightedness, troubled vision, eye fatigue, conjunctivitis, and so on.

## A Short Session of Facial Do-in

This kind of short routine[1] should be performed every morning when you rise, or during the day to help you to relax. It can be carried out standing up or sitting comfortably, as long as you are in a quiet place. Remember to breathe freely and easily during the session.

- Start by rubbing the palms of your hands together for a few seconds to warm them up.
- Then visualize the centerline that goes from the base of the nose upward to the center of the forehead, through the crown and then down toward the neck and ending at the base of the skull. Close your fists and drum softly with the knuckle joints on your skull either side of the centerline, but never on it.
- Bend your fingers and with the knuckles tap your skull on either side of the centerline. Starting from the hairline move to the base of the skull along imaginary parallel lines.
- Now, place the tips of your spread fingers on the scalp on either side of the centerline and make small circles firm enough to move the skin.

This series of exercises favors a good mental function but the beneficial effects do not stop there. They also promote regeneration of the bladder and kidneys, correct functioning of the intestine, and relieve piles or hemorrhoids and problems with the prostate. In women they help with painful periods.

- With the tips of your fingers lightly brush your face from the forehead downward. This stimulates the stomach.
- Now place the spread fingers of each hand above the eyebrow on the corresponding side. Perform tiny rotations on the spot, moving the skin. Recommence with the fingers placed halfway up the forehead, and then again, at the limit of the hairline. Repeat this cycle three

times. This massage has an effect on the circulation of the blood, the nervous system, and the digestion.

- Place the fingertips on either side of an imaginary line going from the root of the nose to the hairline. At the same time as you press with moderate pressure, pull the hands toward the temples as if you were trying to smooth over your forehead or trying to open it up. Repeat this twice. This movement tones up the eyes, clears the sinuses, and helps prevent nervous tiredness.

- Now place your hands on either side of your nose with the fingers pointing upward. Breathe in deeply and then breathe out sharply through the nose while rubbing it vigorously. Do this several times. You will find that you can breathe more easily, even when you do not have any obstructions! This is excellent to use against tobacco smoking and at the same time it stimulates digestion.

- Now turn your attention to the eyes! Start by closing them as tightly as you can and then opening them wide, breathing out. Then rub your hands together and press your palms to your eyelids for a few seconds. These exercises rest and revitalize your eyes when they have become tired from reading or working on a computer. They also prevent wrinkles from forming around the eyes and ugly bags under them.

- Then place your fingers flat on each cheek. Rotate your hands, pushing your cheeks inward over the lower jaw, ears, cheekbones, nose, and corners of the mouth. Repeat this seven times. This relaxes the jaws, which are often tensed up, and protects the health of the teeth and gums.

- Place your fingers slightly apart just above the upper lip in the tiny hollows at the top of the gums. Massage by pressing lightly. Do the same at the base of the teeth on the lower jaw. This massage improves circulation around the gums,

activates the salivary glands, and stimulates the meridians of the stomach and the small and large intestines.

- With your thumbs, massage the zone under the lower jaw, starting from the point under the ears, moving toward and finishing at the chin.

- To terminate this facial massage, place your hands flat on both sides of the face and make sweeping movements upward and backward. Then move to the temples and do the same, ending on the nape of the neck and, finally, repeat from just above the ears.

## KNAP PRESSURE POINTS

Georgia Knap was not Chinese, but French of Alsatian extraction, born in 1866, near Troyes. He dedicated his life to researching what he called the "miracle of Faust," meaning the way of obtaining eternal youth. In doing so, he discovered that stimulating a certain number of pressure points encouraged the elimination of uric acid from the

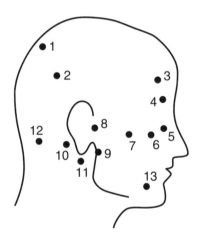

| 1 and 2 | Headaches, arthritis |
|---|---|
| 3 and 4 | Frontal sinusitis, eyesight |
| 5, 6, and 7 | Lateral sinusitis, catarrh, colds, facial neuralgia |
| 8, 9, 10, and 11 | Inflammation of the ear |
| 12 | Headaches |
| 13 | Arthritis of jaw |

Figure A1.2. Knap Points on the head

nerve endings. The points are distributed all over the body. These points—which are usually somewhat tender in a subject in good health—can become really painful in the case of diverse ailments, due to an accumulation of uric and lactic acids and toxins.

Figure A1.2 shows the points located on the face as Knap presented them, with their indications.

He developed a massage of the points that tend to give pain, and he performed this every morning on himself when he woke up. The technique consists in searching for the most painful point and rubbing it using the tip or the joint of a finger. As these points are located on the nerves, unblocking them allows free circulation and improved functioning of the corresponding organs. Knap discovered the very basis of the Chinese energy system and reflexology, using just the means at his disposal!

# Appendix 2

# Japanese Scalp Massage

Just as the face mirrors the entire body, so does the scalp—zones corresponding to the organs of the body can be found there as well. Included here is a simple Japanese scalp massage useful for stimulating the reflex zones and energy pathways on the crown of the head. This massage comes from Japanese author Michio Kushi, a proponent of macrobiotics—a diet and lifestyle that strives to balance yin and yang energies in the body.

Figure A2.1 shows the zones on the scalp that correspond to organs.

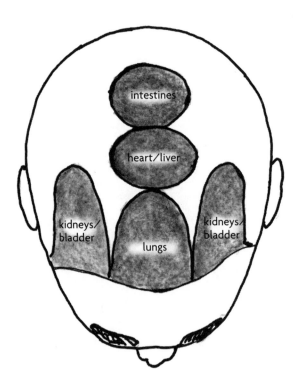

Figure A2.1. Crown reflex zones (as per Michio Kushi)

The crown of the head can also be seen as crossed by fictive lines along which the various acupuncture points can be found.

- The first line, or median, crosses the center of the skull.
- The second line starts at the inner corner of the eye.
- The third line starts at the outer corner of the eye.
- The fourth line starts from the temple.

Figure A2.2 illustrates these energy pathways on the scalp punctuated by specific acupressure points.

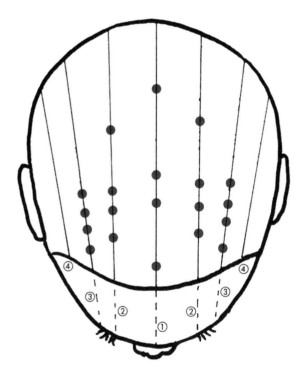

Figure A2.2. Energy pathways (meridians) and acupressure points on the crown of the head

## MASSAGING THE SCALP

It is simple and pleasant to stimulate the following points with the fingers:

- For a few seconds just press quite strongly with four fingers of each hand on either side of the median crossing the crown of the head, then let go.
- Then press down on the second set of lines, which start from the inner corners of the eyes.
- Then move to the third and fourth lines.

This simple massage will stimulate the meridians or energy pathways at the crown and tone up the nervous system and cerebral circulation promoting the diffusion of Chi or Qi.

## MAIN EFFECTS

The main effects of this massage are as follows:

- Helps concentration.
- Improves memory and clears the mind.
- Calms the mind down.
- Relieves headaches, migraines, dizziness, and giddiness.
- Stimulates cerebral circulation.
- Prevents hair-loss and improves the well-being of the scalp.

# Notes

## Introduction

1. See Marie-France Muller, *Colloidal Minerals and Trace Elements: How to Restore the Body's Natural Vitality* (Rochester, Vt.: Healing Arts Press, 2005).
2. Marie-France Muller, *Reflexotherapy Encyclopedia* (forthcoming).

## Chapter 3

1. Method and diagram established following the work of Professor Bui Quoc Chau.
2. Michio Kushi, *Oriental Diagnosis* (London: Sunwheel Publications, 1978).

## Chapter 4

1. See Marie-France Muller, *An Unknown Miracle Cure: Magnesium Chloride* (Saint Julien en Genevois: Éditions Jouvence, 1998).
2. See Marie-France Muller, *Clay Made Easy,* (Saint Julien en Genevois: Éditions Jouvence, 1998).
3. Method and diagram established following the work of Professor Bui Quoc Chau.

4. See Marie-France Muller, *Practical Clay* (Saint Julien en Genevois: Éditions Jouvence, 1998) and *An Unknown Miracle Cure: Magnesium Chloride.*
5. Also see: Dr. Sandra Cabot, *The Liver Cleansing Diet* (Scottsdale, Ariz.: S.C.B. International, 1997).
6. See Marie-France Muller, *Colloidal Minerals and Trace Elements.*
7. Ibid.
8. Ibid.
9. See Marie-France Muller, *An Unknown Miracle Cure: Magnesium Chloride.*

## Appendix 1

1. These exercises are inspired from those described in the book by Jocelyne Aubry and Ho-Han Chang, *Healing By Do-in Self Massage* (Paris: Edi InterEditions, 1995). In this volume a complete cycle of Do-in for use in daily life can be found.

# Bibliography

Aubry, Jocelyne and Ho-Han Chang. *Guérir par l'auto-massage Do-In*. Paris: Edi InterÉditions, 1995.

Blate, Michael. *The Natural Healer's Acupressure Handbook: Advanced G-Jo*. Columbus, N.C.: The G-Jo Institute, 1983.

———. *The Natural Healer's Acupressure Handbook: Basic G-Jo*. Columbus, N.C.: The G-Jo Institute, 1982.

Brelet-Rueff, Claudine. *Les étonnantes techniques chinoises*. Paris: Éditions Retz, 1977.

Chan, Pedro. *Finger Acupressure*. New York: Ballantine Books, 1995.

Chau, Bui Quoc. *Dien Cham Khien Lieu Phap* (Facytherapy). Ho Chi Minh City, Vietnam: Self-published.

———. *Facio Diagnosis – Cyberneto Therapy*. Vietnam: Minh Hai Ed., 1984.

Kushi, Michio. *Oriental Diagnosis*. London: Sunwheel Publications, 1978.

Le Quang, Nhuan. "Massage vietnamien, automassage Dien' Cham'." *Génération Tao* 4, Sept/Oct. 1997.

Long An, Nha Xuat Ban. *So Tay Facy, Bui Quoc Chau*. Vietnam: 1992.

Muller, Marie-France. *Les Réflexothérapies*. Paris: Éditions Retz, 1981.

Ohsawa, George. *Zen Macrobiotics*. Los Angeles: The Ohsawa Foundation, 1965.

Rivière, Françoise. *#7 Diet: An Accompaniment to Ohsawa's Zen Macrobiotics*. Los Angeles: George Ohsawa Macrobiotic Foundation, 2005.

The Group of Researchers and Publishers of Facio Diagnosis and Cyberneto Therapy. "Massage, rubbing, application of balm or medicinal tape at facial points and cure of common diseases." 19 B Duy Tan Street, 3rd District, Ho Chi Minh City, Vietnam, 1985.

Van Sen, Tran and Leon Jones. "Facio Diagnosis and Cyberneto Therapy." *The American Journal of Acupuncture* 13, No. 4, Oct–Dec, 1985.

# Therapeutic Index of Dien' Cham' Point Correspondences

This index lists points given in the Practical Dictionary of Therapeutic Sessions.

Breathlessness, 34, 8, 0
Bronchitis, 3, 17, 26, 8, 61, 37, 51, 73, 38, 14, 0
Bruising, Dislocations, Sprains, 50, 461, 130, 127, 100, 97, 0
Burns, 17, 26, 38, 85, 60, 61, 14, 15, 16, 0
Burping Babies, 126, 19, 0

Cellulitis, 26, 3, 85, 87, 50, 37, 39, 74, 143, 0
   + 85, 87, 22, 0
Cerebral Blood Circulation, 106, 65, 60, 8, 15, 0
Cerebral Functions, 124, 103, 106, 60, 34, 26, 65, 0
Cervical Vertebrae, 8, 34, 26, 65, 106, 16, 0
Chakras, 365, 127, 19, 1, 8, 26, 103
Chi (to provoke its ascent), 126, 103, 1, 19, 127, 22, 6, 37, 50, 0
Chi (to provoke its descent), 26, 3, 51, 87, 14, 15, 0
Chills, 50, 127, 19, 3, 61, 34, 124, 0
Choking or Inhalation of a Foreign Body, 19, 63, 7, 14, 0
Cholesterol Reduction, 41, 50, 37, 113, 7, 233, 0
Coccyx, 126, 143, 0
Cold, the Common, 50, 19, 3, 61, 26, 124, 106, 103, 342, 0
Cold Sensitivity, 15, 17, 60, 61, 1, 0
Colibacillosis, 19, 17, 38, 43, 143, 113, 61, 63, 37, 300, 85, 87, 0
Colitis, Functional Colopathy, 127, 63, 19, 61, 0
   or, 342, 98, 19, 17, 38, 0
Colitis with spasms, 127
   Stress-Related, 124, 34, 8, 61, 3, 0
   With Diarrhea, 103, 50, 37, 63, 127, 22, 365, 19, 0
Conjunctivitis, 73, 180, 130, 100, 16, 51, 50, 38, 17, 7, 0
Constipation, 50, 19, 3, 143, 41, 97, 98, 38, 0
Contraception (see chapter 4)
Cough, 73, 26, 8, 61, 51, 3, 14, 0
Cystitis, 61, 19, 87, 63, 50, 7, 17, 0
   or, 61, 63, 7, 113, 127, 51, 87, 73, 0
Cystitis (simplified for emergencies), 22, 17, 156, 0

Deafness, 14, 15, 16, 45, 65, 74, 0
Deafness, Hearing Difficulties, 65, 3, 45, 300, 14, 15, 16, 0
Decalcification, Demineralization, 85, 87, 43, 45, 20, 300, 0
Depression, Nervous, 34, 124, 22, 127, 50, 1, 19, 103, 0
Detoxification, Drainage, 26, 3, 85, 87, 0
   or, 7, 19, 26, 38, 50, 61, 85, 124, 87, 0
Diabetes, 7, 63, 113, 37, 39, 0
Diarrhea, 50, 127, 19, 61, 0
Digestive Troubles (see Indigestion, Gastritis, Flatulence)
Diuresis (facilitating), 26, 3, 85, 87, 0
Drug-induced Shock, 19, 127, 0
Drug Problems, 34, 26, 19, 50, 61, 85, 124, 127, 0
Drunkenness, 196, 26, 85, 0
Dysmenorrhea (see Periods, Painful)
Dyspnea, 26, 19, 3, 38, 87, 0

Earache, 17, 38, 37, 61, 14, 15, 16, 0
Ears (see Ears, Buzzing in; Earache; and Deafness)
Ears, Buzzing in; Tinnitus, 3, 14, 15, 16, 0
Eczema, 61, 50, 41, 7, 17, 87, 3, 60, 0
   or, 61, 37, 39, 63, 50, 41, 51, 0
   or, 61, 41, 50, 124, 26, 0
Emphysema, Breathing Impairment, 19, 60, 3, 38, 73, 61, 0
Epilepsy, 19, 26, 50, 63, 103, 127, 0
   Epileptic fit, 19, 127, 0
Exhaustion, Nervous, 19, 126, 103, 124, 106, 34, 1, 50, 127, 22, 0
Expectoration (clearing upper respiratory tract), 37, 3, 26, 0
Eyesight Troubles, 3, 6, 8, 16, 34, 50, 97, 98, 130, 0
   Ocular Pain, 130, 100, 0
   + 60, 177, 185, 191, 195, 197, 0
Eye Tiredness or Fatigue, 73, 3, 34, 103, 130, 0

Fainting, 19, 26, 63
   Followed by points for Relaxation, 124, 34, 26

+ Toning Up, 127, 19, 103, 126

or, 19, 127, 61, 1, 124, 103, 34, 0

Simplified procedure, 19, 127, 0

Fatigue, Chronic or General, 50, 127, 19, 26, 103, 0

or, 1, 6, 17, 22, 43, 60, 124, 106, 0

Fever, High Temperature, 26, 3, 8, 38, 85, 60, 87, 180, 14, 16, 15, 0

Fibromyalgia (see Spasmophilia)

Fingers (various problems), 38, 39, 60, 61, 85, 130, 180, 300, 0

Flatulence, Intestinal Gas, 41, 50, 38, 127, 37, 0

Frigidity, 7, 1, 19, 45, 63, 156, 87, 43, 287, 124, 34, 60, 0


Gallbladder, 41, 50, 233, 0

Gallstones (Bile Lithiasis), 41, 50, 233, 124, 0

Gastritis, 39, 37, 50, 61, 45, 63, 19, 127, 0

Gastroenteritis, 14, 17, 22, 38, 61, 143, 127, 0

Gingivitis, 8, 15, 38, 43, 34, 60, 180, 0

Giving Birth, 19, 63, 87, 0

Glands, Swollen, 37, 50, 0

Goiter, Basedow's Disease, 7, 8, 14, 100, 106, 0


Hands, 60, 130, 100, 180, 0

Hay fever, 50, 19, 7, 3, 61, 37, 39, 0

Headaches, 61, 26, 106, 34, 124, 0

Headaches, Crown of the Head, 50, 51, 87, 61, 103, 0

Headaches, Digestive Origin, 50, 19, 3, 61, 26, 106, 103, 34, 124, 0

Headaches, One Side of the Head, 41, 51, 61, 3, 100, 180, 0

Headaches, Temple, 41, 61, 180, 3, 0

Head Injury, 87, 103, 127, 26, 124, 34, 0

Heart Insufficiency, Heart Failure, 1, 3, 6, 19, 73, 100, 106, 156, 60, 191, 0

Heat Stroke, 19, 26, 143, 85, 0

Heat Stroke, Sunstroke, 26, 103, 3, 85, 60, 87, 14, 15, 16, 0

Hemorrhage, Bleeding (from the uterus or elsewhere), 16, 61, 17, 7, 50, 6, 37, 124, 34, 287, 0

Hemorrhage, Bleeding (from the stomach), 16, 37, 61, 50, 0

Hemorrhoids or Piles, 126, 19, 37, 365, 103, 0

Hepatitis, Viral, 17, 19, 38, 41, 61, 74, 50, 0

Hernia, Hiatal, 61, 37, 39, 74, 0

Herpes, 124, 61, 26, 3, 87, 51, 41, 17, 38, 85, 0

Hiccups, 19, 39, 61, 26, 0

High Blood Pressure, 15, 61, 8, 26, 106, 3, 0

Hoarseness, 26, 3, 8, 61, 106, 180, 14, 0

Hot Flashes, 7, 73, 85, 87, 127, 143, 0

or, 7, 113, 26, 14, 15, 16, 0

Hyperactivity in Children, 34, 8, 26, 106, 100, 124, 127, 61, 0

Hypoglycemia, 7, 63, 113, 19, 0


Immune Deficiencies, 63, 7, 6, 22, 113, 127, 37, 0

+ 60, 61, 37, 50, 113, 127, 156, 17, 0

Impotence, 7, 1, 19, 45, 63, 156, 43, 0

Incontinence, Urinary, 124, 34, 103, 37, 19, 1, 0

or, 85, 87, 22, 43, 45, 0

Indigestion, 50, 38, 127, 39, 37, 0

Inflammation, 26, 3, 50, 17, 38, 14, 16, 61, 60, 0

Influenza, Flu, 14, 15, 38, 61, 3, 37, 50, 0

Insect Bites, 16, 17, 124, 34, 26, 3, 0

Insomnia, 124, 34, 26, 0

+ 124, 34, 51, 16, 14, 0

Intestinal Gas (see Flatulence)

Itching and Scratching, 26, 3, 17, 7, 50, 51, 61, 0


Jaws (spasms and problems with articulation), 14, 15, 0


Kidney Stones (Renal Lithiasis), 38, 43, 45, 73, 300, 85, 0

Kidneys, Various Problems, 17, 38, 300, 342, 43, 45, 560, 0

Knees, 17, 38, 197, 300, 156, 1, 45, 37, 0


Laryngitis, Loss of Voice, 14, 8, 26, 106, 61, 38, 0

Legs, Heavy Feeling, 37, 39, 127, 51, 0

Leucorrhea (see Vaginal Discharge)

Lithiasis (see Gallstones, Kidney Stones)
Liver Problems, 50, 103, 233, 197, 0
Low Blood Pressure, 50, 19, 103, 0
Lumbago, 124, 34, 43, 126, 342, 365, 300, 560, 0
Lumbar vertebrae, 19, 1, 45, 342, 126, 300, 0
Lungs (all problems), 26, 3, 61, 73, 60, 0

Malaria, 14, 15, 26, 34, 124, 0
Mastosis, Painful Breasts, 39, 73, 60, 7, 113, 0
Memory, 103, 124, 34, 60, 50, 3, 0
Ménière's Disease (Syndrome), 63, 65, 34, 0
Menopause, 7, 85, 87, 127, 156, 0
Metritus (see Uterine Problems)
Migraine, 50, 127, 19, 3, 61, 124, 180, 0
    or, 124, 41, 50, 61, 51, 180, 0
Motion Sickness (automobiles, aircraft, boats),
    127, 19, 26, 103, 0
    or more simply: 19 + Relaxing (124, 34, 26, 0)
    Seasickness, 63, 61, 26, 0
Multiple Sclerosis, 37, 60, 73, 74, 51, 63, 97, 98,
    64, 0

Nasal Blockage, 50, 19, 3, 61, 26, 34, 0
Nausea, 19, 26, 61, 0
Neck, Stiffness of, 8, 26, 106, 34, 0
    Torticollis, 34, 26, 106, 8, 50, 100, 87, 65, 0
Nervousness, 8, 26, 34, 60, 61, 124, 127, 100,
    106, 103, 0
Neuralgia, 39, 60, 45, 17, 26, 103, 300, 0
Nightmares, 8, 50, 3, 37, 0
Nosebleeds, 16, 50, 61, 124, 17, 0
Numbness (see Paresthesia)
Numbness at Extremities, 1, 19, 17, 51, 127, 60,
    50, 37, 6, 61, 342, 0

Obesity, 37, 85, 87, 50, 124, 34, 26, 0
Ocular Hypertension (high blood pressure in the
    eye), 16, 51, 0
Oppression, Feelings of, 180, 73, 61, 3, 0
Osteoporosis, 1, 8, 20, 43, 45, 300, 342, 0
Ovarian Cysts, 34, 7, 113, 65, 73, 287, 0
Ovaries, 7, 22, 37, 63, 87, 113, 65, 73, 156, 0
    or, 34, 7, 113, 65, 73, 0

Overwork, 19, 124, 103, 34, 45, 127, 22, 0

Pain, 26, 124, 34, 61, 60, 39, 41, 50, 3, 14, 16, 0
Pain, Shooting, 3, 0, 60, 0
Paralysis, 37, 51, 60, 63, 64, 73, 74, 97, 98, 0
    lower limbs, 63, 64, 37, 51
    upper limbs, 97, 98, 51, 37
Paralysis, Facial, 3, 15, 37, 50, 61, 100, 127,
    156, 51, 0
Paralysis, Hemiplegia, 37, 51, 60, 63, 64, 73, 74,
    97, 98, 0
    lower limbs, 63, 64, 37, 51
    upper limbs, 97, 98, 51, 37
Paresthesia (loss of feeling), 19, 37, 51, 60, 50, 0
Parkinson's Disease, 50, 60, 45, 26, 61, 124,
    34, 0
Pectoral Angina, 1, 3, 100, 106, 73, 61, 19,
    60, 0
Periods, Irregular, 124, 37, 26, 63, 50, 7, 0
Periods, Over-abundant, 16, 103, 50, 37, 287, 7,
    127, 1, 0
Periods, Painful, 127, 156, 63, 7, 61, 1, 50, 37, 0
    Simplified procedure, 37, 7, 113, 0
Perspiration, Excess, 124, 34, 60, 19, 61, 50,
    127, 87, 51, 16, 0
Pneumonia, 26, 3, 61, 7, 8, 73, 60, 14, 0
Pregnancy, 7, 113, 63, 127, 0
    + 127, 156, 87, 50, 37, 65, 0
Premature Ejaculation, 19, 63, 300, 0
Prostatitis, 7, 113, 65, 73, 156, 87, 0
    + 22, 37, 63, 0
Pruritis, 17, 50, 3, 60, 0
    + 26, 3, 61, 60, 50, 87, 0
Psoriasis, 34, 124, 19, 50, 26, 61, 3, 41, 38, 0
Psychological Troubles, 87, 103, 106, 124, 34,
    26, 0
Ptosis of the Bladder, 22, 87, 126, 0
Ptosis or Prolapse of the Uterus, 22, 87, 103, 19,
    63, 156, 127, 0

Rectum, 19, 126, 365, 0
Relaxation, 124, 34, 26, 0
Resuscitation, 19, 127, 26, 124, 34, 0

Salivation, Insufficient, 14, 0

Scapulohumeral Periarthritis, 98, 180, 61, 34, 65, 97, 156, 0

Sciatica, 17, 1, 126, 342, 0
    and, 461, 43, 63, 365, 64, 74, 113, 127, 143, 0

Secretions (decreasing), 103, 126, 63, 7, 17, 1, 50, 61, 15, 16, 51, 22, 0

Secretions (increasing), 26, 3, 39, 85, 19, 87, 0

Sexuality, 1, 7, 19, 43, 45, 63, 300, 0

Shaking, 45, 1, 50, 60, 124, 34, 0

Shingles, Herpes zoster, 17, 300, 124, 64, 61, 60, 3, 38, 50, 0

Shock, 19, 26, 124, 34, 43, 0

Shoulder (see Scapulohumeral Periarthritis)

Shyness, Fright, 124, 34, 8, 0

Sinusitis, 26, 50, 61, 65, 8, 124, 126, 106, 0

Skin Problems, 26, 61, 3, 19, 0

Sleepiness, 19, 0
    Following a meal, 19, 50, 0

Smoking (stopping), 50, 19, 3, 60, 85, 127, 300, 61, 14, 124, 34, 26, 0

Solar Plexus, 180, 73, 61, 3, 0

Sore Throats, Pharyngitis, 14, 3, 61, 8, 0

Spasmophilia, Spasms, Fibromyalgia, 61, 16, 19, 20, 63, 87, 0
    or, 65, 60, 50, 45, 34, 26, 0

Speech Difficulties, 8, 14, 60, 65, 0

Spinal Column, from 19 to 126

Sprains, 61, 127, 51, 34, 26, 103, 106, 0
    or, 127, 124, 106, 26, 0

Stiffness, Aching, and Muscle Cramps, 34, 127, 19, 61, 342, 50, 37, 0

Stomach (see Appetite; Gastritis; Flatulence; Ulcer, Gastric)

Stomach Acidity, 124, 34, 26, 39, 19, 0

Stress, 17, 6, 19, 180, 124, 34, 26, 0

Suffocation, Feelings of, 19, 60, 14, 3, 85, 87, 0

Tachycardia (fast heartbeat), 34, 124, 3, 8, 26, 0

Teeth, 39, 3, 16, 43, 51, 57, 61, 8, 34, 106, 124, 180, 0
    simplified procedure, 124, 180, 61, 127, 22, 0

Tennis Elbow, 97, 98, 17, 0

Testicles, 7, 113, 65, 73, 287, 0

Tetany, 50, 19, 63, 26, 61, 103, 0

Throat Inflammation (see Sore Throat and Cold, as well as Cough, Laryngitis, and other ENT problems)

Thyroid Regulation, 7, 8, 14, 39, 100, 0
    + 14, 15, 26, 8, 20, 0
    Hypothyroidism, add 15 as well as Toning Up points

Tinnitus (see Ears, Buzzing in)

Toes, 365, 0

Tongue cramp, 7, 60, 3, 8, 14, 0

Toning Up, 127, 19, 26, 103, 126, 1, 0

Tonsillitis (see Sore Throat)

Torticollis (see Neck, Stiffness of)


Ulcer, Gastric, 61, 64, 74, 39, 34, 17, 0

Ulcer of the Mouth, Thrush, Aphtha, 8, 14, 15, 0

Uterine Fibroids, 7, 19, 63, 16, 17, 22, 87, 0
    + 7, 113, 63, 38, 50, 37, 61, 0

Uterine Problems, 63, 19, 22, 87, 287, 0
    or, 7, 37, 65, 113, 156, 0


Vaginal discharge, Leucorrhea, 1, 3, 7, 43, 61, 37, 63, 87, 127, 22, 287, 16, 0

Vaginal Dryness, 287, 0

Vaginal Inflammation, 61, 60, 37, 50, 17, 38, 63, 7, 87, 0

Vaginitis, Vaginismus, 19, 63, 50, 156, 127, 0

Varicose Veins (see Legs, Blood Circulation)

Vertigo, Dizziness, 63, 34, 106, 65, 60, 8, 0

Voice, Loss of (see Laryngitis)

Vomiting, 50, 19, 34, 124, 0


Warts, 26, 20, 50, 3, 51, 0

Water Retention (see Cellulitis)

Worms, Intestinal; Tapeworms, 19, 41, 43, 45, 3, 38, 39, 126, 127, 130, 365, 0

Wrinkles, 124, 34, 26, 103, 106, 0

# Books of Related Interest

**Colloidal Minerals and Trace Elements**
How to Restore the Body's Natural Vitality
*by Marie-France Muller, M.D., N.D., Ph.D.*

**The Reflexology Atlas**
*by Bernard C. Kolster, M.D. and Astrid Waskowiak, M.D.*

**The Reflexology Manual**
An Easy-to-Use Illustrated Guide to the Healing Zones of the Hands and Feet
*by Pauline Wills*

**Gemstone Reflexology**
*by Nora Kircher*

**Sexual Reflexology**
Activating the Taoist Points of Love
*by Mantak Chia and William U. Wei*

**Reflexology Today**
The Stimulation of the Body's Healing Forces through Foot Massage
*by Doreen E. Bayly*

**Trigger Point Therapy for Myofascial Pain**
The Practice of Informed Touch
*by Donna Finando, L.Ac., L.M.T., and Steven Finando, Ph.D., L.Ac.*

**Trigger Point Self-Care Manual**
For Pain-Free Movement
*by Donna Finando, L.Ac., L.M.T.*

**Acupressure Techniques**
A Self-Help Guide
*by Julian Kenyon, M.D.*

**Thai Yoga Massage**
A Dynamic Therapy for Physical Well-Being and Spiritual Energy
*Kam Thye Chow*

Inner Traditions • Bear & Company
P.O. Box 388
Rochester, VT 05767
1-800-246-8648
www.InnerTraditions.com

Or contact your local bookseller